THE SINGER'S GUIDE
TO COMPLETE HEALTH

The Singer's Guide to Complete Health

EDITED BY Anthony F. Jahn, MD

OXFORD
UNIVERSITY PRESS

OXFORD
UNIVERSITY PRESS

Oxford University Press is a department of the University of Oxford. It furthers the University's objective of excellence in research, scholarship, and education by publishing worldwide.

Oxford   New York
Auckland   Cape Town   Dar es Salaam   Hong Kong   Karachi
Kuala Lumpur   Madrid   Melbourne   Mexico City   Nairobi
New Delhi   Shanghai   Taipei   Toronto

With offices in
Argentina   Austria   Brazil   Chile   Czech Republic   France   Greece
Guatemala   Hungary   Italy   Japan   Poland   Portugal   Singapore
South Korea   Switzerland   Thailand   Turkey   Ukraine   Vietnam

Oxford is a registered trade mark of Oxford University Press in the UK and certain other countries.

Published in the United States of America by
Oxford University Press
198 Madison Avenue, New York, NY 10016

Library of Congress Cataloging-in-Publication Data
The singer's guide to complete health / edited by Anthony F. Jahn.
    p.   cm.
Includes bibliographical references and index.
ISBN 978-0-19-537403-2 (pbk.)
1. Voice—Care and hygiene. 2. Singers—Health and hygiene. I. Jahn, Anthony F.
MT821.S57 2013
612.7′8024782—dc23   2012023864

Contents

Foreword

BY FRED PLOTKIN

To be a singer is to be born with many rare gifts—and then to have the wisdom and courage to enable them to survive and flourish. You have been given a special privilege and a huge responsibility.

The most successful singers I have known often tended to be the smartest and most practical. I sometimes wonder to what degree their success is based on innate behaviors, and what has come thanks to having learned how to do things right. Can you be self-protective without being phobic? Mindful without being narcissistic? Do you feel free enough—mentally and physically— to fully inhabit a character you will perform?

If you are reading this, I am sure you have heard the oft-repeated nugget that the most important word in a singer's vocabulary is *no*. Or, at times, *NO!!!* If you have not come across this concept, then you have heard it here first. And it's about time. You can go far, but only so far, without knowing what is right for your voice, your body, your repertoire (aka *fach*), and your spirit. To be able to say no at the right time is to have the self-knowledge and fortitude to know what is right for you and your voice. It can also be courageous to say no when you really want to work for this opera company, or with that colleague, or frankly, just really need the paycheck.

Singers want to be paid for singing, but they also need to sing without being paid. This is called practice and study, and they are things you must do not only at the start of your career but throughout your life. It keeps the mind fresh, as well as the voice. The most successful people in all fields apply themselves every day to honing their craft. It is like the writer who faces the computer screen every morning, the chef who again faces the cutting board and the stove, or the doctor who quickly engages when presented with a new case. Every one of these people is given gifts that have been developed, but the best ones also have something else: joy in work. They cannot imagine not doing it.

You have landed in a profession that should not only give you heaps of joy but enable you to give joy to others. What an honor that is! You only need to listen to recordings of Leontyne Price or Joan Sutherland to understand what joy in singing is all about. These two artists were given amazing gifts. Price often referred to her instrument as "the voice," as if it were some foreign object that God or Nature determined she should be the custodian of. She studied very hard and was remarkably disciplined when necessary, but also sang with great freedom. I have heard her, Sutherland, James Levine, and other artists emphasize the same basic concept in different ways: "If you do all the hard work in the study and the rehearsal, then you are free during the performance." In other words, if you cut corners on study, thought, rest, and maintenance of your health, you will in one way or another pay for it during the performance.

Another of Price's beliefs is to "only use the interest and never touch the principal." This is wise in all pursuits, and not just singing. I believe it is a corollary to the concept of how to be free during performance. Your anatomic and physiologic attributes and your innate musicality are the basis of your principal. Ceaseless study and intense rehearsal build your interest. In certain ways, as you age, some of the principal will evaporate. You will need to learn how to do a full performance on less energy. There might be outside stresses in your life, beyond your control, that seem to nick into the principal, though you want to have built up enough interest to see you through. Attentive care to your health is a big part of this.

There will be those rare days when the voice just does not kick in as you want it to. A singer friend who is one of the world's great artists has an expression for when this occurs: "The store is closed today." He almost never cancels, but he is also very smart. He knows that if the voice is not happening he must not force it. And he respects his colleagues and audiences too much to fake it.

You may be the custodian of your voice, but there are many people along your professional road who will have an impact on it. Your teachers and coaches, for example. The best ones are those who have the experience and humility to treat it as a rare gift and educate you on how to use it. Learning and maintaining a rock-solid technique is essential, but there probably is more than one way to get to it. A teacher who imposes one method across the board does not recognize the differences in biology and temperament that exist among singers. If you have been given the gift of wisdom, you will know when a teacher is right for you.

Another relationship as rewarding as it is delicate is between singer and conductor. He or she is, after all, a *maestro*, a word that signifies both teacher and master. The conductor is responsible for the overall musical content of a performance, which includes you, your colleagues, the orchestra, and the chorus. Sometimes, to achieve an effect, the conductor will play too fast or slow, too loud or soft to suit your needs. Levine is the gold standard, I think, in shaping a performance that enables the singers to do their best while also achieving his vision of what a performance should be. Every singer I have ever conversed with on the topic smiles glowingly in reflecting on Levine's skill and willingness.

Other conductors, typically those who are not as capable, are also less compliant. They arrive with their concept and expect singers to conform. One lyric soprano I know, who has had a very long career because she wisely chose roles that suit her gifts, refuses to sing louder if her conductor blasts the orchestra. I have seen her onstage often, and she will simply smile and keep singing when the conductor pumps up the volume. Listeners who don't recognize this think she is losing her voice, which is not true. She is protecting her voice, and her conductor colleague is being unhelpful.

This is an example of a decision you might have to make: dip into the principal to get through the performance and ingratiate the management of the theater (and the maestro), or sing beautifully and prolong your working life. In the best of all possible worlds, all of these issues are sorted out in rehearsal. But in the real world, there sometimes is no stage rehearsal with orchestra, perhaps because the production is frequently revived or because you have been asked to step in for an ailing colleague.

A marvelous dramatic soprano I know becomes justifiably irritated when a conductor paces her big aria too slowly. She feels it loses impact and continuity and makes her need even more breath than the considerable resources she has at her disposal. Again, this is an accord that must be reached with a maestro, who might grumble that his vision is being hindered or that the singer needs a better teacher. One or both might be true, but when the show has to go on, it is about service to the *music* and to the *audience*. Without both of these, you would need to be in another line of work.

All of what I have discussed here will only get you so far without practical and vigilant (but not obsessive) attention to your health. As Dr. Anthony Jahn points out in these pages, a sound mind and a sound body are fundamental for a sound voice. And for good singing. You will find that you, as a singer, will develop a special team of doctors, practitioners, trainers, and perhaps healers, psychologists, and the occasional hand-holder. The best of these are all professionals, just as you are, and become partners in your well-being.

Because singers travel so much for their work, they often need care in other cities. You learn from colleagues, and from the theaters where you perform, who the good people are. A wonderful European soprano I had the honor to work with had severe back problems that worsened as she aged and took a psychic as well as physical toll. Because she was such an artist, she channeled her pain into performances, but this is not something I would recommend to you. That is *too much* service to art. I helped her find the right doctor, an acupuncturist, and an excellent massage therapist in New York, which made her more inclined to go there. As a result, in the latter stage of her career this artist appeared at the Metropolitan Opera more than any European opera house, even though it meant flying nine hours to get to New York.

You will likely have a general practitioner in the town where you live. He or she will coordinate your care, referring you to specialists. This is a relationship as important as the ones with your teachers and conductors. This doctor should be someone you can speak frankly and openly with on any topic. You will likely also need a specialist in ear, nose, and throat care. Some singers I know regularly consult with a pulmonary specialist about their lungs and breathing.

Dental care is also very important. Although a dentist looks after the health of your mouth, she or he also is concerned with your bite and alignment of teeth, which are essential for proper diction in performance. My dentist specializes in singers, actors, and speakers and understands their special needs and requirements.

The issue of psychological and psychiatric care is delicate but worth discussing. Birgit Nilsson, in talking about the working environment of an opera house, once remarked, "If the birdies are not happy, they do not sing!" This also applies to general mental health. All of us face challenges in life, many of which are resolved with time or proper responses. But certain burdens interfere with work. Some of them can be ameliorated with the right psychological care, though if a psychiatrist recommends medication it probably would be smart to bring this up with your general practitioner. Many creative people I know, including singers, want an "edge" to make their work more compelling and are able to forgo certain mental health treatments. Each case is distinct, and in all circumstances, self-knowledge and honesty serve you best. When it comes to a singer's health and well-being, there is so much more to think about that you might never have a chance to learn your roles! This is why you, the singer, need a support staff for these issues. But the top practitioners are hard to locate. And that is the beauty and the value of the book you are now holding.

Dr. Anthony Jahn and his colleagues are all experts in their specialties, and all have long experience dealing with singers. In their essays here on a wide range of topics of concern to you, they offer precious wisdom and insights. Many of the questions and concerns you have are addressed in these pages, and I am sure you will learn a great many valuable things you never even thought of.

I suggest you show this book to your general practitioner, to colleagues and to your teachers, all of whom will benefit from its contents. I have no doubt that you, and all who read these pages, will make beautiful music, deriving great joy and giving it to others.

Fred Plotkin
New York City
April 2013

THE SINGER'S GUIDE
TO COMPLETE HEALTH

1

Good Health and Singing

An Overview

ANTHONY F. JAHN, MD

The Romans expressed their ideal of good health as *mens sana in corpore sano*, a healthy mind in a healthy body. Implicit in this phrase is a duality that has characterized Western medicine since ancient times. With the increasing appreciation and integration of other, non-Western, medical paradigms, we are coming to realize that this is a duality in appearance only: the mind and the body are just two aspects of the same human being, and they reciprocally interface and shape each other. To sing well—indeed, to perform any task well and live as a fully actualized human being—a person needs to be as healthy as possible. That health is then reflected in multiple manifestations, which in the West we have traditionally (and some would say misleadingly) divided into physical and mental.

Although the overall purpose of this book is to deal with the specifics of good health that lead to a successful and long singing career, there are some general principles that influence everything we do, as singers and as humans. First, our life, in all its aspects, is primarily determined by our genes. The DNA material that has been passed down from our predecessors determines not only our hair color and our musicality but also how long we live, and what we are likely to die from. No one can outlive this genetic prescription. Our cells renew themselves daily, but if our genes have predetermined a certain maximum number of years for us, we cannot live beyond that.

The problem is, almost all of us live *less* than we potentially could—fewer years, and with more health problems. Instead of doing everything we can to allow our genetic program to run its full course, we thwart it through harmful behavioral habits: lack of exercise, lack of sleep, poor diet, and negative feelings. The good news is, unlike our DNA-determined life span, these negative factors are for the most part within our control! So our job, simply put, is just to get out of the way, let our bodies do their job, and not sabotage the normal course of life.

Recipe for a Healthy Life

Here is a typical prescription for good health, penned five hundred years ago:

To keep in health this rule is wise
Eat only when you want, and sup light.
Chew well, and let what you take be well cooked and simple.
He who takes medicine is ill advised.
Beware of anger and avoid grievous moods.
Keep standing when you rise from the table.
Do not sleep at midday.
Let your wine be mixed (with water), take little at a time,
Not between meals, and not on an empty stomach.
Go regularly to stool.
If you take exercise, let it be light.
Do not be with the belly upwards, or the head lowered.
Be covered well at night.

Rest your head and keep your mind cheerful.
Shun wantonness, and pay attention to diet.

The author of these lines was Leonardo da Vinci (1452–1519), the Renaissance genius aptly described as "the last man who knew everything in the world."[1] This is a remarkably relevant document with a surprisingly modern and commonsense feel. It addresses diet and exercise, as well as how to avoid indigestion, reflux, and sexually transmitted diseases, among other things. Most significantly, it recognizes the importance of the emotions for health. There have been many such recipes, both in the East and the West. Apart from regional and cultural differences, they all convey the same message: use your body wisely, and respect your body's needs. Above all, obey the ancient Greek maxim: all things in moderation.

From a more modern medical perspective, a healthy and maximally lived life requires that we pay attention to three things: our body's circulation, our immune system, and the effect of our mind on the physical body.

Circulation

There are only a few fundamental things we need to do in order to allow our genes to convert their potential into actuality, to live out our full, healthy life. Perhaps the most important task is to allow our cells to work to their best capacity. To do this, they need nourishment, oxygen, and the ability to get rid of metabolites and waste. And this, in turn, requires good circulation. Think of the organs of the body as a vast archipelago, connected by a complex of waterways and blood vessels that bring food and oxygen and remove waste. Every cell in every organ has evolved to perform specific functions, its unique contribution to the general well-being of the body. For good contraction, good digestion, and good absorption and excretion (to single out muscles, stomach, intestines, and kidneys as examples), the cells in those structures must be generously supplied with nutrients, oxygen, and waste removal services, a vast catering service that requires good circulation.

So the first order of the day is to avoid anything that will narrow, block, or damage those blood vessels. Common culprits include unhealthy diet, smoking, and stress. To keep the vessels open and flowing, exercise! The circulatory system is dynamic, and highly sensitive to the needs of the body. New vessels form constantly to meet the demands of specific parts of the body, whether in response to exercise or healing. Eating foods that minimize atherosclerosis or diabetes also keeps the circulation healthy. Stress and smoking both lead (in differing ways) to narrowing of the arteries; the first should be minimized, and the second entirely avoided.

Immune Defense

Also of cardinal importance is your immune system. The immune cells, and the organs that generate them, defend the body from aliens, whether external (bacteria, viruses, etc.) or internal (mutant cells). The eminent Australian bacteriologist Sir MacFarlane Burnet once remarked that, unbeknownst to us, our bodies produce and destroy hundreds of potential cancer cells every day. A healthy immune system therefore protects us both from infections and (logically, but less explicitly) from cancer.

As the world grows smaller, pathogens cross oceans and continents daily. Infections and potential epidemics travel from one part of the world to another at the speed of a jet plane. They travel attached to food, manufactured goods, and your fellow passengers. Our body must deal with potential invaders it has never seen before, bugs for some of which effective medications are yet to be invented. HIV and SARS are but two of many such acronymic diseases, and there are likely more to follow.

Again, a healthy immune system is the key. Whatever medications we may take, they can tip the balance in our favor only if our immune system is functional. Antibiotics, no matter how potent, cannot do the job alone. Furthermore, routine overuse of antibiotics, both in our food supply and in medical care, renders them ineffective more rapidly than was the case in the past, as bacteria evolve resistant strains. An antibiotic may destroy most bacteria of a certain kind, but the few survivors reproduce and thus give rise to resistant strains. Since all living beings potentially adapt to changes in the environment with every succeeding generation, there is no possible way that our scientists can stay ahead of these bugs: we reproduce every twenty-five to thirty-five years, they every thirty minutes, and so the evolutionary odds are clearly on the side of the microbes.

My message here is twofold. First, don't be irrationally germphobic. We are all covered with billions of bacteria, inside and out. From the bugs' eye view, we are vast continents of diverse ecological systems, to be colonized and exploited. And those microbes have subspecialized to live and thrive in those ecologic niches, whether on our heads, our armpits, or our intestinal tract. Most are harmless, some are beneficial, and even the potentially harmful ones don't usually make us sick unless they are present in overwhelming numbers or our immune defenses are compromised. Normally, their presence forms a stimulus, a challenge to our immune system, and a call to arms that our bodies are prepared to meet. If we hunt them down indiscriminately and obsessively, with unnecessary antibiotics, mouthwashes, gargles, douches, and other interventions, an undereducated and incompetent immune system may become the unintended result. Stay healthy, stay strong, and for the most part let those bugs fall where they may. Your body is armed with millions of years of immune knowledge to deal with most potential invaders.

At the same time, however, take reasonable care to avoid the avoidable: wash your hands, cover your mouth, and drink plenty of water, which is the most abundant material in our bodies and the common currency for all bodily transactions. The solution to pollution is dilution: your body can wash out most contaminants over time, given adequate hydration and a healthy excretory system. Avoid drugs and chemicals, which can weaken the body. Practice safe sex. Monitor and treat any chronic illness or infection, which can tax your body unnecessarily. You can slow aging with regular exercise, healthy diet, reduced exposure to UV and other radiation, and antioxidant vitamins.

Conscious Awareness of the Body

And finally, the mind-body connection. Develop awareness of it, gain control, and you will master your body. Yoga recognizes and uses the breath as the great bridge between the conscious and unconscious, the voluntary and the reflexive.

By happy coincidence, mastering the breath is also one of the singer's main tasks. Singing, like any other learned task, is, on a certain level nothing more than gaining conscious awareness and voluntary control of actions that are normally unconscious and reflexive. The normal movements of the larynx and rhythmic movement of the diaphragm happen unconsciously for most of us, but not for the trained singer. In the same way, using relaxation and meditation techniques, yoga, Qi Gong, and others, you can live with greater awareness of other parts of your body. The mind-body interface doesn't separate one system from the other (as the Romans would have said) but joins and unifies two aspects into a healthy and fully actualized whole.

So, take care of your circulation, keep your immune system strong, master the mind-body connection, and then, as a singer, you will have achieved your goal, which is also the motto of this book: a healthy voice in a healthy body, *vox sana in corpore sano*!

Notes

1. Leonardo da Vinci, *Notebooks*. Edited by Thereza Wells. Oxford University Press, 2008.

2

The Vocal Apparatus

Structure and Function

ANTHONY F. JAHN, MD

Although we conventionally equate the larynx with the voice, singing in fact involves a complex and coordinated series of activities that begins in the lower abdomen (even the pelvic floor), extends to the thorax, and then continues, through the larynx, to the pharynx, mouth, and nasal cavity. If we add in the importance of proper posture and relaxation of the body, as well as the indescribably complex mental activity required to produce and monitor the voice, you could fairly say that almost no part of the body is *not* involved in the act of singing.

The anatomic description of voice production is normally divided into three components: the *power source* for the voice (abdomen, thorax, and lungs), the *sound generator* (larynx), and the *sound modulators* above the larynx (supraglottic resonators).

The Larynx: Organ of Voice or Retrofitted Sphincter?

Before describing these in detail, it is important to consider that, as much as we think of the voice as fundamental to human expression, the larynx did not originally evolve for speaking or singing. Perched on top of the trachea and separating the upper common passage for respiration and food (pharynx) from the lower airway (trachea, bronchi, and lungs), the larynx's main function is to protect the lungs from aspirated food and liquids (Figures 2.1 and 2.2).

When we swallow, the powerful elevator muscles of the larynx contract, lifting the larynx up and forward, and pulling it (and the attached trachea) out of the way of the swallowed food bolus, which passes around and behind it, into the esophagus. At the same time, the vocal folds reflexively squeeze together, along with two other sphincters, the false vocal folds and the aryepiglottic folds.

Once the swallow is completed, the weaker depressor muscles pull the larynx down and back, and the larynx opens again, ready to take the next breath.

This triple sphincter mechanism, as well as powerful contraction of the muscles that pull the larynx out of the way, acts instantaneously and reflexively every time we swallow. It prevents aspiration, pneumonia, and possible death, which would occur if we soiled our lungs repeatedly. The fact that nature has evolved not one but four separate mechanisms to do the same thing is proof of how vital this protective action is.

The second main function of the larynx is to close tightly when we lift or exert ourselves. By squeezing the vocal folds together so tightly that no air escapes and pushing, we raise the intrathoracic pressure and brace and stiffen the thoracic walls and the diaphragm. Many muscles originate from the outer surface of the thoracic wall, and this action (known as the *Valsalva maneuver*) allows the muscles to work more effectively during exertion. The bracing of the diaphragm also means that, when the muscles of the abdominal wall contract, their force is directed downward, into the pelvis. The need to do this becomes clear during childbirth or evacuation of the bowels. You probably never

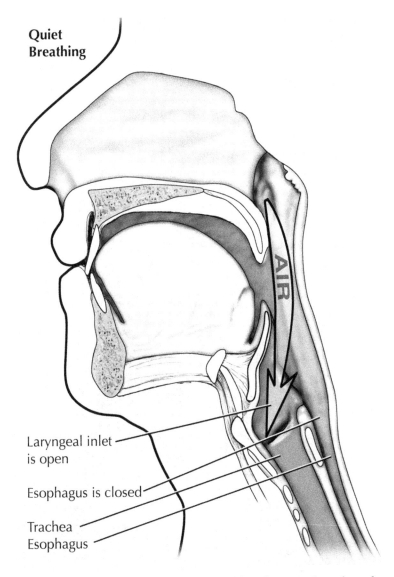

Quiet Breathing

AIR

Laryngeal inlet is open

Esophagus is closed

Trachea
Esophagus

FIGURE 2.1 The throat during quiet nasal breathing. Air flows from the nose, through the nasopharynx, and into the open lowered larynx and trachea. ©2011 Carolyn R. Holmes, CMI

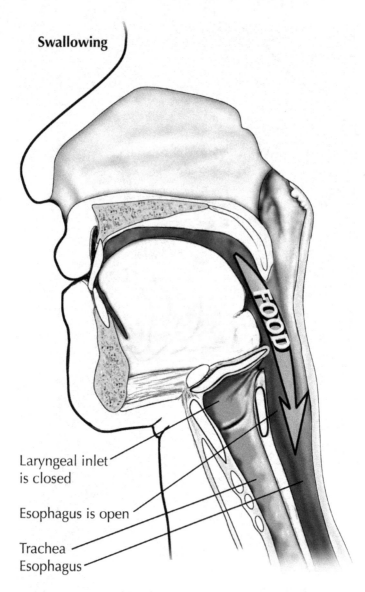

Swallowing

Laryngeal inlet is closed

Esophagus is open

Trachea

Esophagus

FIGURE 2.2 The throat during swallowing. Food enters through the mouth, and passes into the open esophagus. Note that the larynx is elevated, pulled out of the way. The epiglottis flips down, covering the laryngeal opening and further protecting the airway. ©2011 Carolyn R. Holmes, CMI

thought about it, but your larynx is responsible not only for success on the concert stage but also success in the bathroom!

A third important item in the repertoire of the larynx is the cough. A cough also begins as a squeezing together of the vocal folds while exerting upward pressure from the abdomen. This builds up intrathoracic pressure. The vocal folds are then suddenly pulled apart, producing an explosive release of air up the trachea and into the pharynx. The flow of air (as fast as 70 mph) carries with it bits of mucus or other debris in the tracheobronchial tree. The airway is cleared by the cough and can resume its vital function of respiration. The entire event takes less than a second, and occurs (and repeats) as a reflex response to irritation.

What about the voice? One might speculate that phonation may have begun as a grunt during an imperfectly controlled Valsalva maneuver: the muscular effort of the "ancestor" exceeded her ability to hold the vocal folds together and some air escaped, causing an audible sound. Since moments involving effort are often moments of emotion or a need to communicate, the involuntary grunt over time became a voluntary one, signaling information to others. How this original vocal utterance evolved into speech and singing is a topic for another book, not this one. But it is enough for now just to consider that the larynx—a complicated sphincter, defender of the airway, master of the bowels and childbirth—came rather late (in evolutionary terms) to be an organ of the voice. Like sound-producing structures in other species (such as the syrinx of birds or the wings of crickets), the larynx has been adapted from its original evolved role to become the organ of voice. Perhaps this is why learning to sing well is so laborious, and why singing "naturally" is so difficult.

Power: Abdomen, Pelvis, Thorax

The voice is generated as a stream of air, which is pushed from the chest, goes through the larynx, and rushes past the vocal folds. The air originates from the lungs: it is inhaled and then exhaled again through the trachea and larynx, into the pharynx. The loudness, and to a lesser degree the pitch, of the sound is determined by how rapidly and effectively the air is expelled. This, in turn, is controlled by contraction of the thoracic cavity, which squeezes the air, like a bellows, from the lungs, as well as the degree of vocal fold abduction or adduction at the laryngeal opening.

The chest is descriptively termed the thoracic cage. Like an old-fashioned bird cage, it has curved walls, formed by the rigid ribs and their connecting intracostal muscles. Unlike a bird cage, however, its floor, formed by the diaphragm, is soft and moveable. As well, the walls of the thoracic cavity (formed by the ribs) also move. The ribs are hinged to the spinal column in the back, and attached to the breast bone in the front, and they can swivel like a bucket handle. When the breast bone is pulled up, the inside expands; when it is lowered, the volume decreases. This form of breathing, termed thoracic breathing, is more common in women (Figure 2.4).

It requires relatively greater muscular effort, doesn't expand the chest significantly, and is not used in effective singing.

To optimally expand the thoracic cavity and fill and empty the lungs effectively, the diaphragm and abdomen are required. Abdominal breathing, more natural to men, must be mastered by singers of both genders for effective control of the breath during singing (Figure 2.3).

The diaphragm forms a partition that separates the thorax from the abdomen. It consists of a central dome of fibrous tissue

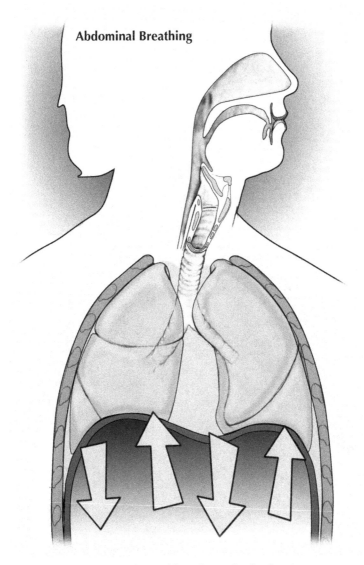

FIGURE 2.3 During abdominal breathing, the diaphragm contracts and moves down, then is pushed up by contracting abdominal muscles. This fills and empties the lungs. ©2011 Carolyn R. Holmes, CMI

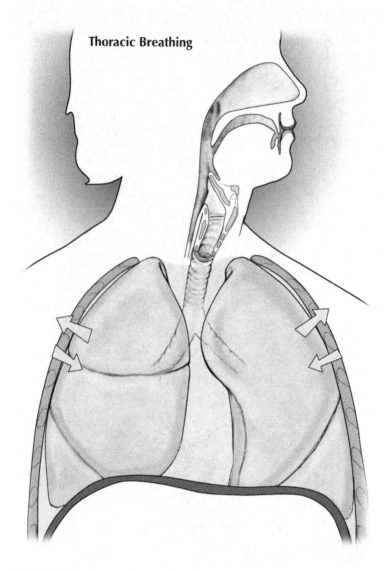

Thoracic Breathing

FIGURE 2.4 During thoracic breathing, the ribs move in and out, enlarging and dreasing the size of the thorax, and filling and emptying the lungs. ©2011 Carolyn R. Holmes, CMI

that arches upward and is anchored all around to the inside of the thorax by muscles. On inspiration, these muscles contract, the diaphragm is pulled down, the thoracic cavity expands, and the lungs fill with air. When the diaphragm relaxes, the contents of the abdomen push upward, the floor of the "cage" rises, and air is pushed up the trachea.

From this description, one thing is obvious: contraction of the diaphragm can only fill the lungs, i.e., on inspiration. Expiration must take place with a relaxed diaphragm, which is passively pushed upward.

On the abdominal side, expiration is either passive or, importantly during singing, actively assisted by the muscles in the abdominal walls. These muscles (which include the recti anteriorly and the obliques laterally) tighten to squeeze the walls of the abdomen, forcing the abdominal contents upward.

To effectively empty the lungs of air, the abdominal contents must be pushed up. Think of the thorax as an air-filled syringe, and the abdominal contents as the plunger: to push air out of the syringe, you must push the plunger up into the barrel. The push comes from the muscles in the walls of the abdominal cavity. This is abdominal breathing. It moves more air and is more effective than thoracic breathing.

When discussing the parts of the abdominal cavity, we focus on its roof (the diaphragm) and its muscular walls. We should, however, not neglect the floor, which is the floor of the pelvis. To direct the force of contraction from the abdominal walls upward, the floor must be firm; otherwise energy is lost downward. Maintaining muscle tone in the pelvic floor is an important part of abdominal support, and it needs to be addressed during singing.

To power the voice effectively, several attributes are important. The thoracic cage should be capacious, its walls mobile. The lungs must be flexible, the airways (bronchi, bronchioles, alveoli) open.

The plunger must also be in good working order—strong muscles in the abdominal walls, with the ability to fully contract under voluntary control. Finally, mastery of the coordination among intra-abdominal pressure, intrathoracic pressure, and laryngeal contraction is the ultimate key to good breath control.

The Larynx

The larynx sits on top of the trachea, the guardian of the airway. Its outer walls are made of two rigid cartilages (Figure 2.5).

The larger of the two is the thyroid cartilage, shaped like a shield that is open posteriorly. The thyroid cartilage hinges on the ring-shaped cricoid cartilage below and tilts forward and backward, like the visor on a knight's helmet. This tilting motion is caused by the contraction of the two cricothyroid muscles, which are attached on each side to the outer surface of the thyroid and cricoid cartilage. Inside the laryngeal framework, there are several valves of muscle and soft tissue. The two (true) vocal folds are the lowest of the three, and of course essential for singing. In the front they meet at a common attachment to the inner surface of the thyroid cartilage. In the back, each is attached to one of two arytenoid cartilages. The arytenoids are controlled by several muscles, and they slide and swivel in a complex fashion. They come together (adduct) and rotate in to bring the vocal folds together for phonation. During quiet breathing, the arytenoids pull apart (abduct) and rotate outward, pulling the vocal folds apart to let air flow through the laryngeal inlet (Figures 2.6 and 2.7).

Vocal sounds are normally generated by the true vocal folds, but it is of interest that sound can also be generated by the false vocal folds, two thicker structures that sit above the true folds. False vocal fold phonation is usually a raspy, pathologic sound, a growl. It is, however, occasionally used in singing—most notably

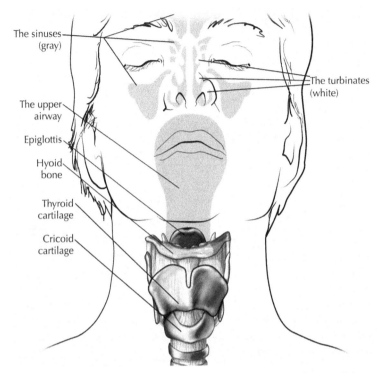

The sinuses (gray)

The turbinates (white)

The upper airway

Epiglottis

Hyoid bone

Thyroid cartilage

Cricoid cartilage

FIGURE 2.5 Frontal view illustrating the various cartilage and bony components of the larynx. They are connected to one another by ligaments, muscles and membranes. This allows for flexibility of movement during breathing, swallowing and phonation. ©2011 Carolyn R. Holmes, CMI

by the "throat singers" of Tuva in Central Asia. In conventional Western singing, only the true vocal folds produce sound.

How the Vocal Folds Produce Sound

The sound produced during singing is the result of vibration in the vocal folds triggered by airflow from the lungs and trachea below. The rate of flow and force of this air stream is in turn con-

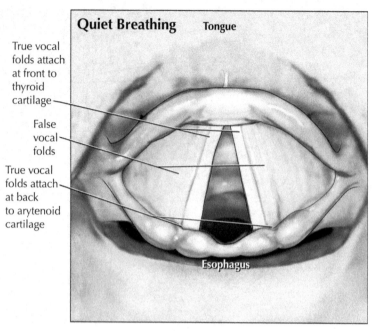

FIGURE 2.6 The larynx, viewed from above, during quiet breathing. The vocal folds are abducted (drawn apart), and the trachea is visible. ©2011 Carolyn R. Holmes, CMI

trolled by two main factors. First is the pressure of the abdominal contents up against the diaphragm, which compresses the thoracic cavity and pushes air up below the vocal folds. Second is the degree and force with which the vocal folds are pressed together (adduction). If intrathoracic pressure is greater than the force compressing the vocal folds together, a stream of air will push the vocal folds apart, and escape into the pharynx. For a moment now, intrathoracic pressure drops, allowing the vocal folds to close. Air pressure builds again, and the vocal folds are once again blown apart. With repeated opening and closing, the edges of the vocal fold are brought into vibration, and sound is produced.

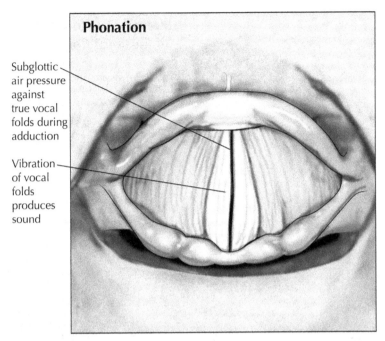

Phonation

Subglottic air pressure against true vocal folds during adduction

Vibration of vocal folds produces sound

FIGURE 2.7 The larynx during phonation. The vocal folds are approximated (adducted), and as exhaled airppasses between them, the fold edges vibrate, producing sound. ©2011 Carolyn R. Holmes, CMI

The vocal folds are not simple ledges of tissue. They have a multilayered internal structure that allows great finesse in vibration (Figure 2.8).

Their underlying strength comes from a slip of muscle (vocalis, or thyroarytenoid muscle), which can tense or relax, controlling both the firmness and the bulk of the fold. This muscle is covered by the vocal ligament, a somewhat flexible sheath that has no intrinsic power of movement. Muscle and ligament are tightly connected and form the "body" of the vocal fold.

The truly remarkable feature of the vocal fold, however, is its surface cover, the superficial layer. This is a modified mucous

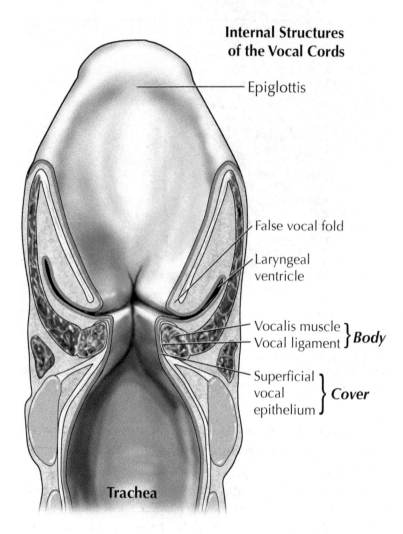

Internal Structures of the Vocal Cords

- Epiglottis
- False vocal fold
- Laryngeal ventricle
- Vocalis muscle } **Body**
- Vocal ligament }
- Superficial vocal epithelium } **Cover**

Trachea

FIGURE 2.8 Coronal cross-section of the larynx. Note the false vocal folds above, which partially cover the true vocal folds. Note also the multilayered structure of vocal folds. ©2011 Carolyn R. Holmes, CMI

membrane loosely attached to the underlying vocal ligament. It rides on a thin layer of gel (Reinke's space) and is firmly anchored only anteriorly and posteriorly. Since this covering layer is for the most part only tenuously attached, it can slip and slide, and it vibrates with the slightest flow of air. The flow of air past the vocal folds is a finely tuned balancing act between subglottic air pressure and the muscular squeeze that pushes the vocal folds together (glottic pressure). To initiate the voice, the vocal folds are approximated, and then intrathoracic (and subglottic) air pressure is increased until it is just greater than glottic pressure: the vocal folds are momentarily blown apart, a bit of air escapes up, which reduces subglottic pressure. Now, glottic pressure is momentarily greater, and the vocal folds close again. With continued expiration, the subglottic pressure rises again, and cycle repeats. As the air flows past the adducted vocal folds, it is released into the pharynx in rhythmic puffs. How quickly does the process repeat itself? When singing a high C, this sequence of events occurs 1,024 times per second!

Imagine you could isolate a larynx, and listen to the sound produced by the vibrating folds. What does this first, raw, "voice" sound like? It is like a buzz, a Donald Duck-like quack, not very loud and lacking musical quality. This initial sound is of course modified by the various resonating cavities above the larynx, which are described below.

Chest Voice, Head Voice, Passaggio, and Belt

Although the terms "chest voice" and "head voice" probably originated from the place where singers feel maximal resonance, the difference is clearly not only one of pitch, but also of quality. Two different muscle mechanisms are used to produce these two types of voice.

The main mechanism used in producing chest voice is an increasing contraction of the muscles attached *within the larynx*, the vocalis muscle, and the arytenoid adductors. There is, of course, a limit to how hard you can push the folds together, a physical limit to this laryngeal squeeze, which is determined by how hard the muscles inside the larynx can be contracted, how bunched up the vocalis muscle can be, and still vibrate. Once this limit has been reached, a second mechanism can be brought into play, one that produces head voice. Instead of increasing tightening the muscles of the vocal folds and the arytenoid adductors, the two larger cricothyroid muscles attached to the *outside the larynx* begin to tighten. Simultaneously, the vocalis muscles relax somewhat. This tilts the thyroid cartilage forward and elongates the vocal folds.

Contraction of the cricothyroid muscles is the mechanism involved in head voice. Functionally, this contraction has several consequences: (1) it elongates and thins the vocal folds by tilting their anterior attachment (inner surface of thyroid cartilage) away from their posterior attachments (arytenoid cartilages); (2) it transfers the muscular contraction from several smaller muscles (vocalis, arytenoids adductors) to two larger muscles, with the result that overall muscle effort used in head voice phonation is reduced; and (3) finally, by pulling and tightening the vocal fold "body" (vocalis and vocal ligament), it decouples the connection between these deeper structures and the overlying vocal epithelium ("cover"). The result is a longer, thinner vocal fold with a covering layer that is functionally more detached, hence more responsive, and vibrates easily with less air and effort.

Since the two mechanisms are quite different, a smooth transition from the muscles used in chest voice to those used in head voice is essential for good singing. This transition, the *passaggio*, is analogous to shifting gears in a car. One set of muscles is gradually released, and the second set gradually engaged. With a car, the driver can shift when the engine is revving at a range of speeds. Similarly, the singer can choose to make the shift within a limited range of frequencies, although there is obviously an optimum frequency where this is most easily done (often around E or E flat for sopranos). If properly done, the transition is seamless. If improperly done (for any of several reasons), the shift is bumpy and obvious. If the transition is accentuated rather than smoothed, the result is a yodel, which is also used in certain types of singing.

As was already mentioned, the exact point of transition is somewhat optional. There is a vocal range where a singer has the option to stay in chest voice or move to head voice. For some types of singing, the singer may choose not to transition, and to push the voice into the higher "head" range while keeping the chest mechanism. This is the belted voice. Like the sound of a motor when driving a car fast in a low gear, the belt voice conveys energy, urgency, and emotion, relying more on muscle power than resonance. Belted singing is more effortful and leads to greater wear and tear on the vocal mechanism. It should be used only when necessary, and never as a substitute for an undeveloped head voice.

The Modulators

We have alluded to the raw, unprocessed sound originating from the vocal folds. This soft, rough bleat is transformed into "the voice" by the structures above the vocal folds. It is in the upper airway that the voice acquires power, color, and ring, as well as expression and emotion. These structures of resonation and articulation include the supraglottic larynx, pharynx, nose, palate, tongue, mouth, and teeth.

The sung sound generated by the larynx, even though centered around a specific pitch, contains many frequencies. The color and power of the voice comes from selective amplification of different frequencies and the resulting alteration of the ratio between them. The fundamental frequency conveys pitch, but the amplification of the various overtones, and their ratio to one another, produces color and "quality." The size, shape, and flexibility of the resonators in the upper vocal tract are some of the parameters that distinguish the voice of one singer from another.

Acoustic resonance, which is the sympathetic vibration and amplification of a sound, depends first on the size and shape of a resonating chamber. Furthermore, the frequencies that are amplified also depend on whether the resonator is closed (like a box), or open, either on one end or both. By changing the size and shape of the resonating cavities, the singer is able to selectively emphasize certain overtones, and convey color and emotion in the voice.

As we look above the vocal folds, we see the first resonating chamber immediately above the glottis. It is in the supraglottic larynx that the "ring" of the voice (a frequency of around 2,700 Hz) is generated. This ring, also called the singer's formant, is not natural and develops as the singer learns to posture the larynx properly. It allows the voice to project above most instruments of the orchestra.

The entire pharynx, from vocal folds to the nasopharynx, is a cavity and has resonant properties. The shape of the pharyngeal air column can be varied almost endlessly. You can close the top, by lifting the palate. You can partially cover it with the back of the tongue. You can narrow it by constricting the lateral pharyngeal walls. You can elongate and enlarge it by lowering the larynx. All of these activities are initially learned by proprioception and sound imitation. During a trained vocal performance they go on seamlessly and unconsciously, in an ever-changing fashion. So, even though the voice originates from two vibrating slips of soft tissue, it develops its secondary qualities from a complex array of constantly changing resonating cavities, some fixed in dimension (the nose) but other cavities with moveable walls and baffles that shape the voice by selecting specific frequencies in that basic laryngeal emission.

We have seen how the larynx moves up and forward in the neck, up with every swallow and back and down with every breath. The larynx is pulled up and down by two sets of muscles, the elevators and the depressors. As protectors of the airway during swallowing, the laryngeal elevators are necessarily greater in number (and strength) than the depressors. Figure 2.9, redrawn after Negus,[1] illustrates the vector forces of various muscles acting on laryngeal position. If one were to maximally contract all of the elevators and depressors at the same time, the resultant movement of the larynx would be in an upward direction. In fact, this tug-of-war does occur in singers who sing with excessive and uncontrolled laryngeal muscle tension.

The elevators of the larynx attach to the hyoid bone, which in turn is connected to the tongue. In the vocally untrained person, the larynx, hyoid, and tongue usually move reflexively and *en masse*. Part of good vocal technique involves learning to contract or relax these muscles separately and at will, in a way that the normally weaker depressors win. Inadequately trained singers may try to lower the larynx by pushing back the tongue. This, however, doesn't achieve the intended result of lowering the larynx in isolation, and it increases the covering effect of the tongue in the back of the throat. When properly done, the larynx is pulled down at will by the laryngeal depressors with simultaneous relaxation of (antagonistic) laryngeal elevators, and no change in tongue position. The resultant lowering of the larynx elongates and opens the pharynx and adds strength and resonance to the voice.

Much is made of the soft palate. This is a thin muscular partition that separates the nasal area from the mouth and lower

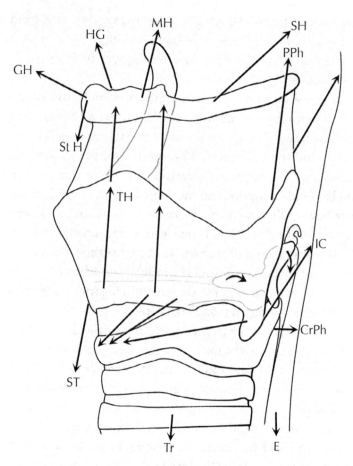

Key

St H= Sternohyoid	E= Esophagus
HG= Hyoglossus	Tr= Trachea
GH= Geniohyoid	MH= Mylohyoid
SH= Stylohyoid	IC= Inferior constrictor
TH= Thyrohyoid	ST= Sternothyroid
Cr Ph= Crycopharyngeus	PPh= Palatopharyngeus

FIGURE 2.9 Diagram showing the direction of pull of the various muscles attached to the larynx. Note that the elevators (protecting the airway during swallowing) greatly outnumber the depressors (which lower the larynx back into breathing position) ©2011 Carolyn R. Holmes, CMI

pharynx. To direct the sound into the mouth, the palate must lift and close off the nasopharynx. Although resonance in the nose and mask is an undeniable part of singing, that resonance is transmitted through the bony structures (hard palate, facial bones), and not through the nasopharynx.

The tongue is one of the most important components of the vocal mechanism. It is a bulky muscular organ that changes size, shape, and location constantly. It is responsible for the shape of the upper pharyngeal air column, for the volume and dimensions of the resonating chamber of the mouth, and for articulation, as it touches the anterior hard palate and the teeth.

There is no instrument that works exactly like the vocal apparatus. The closest comparison might be to the trombone: the two lips[2] generate a buzz into the mouthpiece, and this buzz is selectively amplified by a complex set of resonating tubes whose dimensions are constantly adjusted by the performer.

The Path from Voice to Singing

Many words have been expended trying to explain the vocal mechanism (including what you have just waded through), but no description can begin to touch the complexity of the act of singing.

A preliminary but important consideration is the degree of musical and vocal aptitude that a singer brings to the task. Some have favorable anatomy, others deeply intuitive musicality, and yet others great ambition and persistence. And occasionally, a singer is blessed with all of these talents.

But the reality is that, in listening to two singers of similar quality, you may not appreciate that they have traveled very different paths to get to the same place. One may have started with a great natural ability that required only a bit of fine tuning, while the other arrived at the same level of performance only after many years of expensive tuition, painstaking hard work, and psychotherapy.

The actual task of learning to sing can be divided into three phases. First, the singer must gain conscious sensory awareness of parts of the body that for most people function automatically and unawares. An acute sense of the breath, the proprioceptive perception of expansion and contraction of the chest, the physical sensation produced by sound vibration in different parts of the body . . . these are all phenomena that for nonsingers remain below the radar.

Second, this sensory awareness is used to gain conscious motor control over muscles that normally contract and relax reflexively. Learning to lower the larynx at will, to shape the tongue, to lift the palate, are just some of the many motor tasks over which the singer must gain consistent voluntary control. These movements usually occur as components of phylogenetically ancient lower-brain reflexes such as swallowing and coughing. Table 2.1 sum-

TABLE 2.1 Singing Naturally vs. The Art of Singing

Natural (Reflexive):	Artificial (Voluntary):
Laryngeal position high	Laryngeal position low
Pharynx moderately constricted	Pharynx open
Palate low	Palate raised
V.F. pressure: open or closed	V.F. pressure: moderated
No vibrato	Vibrato
Yodel	Passaggio
Normal insp/exp ratio	Reversed insp/exp ratio
Passive expiration	Active expiration
Thoracic breathing	Abdominal breathing
Mass reflexive movement of muscles	Individual controlled movement of muscles

marizes some of the technical differences between the untrained vocal apparatus attempting to sing and the vocal technique of a trained vocal performer. Considering this list, you can see that the exhortation to "sing naturally" is somewhat misleading.

But how do we get from producing a controlled, modulated and projected voice to actually singing? As with most musical performance, mere strengthening of the appropriate muscles is only part of the task. As the third step, once the singer has gained conscious and voluntary control over these involuntary movements, she finally renders them "reflexive" again, but this time at the service of the highest brain centers. Singing is about conveying emotion, and technique becomes the toolkit of the artist. Certainly a performer does not monitor in real time what her vocal apparatus is doing during an aria. Color, drama, projection all result from how these structures of the vocal tract, evolved for basic survival and once humble servants of the brainstem, perform in the service of their new master, the musical cortex.

Notes

1. Sir Victor Ewings Negus, MS, FRCS (6 February 1887–15 July 1974), was a British surgeon who specialized in laryngology and also made fundamental contributions to comparative anatomy with his work on the structure and evolution of the larynx. The diagram is based on his illustration in *The Mechanism of the Larynx*, published in 1929.

2. The German word for "vocal folds" is actually "voice lips" (*Stimmlippen*).

3

Pulmonary Medicine for Singers

LEN HOROVITZ, MD

Although much is written in singing literature about abdominal support, posture, and other issues, it is the respiratory system that forms the core of the singer's being. Imagine that your respiratory system is like a tree. The sinuses and throat might be thought of as leaves and branches; the larynx would represent where the branches converge; and the trachea, lungs, and muscles of breathing would be the trunk and roots. The entire system is interconnected, and its lining forms topologically one surface. No part functions well without working in concert with the others (Figure 3.1).

When you look at the picture of the respiratory tree, you notice that each of your lungs has divisions (lobes), which contain the branching breathing tubes (bronchi and then bronchioles). The budlike sacs (alveoli) are the ultimate destination of the inhaled air. The two lung cavities are separated by a partition (mediastinum), which contains the esophagus, trachea, and the heart.

Most people who aren't cardiologists don't need to think much about how the heart works. But it occupies a rather substantial space in the chest between the two lobes of the lung. Singers don't have to think about their heart, and they rarely do unless there are dramatic symptoms. But the heart is surrounded by the

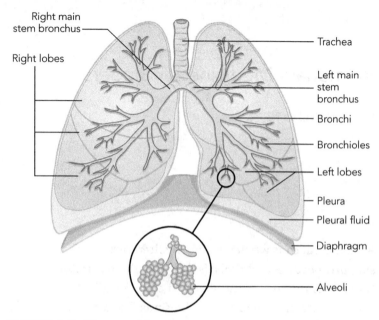

FIGURE 3.1 Diagram of the respiratory system.

lungs and sits right on the diaphragm. Perhaps this is why some are said to "sing with heart." Even at rest, there is constant movement in the chest. Inhalation and exhalation alternate continuously, just as the heart functions by filling and pumping in continuous cycles.

Your voice teacher has already made you aware that you must understand how, during singing, air goes into and out of the respiratory structures. You may never have thought of what happens during "normal use" breathing: talking, exercising, sleeping, or yelling. But you already know that understanding "abnormal use" breathing—singing—is critical to your foundation as a singer. No matter what the activity, from swimming to yoga, it all comes down to breath. And robust general health.

Every singer has to learn and understand the function of the muscles of breathing (Figure 3.2), and the requisite posture and

Respiratory system

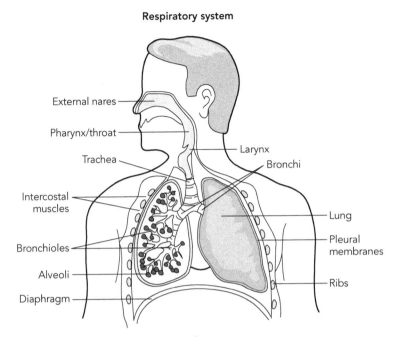

FIGURE 3.2 The muscles of breathing.

positioning of the chest and pelvis. The head, the shoulders, and the spine must be in alignment for the breathing required in singing. The Alexander technique addresses this well and should be reviewed and practiced.

When breath is taken, the diaphragm descends while contracting, causing the abdomen to move outward, and the lower intercostal muscles pull the ribs outward (Figure 3.3). The resulting expansion of the thoracic cavity creates a vacuum in the chest so that air simply rushes in and fills the lungs.

Once a good inhalation breath is accomplished, the expiration part of the cycle begins. This is due in part to the natural elastic recoil of the muscles that have "pulled in" the air, and their attachments, including the chest wall, trachea, and the lungs themselves, which have inflated. If the glottis is closed, there will

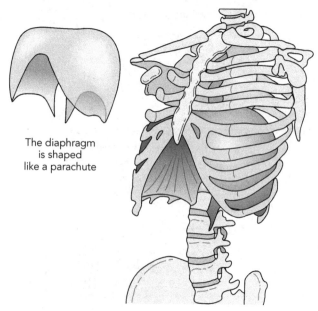

The diaphragm
is shaped
like a parachute

FIGURE 3.3 The diaphragm.

be positive air pressure in the system, from the lower pelvis right up to the trachea and vocal cords.

A simple way to see this phenomenon is to blow up a balloon to maximal volume. If you squeeze the neck of the balloon tightly, without letting any air escape, you can feel the pressure of air inside the balloon. The natural tendency of rubber or latex to recoil will cause tension at the neck where your fingers pinch off the opening. Using both hands at the outlet, you can actually "phonate" the balloon and observe the tendency for air to flow out between your fingers. Pushing on the bottom of the balloon (as a singer does, by actively exhaling and pushing the air out with the abdominal muscles) creates additional pressure at the outlet, sometimes changing the pitch or airiness of the vibration. The rate of air flow, and the sound produced, is affected by both the natural elastic recoil of the balloon (respiratory system) and

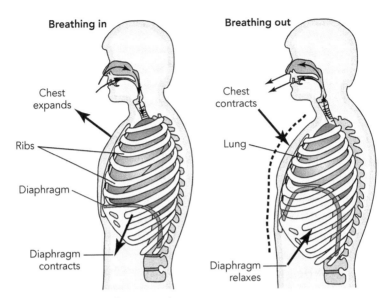

FIGURE 3.4 Breathing in and out.

the pressure applied by your second hand (abdominal muscle contraction, or "support"). This is a simplistic way to understand what happens in the compression of singing, and to imagine the experience of what happens in your body (Figure 3.4).

In singing, a breath is "taken"; then the vocal fold edges adduct (are brought together by the laryngeal muscles) and close for phonation. This creates a buoyancy that many teachers refer to as the *appoggio*. The great mezzo-soprano Dolora Zajik once explained: "Think of a garden hose turned on, with a nozzle to create spray on the end. That's your compression, your appoggio."

The regulation of airflow through the vocal folds, and of the compression that exists in the system, when correctly used, can result in good technical singing. If your "support" is improperly regulated, it can give the impression to a listener (or to a viewer) of "pushing," "sitting down on a depressed larynx," breathiness, straining, "cracking," and limiting the tessitura of the voice.

Flat or sharp singing can be the result of problems with compression.

Optimal breath support avoids faulty negotiation of register breaks (crucial to an even column of sound). For many singers, good breath control is the key to successfully navigating the passaggio between registers, resulting in an even voice, top to bottom.

A few breathing exercises are well known, such as panting, which gives an awareness of the diaphragm. Another exercise, done with hands on the rib cage and hips, emphasizes expansion of the rib cage. Lying on the floor with a heavy book on the abdomen will activate the diaphragm and simulate appoggio when air is expelled with a slow, hissing sound.

As if all that weren't enough to master, it still does not address the articulators (mouth, tongue) and resonators (pharynx, sinuses) and coordination of the soft palate's ability to contract upward, as in the highest registers of the singer. Vowel purity, breathing, and "having the energy under the voice" all need to work in concert. Although some singers seem to have naturally good technique, even great voices need constant scrutiny, as well as the ears of others to hear what a singer cannot hear.

Many singers can identify positive physical sensations when they are singing well, such as vibration in the sinuses, a feeling of elasticity in the solar plexus, or buzzing in the ears. Curiously, some of the most beautiful voices are the most difficult to train well, since the beauty of sound may obscure subtle technical flaws that, if not corrected, will lead to future problems. An expert voice teacher is the best medicine you have. One thing has been made clear to me over the years: singers with good breath control rarely develop vocal problems (unless ill) such as vocal fold edema or nodes.

There is no substitute for good technique when it comes to vocal consistency and longevity, and control of the breath is the cornerstone of good technical singing. So find the best teacher you can, and sing for anyone who can comment on your progress.

Disorders of the Respiratory System

The Common Cold

The average adult will catch two or three colds a year. For a singer, a common cold is a lot more than an inconvenience. Rehearsal time, coaching schedules, and possibly performances may be demanded at a critical time when "just a cold" can threaten not just vocal health but the quality of a performance in an audition, or on stage.

It is important not to confuse colds and allergies. The presence of fever, chills, sore throat, sneezing, body aches, and coughing clearly points to infection—most often the common rhinovirus or adenovirus, usually a simple cold. Other more serious viruses, such as influenza, are more dramatic, debilitating, and abrupt in their onset and clearly send the message that I get so often: "I've come down with something." Since flu is a more serious condition, I generally recommend that singers consider getting a flu shot every fall, unless allergic to eggs.

Allergies are usually perennial (dust, animal dander) or seasonal (ragweed, tree pollen), although we are all somewhat allergic to dust mites. The difference between a cold and an allergy is that the symptoms of inhaled allergy are generally limited to the eyes, throat, nose, and sinuses. These symptoms include itchy palate, watery and itchy eyes and nose, sneezing with clear mucus, and bogginess of the sinuses; but they do not evolve into fever, colored discharges, or coughs productive of colored mucus. Unless asthma is present, there are no pulmonary symptoms except cough, which is usually due to allergic sinusitis with its accompanying postnasal drip.

Colds caused by simple viruses do not respond to antibiotics. A doctor cannot "nip it in the bud" with inappropriate administration of antibiotics. Frequent and unneeded use of antibiotics will not only be useless but may cause yeast infections, allergic reactions to the drug prescribed, or antibiotic-associated colitis.

On the other hand, a persistent sore throat with swollen cervical lymph nodes and fever may be indicative of strep throat, a bacterial infection that does require antibiotics. A throat culture can easily detect this. Mere inspection of the throat leads to the wrong diagnosis in about half of cases! It's always best to be seen and examined when ill, and not to assume that you know the diagnosis. Cultures of the sinuses, throat, or sputum can help determine whether bacterial infection is playing a role. Only then should antibiotics be prescribed.

A simple cold should be treated supportively, with time-honored remedies such as hydration, sleep, reducing fever with acetaminophen, humidification, gargling, and good nutrition with fresh fruit juices.

Inhalation of warm (not hot) steam, with small amounts of herbal extracts such as eucalyptus oil added to the steam, is soothing. Slippery elm tea coats the throat well, as do honey and lemon brews. Ginger tea or ginger root used in any form is popular with some singers. Freshly blended fruit smoothies provide hydration, and plenty of vitamin C. As well, B12 and beta-carotene can be added in higher quantities to your daily multivitamin supplement.

If a cold is detected quickly, application of zinc, via nasal swabs, and zinc lozenges can shorten its duration. It is important to remember that these remedies are optimal only if used within the first twenty-four hours of onset of the infection. Expectorants such as guaifenesin and licorice tea can loosen thick mucus and help expectoration. A humidifier or vaporizer is an essential appliance that is mandatory anytime indoor air is dry, and all the more so with a cold. Black pepper used generously on food can serve as an excellent natural expectorant.

Cough suppressants given at night, especially those containing codeine, are a boon to the sufferer of the dry, hacking, and nonproductive coughing that causes loss of sleep, and they avoid the swelling of the vocal cords that can occur with explosive coughing. Sometimes daytime use of a cough suppressant is indicated as well. Allergy to codeine might lead to use of promethazine instead. Occasionally both are used. Valerian root is a natural remedy for quieting down a nighttime cough, and inducing sleep.

Generally speaking, I avoid most decongestants, for several reasons. They cause jitteriness and wakefulness, and they give many singers a "dried-out" sensation. In certain situations, such as for airplane flights, they can help avoid severe sinus and Eustachian tube congestion, which in turn can cause middle-ear problems. Flying with a cold is never a good idea.

Nasal irrigation can be repeated several times daily if necessary, and nasal topical steroid sprays can be useful after irrigation. These sprays are most beneficial for nasal allergy, or for nonbacterial nasal congestion. In the presence of bacterial infection, steroids may actually inhibit the body's normal healthy inflammatory response. In spite of the fact that a cold is not an allergy, some studies have found antihistamines helpful with symptom relief, because viruses can activate a histamine response.

Should you sing with a cold? It is inevitable that you will have to endure a cold at some point in your career. It is sometimes possible to sing with a cold without risk of damage, especially if the larynx and soft palate are relatively spared from the swelling and inflammation. In fact, many singers have told me that they felt they really learned to sing well after having the experience of singing with a cold. Because they could not "place" the voice, they "allowed" it to "find" resonance, and they came to trust that feeling. They found the experience pivotal and valuable, feeling a new sense of professional reliability. After examining your larynx, your otolaryngologist can give you the clearance to go ahead with a performance. In the professional vocal world, where consistency is critical, you need to learn to deal with a cold before the stakes become high. It can be actively managed by you in concert with your doctor.

An old adage states that if left unattended, a cold lasts a week; if well treated, it lasts seven days! My experience differs. Patients who respond to a viral upper respiratory infection by reducing activities, sleeping more, and following closely the suggestions previously covered will definitely fare better than those who try to plod through their usual schedule. Denial of illness often leads to a complication of a cold, such as bronchitis or pneumonia, or it may trigger asthma. Specifically, a common cold can progress to involve the entire respiratory tree, resulting in tracheobronchitis (Figure 3.5).

Although most colds do eventually end up in the chest, hopefully without much coughing and mucus, after a week or so they normally just fade away. Less commonly, some viruses have a predilection for lodging at particular sites such as the trachea. For singers, isolated or associated laryngitis is an especially troublesome scenario.

When a chest cold doesn't follow its normally limited and benign course, the pulmonary airways (bronchi) persist in being inflamed, and a secondary bacterial infection can develop. Symptoms will then change for the worse. Sputum may become thick, yellow-green, brown, or rust-colored, sometimes with small amounts of blood. Fever may return, and cough worsens. At this point your physician will decide whether bacterial bronchitis is present. Other symptoms such as shortness of breath or chest pain that occurs with simple breathing may suggest pneumonia. A chest X-ray will determine if pneumonia has developed.

Both bacterial bronchitis and bacterial pneumonia require antibiotics. Since a severe viral infection can often mimic a bac-

Normal bronchi | Bronchitis

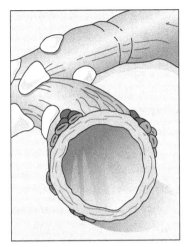 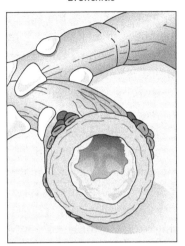

FIGURE 3.5 Bronchitis.

terial infection, and—once again!—viruses should not be treated with antibiotics, my treatment plan is to obtain a sputum culture before the first dose of antibiotic. The culture will demonstrate the presence (or absence) of abnormal amounts of the particular bacteria, and also the sensitivity of the bacteria to various antibiotics. If the culture grows "normal flora," then the antibiotic can be stopped.

If the chest infection is viral, management is mostly supportive. One exception to this rule is the influenza virus, which can be treated with a specific antiviral medication, oseltamivir (Tamiflu). For best effect, the medication must be initiated within twenty-four to forty-eight hours of the onset of the flu.

Asthma

Asthma is a fairly common disorder, particularly in urban areas. Most people think of asthma as a pediatric disease that children outgrow, but the fact is that adult-onset asthma is a common presentation. Symptoms include wheezing with chest tightness, shortness of breath, coughing, and scanty mucus production. Triggers of asthma can be exposure to chemical irritants such as smoke, paints and "fog" used for the stage, and allergens such as mold, as well as cold weather, exercise, and the common cold. Stress can also cause exacerbation of asthma.

The problem in asthma is not with getting air into the lungs, but rather the inability to expel air that is trapped in the lungs by constricted airways. In addition to narrowed bronchi and bronchioles these breathing tubes also produce reactive, inflammatory mucus that further blocks the ability to exhale. This air trapping or "hyperinflation" causes the wheezing sound so typical of asthma. Since some cases of asthma are not obvious, a simple office-based test called spirometry can determine the presence of the condition, and whether asthma is mild, moderate, or severe.

Even though the exact cause of asthma is not completely understood, it is clear that two pathologic issues exist. The first is bronchoconstriction, wherein the involuntary muscle around the bronchial tubes tightens and narrows the airways. This can be treated with bronchodilator inhalers, and relief can be rapid. This is the mechanism of "rescue inhalers" such as Albuterol. Incidentally, caffeine is an excellent, natural bronchodilator.

The second issue is inflammation of the bronchial lining. The best treatment for inflammation in asthma is use of corticosteroids. These are various forms of cortisone—not the anabolic steroids used for "doping" in sports.

Corticosteroids can be given in various dosages and by various routes, but doctors generally prefer using the least amount necessary to achieve relief. For this reason, inhaled steroids are used most frequently, since oral doses will result in a higher systemic steroid level, and a greater incidence of side effects to other parts of the body.

There are many formulations of steroid inhalers, and they are considered to be the mainstay of asthma management. The problem with the use of inhaled steroids is that dysphonia (hoarseness or breathiness) can occur. Even in nonsingers, whose vocal demands are less exacting than those of the vocalist, dysphonia is reported about 4 percent of the time. There are some physicians (and patients) who are not bothered by this risk, but most singers are reluctant to use steroid inhalers when they learn this fact. For this reason I do not prescribe aerosolized steroids for singers because of this possibility, however infrequent.

There are alternative anti-inflammatories that can be given that block the biological pathways of inflammation, such as montelucast (Singulair). Occasionally steroids are given by mouth in small doses, but in long-term management of asthma the less steroids are used, the fewer side-effects will be induced. It should be mentioned that the anti-inflammatory drugs used for asthma differ from conventional over-the-counter anti-inflammatories. These OTC drugs, such as ibuprofen and aspirin, should not be used by singers because of the risk of vocal cord hemorrhage. In fact, some asthmatics may actually experience an asthma attack from these drugs. Always ask your doctor about medications you are tempted to take on your own.

Some asthma medications can be taken through inhalation by a nebulizer, a machine that mixes air with the liquid version of the medication. Though this may have an obvious advantage over dry-powder formulation, especially for a singer, the machine must be taken everywhere you go, and if not battery operated it must be plugged in. Moderate or severe asthmatics are candidates for this route; most others will do well with standard inhalers.

Having asthma need not be an impediment to a singer if it is well controlled. In fact, many asthmatic singers have told me that they learned a better sense of compression because of the air trapping of asthma, and that it prevented them from "blowing too much air" in singing! As a pulmonary specialist, I usually take an approach to asthma that combines a traditional medical approach with homeopathy and acupuncture in selected cases.

A few final words should be said about general health concerns for singers. Obviously, maintaining good pulmonary, vocal, and general health is better than dealing with potentially avoidable medical problems. General measures that must be adopted by singers include good nutrition, maintenance of an approximately ideal body weight, and regular exercise—cornerstones of general health. They cannot be ignored. Sleep—at least seven hours nightly—is a must. There is no better vocal rest than sleep. Although few singers smoke, this activity is obviously harmful. It is hard enough for singers to deal with air pollution, stage fog, and chemicals used in set design. Secondhand smoke is also a pulmonary irritant that must be avoided.

Many professional singers have never been told about the importance of nasal irrigation, which is critical in maintaining clear and open sinus passages, just as brushing the teeth and gargling with salt water ensure proper hygiene of the oropharynx. Whether by "Neti pot" or another device, saline irrigation must take the form of "power washing." Merely sniffing and moisturizing the sinuses with saline nasal drops or sprays will not loosen the excess mucus that can interfere with resonance—mucus that compromises taking a proper breath for singing. Nasal irrigation should be a daily activity, best done in the shower, and not something done only when there is congestion or swelling of these membranes. Prevention is easier than treating problems. If there is an indication, nasal douching can be followed by instilling topical steroidal sprays. Over-the-counter nasal decongestants are for emergency use, as on an airplane, when changes in barometric pressure affect the ears.

Inhaling steam has benefits for loosening secretions, but caution must be taken not to cause a thermal injury by getting too close to the jet of steam, which would compound swelling. Mucous "thinners" such as guaifenesin are popular with many singers when mucus feels thick and viscous. Again, humidification is a ground rule.

Most singers come to realize that excessive rehearsing, performing, or just talking (especially above ambient noise) will fatigue the voice. The "opening night party" can be especially dangerous in this regard. Speaking should use the same technique as good singing. Leontyne Price once said, The less you engage in unnecessary talking, practicing, and "testing" of the voice, the more your vocal reserve will remain. Fortunately for our electronic culture, texting and e-mail can help with maintaining vocal rest.

Apart from specific pulmonary or vocal issues, is important to have annual checkups with an internist to monitor overall health. Your otolaryngologist can coordinate care with your internist or pulmonologist. As a general rule, whether your "go-to" doctor is your internist, pulmonologist, or otolaryngologist, as a singer you need to find a doctor who listens to all your concerns, asks questions, thinks globally, and spends as much time with you as is necessary to solve whatever medical or emotional issues you need to explore.

4

Allergy Basics

BOYAN HADJIEV, MD

In my practice as an allergist and immunologist, I get to see a wide variety of patients. Because we are located in New York, I consult on singers, actors, and anyone and everyone who is in show business. Performers present a particular challenge, with management of their nasal allergies and sinus disease because they use their upper respiratory system to make their living. They have to be in tip-top shape at all times. They cannot afford to sound nasal, have a persistent cough, or have so much mucus that they constantly need to clear their throat.

Unfortunately, most patients, including professional performers and entertainers, have a misconception that allergies are only about sneezing, when in reality they are responsible for so many more symptoms. As allergies can affect your nose, throat, ears, and eyes, the symptoms they produce can be quite varied. The nose, the throat, the ears, and the sinuses are all anatomically interconnected, covered by the same mucous membrane; in fact, they consist topologically of one single surface. Imagine having a finely tuned orchestra: if the wind section is not performing well, the whole orchestra's performance suffers. The same thing can happen with the upper airway. If the nose is congested, the voice sounds nasal. If you have chronic indoor allergies, a sinus infection, or a cold, then your ears can feel clogged. As I said, everything is connected.

So how does one know if one has a cold, or a sinus infection, or allergies? I hope to explain all this without sounding too scientific and boring. As always, keep in mind that this chapter is meant as a general aid and educational material. It is not meant to diagnose or cure anyone. So please, read this chapter as a general aid, but do not try to diagnose yourself. Leave that to your physician or health professional.

Rhinitis

Rhinitis simply refers to inflammation of the nasal passages. From a practical standpoint, rhinitis symptoms include sneezing, itching, nasal congestion, runny nose, and postnasal drip (the sensation that mucus is draining from the sinuses down the back of the throat). Note that these symptoms all originate in the nose only and are not "sinusitis," as some patients believe.

Chances are, you have already experienced rhinitis at some point in your life. Brief episodes of rhinitis are usually caused by respiratory tract infections with viruses such as the common cold virus. Chronic rhinitis, by contrast, is most commonly caused by allergies. For many people, rhinitis can be a lifelong condition that waxes and wanes over time. Fortunately, symptoms of rhinitis can be controlled with medications, environmental measures, and immunotherapy (also called allergy shots).

Allergic rhinitis, which some also call hay fever, affects up to 20 percent of people of all ages. Historically, *hay fever* was the term given to fall-time seasonal allergy symptoms. When they hay was collected, people experienced an itchy and runny nose, sneezing, and itchy eyes, which was then called hay fever. In the springtime, those same symptoms were called "rose fever." Over time, the term *rose fever* fell out of favor, and the term *hay fever* stuck for both spring-time and fall-time allergies. The reason people suffer from hay fever is that tiny pollen particles from plants become airborne and stick to one's mucous membranes— the lining of the nose, and eyes, in particular. Once the pollen sticks, it causes a local inflammatory reaction and triggers the symptoms familiar to every sufferer. The exact timing of pollination of plants varies by geographical location, but generally speaking trees pollinate in March, April, and May; grasses in May, June, July; weeds in July, August, September; and ragweed in July and August through the first frost. For more information on your particular area, visit **www.pollen.com** and see your local allergy forecast.

Let us look at the science behind allergic rhinitis/rhinoconjuctivitis (conjunctivitis refers to inflammation of the mucous membrane lining of your eyes, also known as conjunctiva).

Allergic rhinitis, or nasal allergies, can begin at any age, though most people first develop symptoms in childhood or young adulthood. The symptoms are often at their worst in children and in people in their thirties and forties. Severity of symptoms can vary throughout life, and many people experience periods of remission.

Remember the local inflammatory reaction that pollen causes? This reaction can occur in the nose, the skin, the eyes, or anywhere else in the body. The same underlying mechanisms are valid, whether the allergen is pollen or a food particle.

An allergen (a substance that provokes an allergic reaction) is recognized by the immune system. The immune system, acting through two types of cells called mast cells and basophils, releases inflammatory substances such as histamine. If this reaction occurs in the nasal tissues, a person with allergies will experience nasal congestion, itching, sneezing, and runny nose. Similar reactions can occur in the lungs (asthma) and eyes (allergic conjunctivitis). Over several hours, these substances activate other in-flammatory cells, which can cause persistent symptoms. Of course, this is an oversimplification, yet a useful one to keep in mind.

To keep things organized, doctors like to separate nasal aller-gies (allergic rhinitis) into seasonal (occurring during specific seasons) or perennial (occurring year round). As mentioned ear-lier, the allergens that most commonly cause seasonal allergic rhinitis include pollens from trees, grasses, and weeds, as well as spores from fungi and molds.

The allergens that most commonly cause perennial nasal al-lergies are dust mites, cockroaches, animal dander, and fungi or molds. A note: mold spores can be both seasonal and perennial; it all depends on one's environment. Yearlong nasal allergies tend to be more difficult to treat.

The symptoms of allergic rhinitis vary from person to per-son. Although the term *rhinitis* refers only to the nasal symp-toms, many people also experience problems with their eyes, throat, ears, and sleep. It all depends on which organ, or mucous membrane, is involved in the allergic reaction. Here are some symptoms:

- Nasal: watery nasal discharge, sneezing, congested or blocked nasal passages, nasal itching, postnasal drip, loss of taste, and also facial pressure or pain
- Eyes: itchy, red eyes, swollen eyelids, sensation of "gritti-ness" in the eyes, swelling and dark-looking circles under-neath the eyes (called allergic "shiners")
- Throat and ears: chronic sore throat, voice hoarseness, con-gestion or popping of the ears (called Eustachian tube dys-function), itching of the throat, roof of the mouth, or ears
- Sleep: mouth breathing, frequent awakening, daytime fa-tigue, difficulty in performing work

Generally speaking, seasonal allergies usually cause sneezing, itching, a sore throat, and a runny nose. It feels almost as if one has a cold, except fever is usually absent. It is not unusual for a patient to come into the office and complain of getting "colds" in the spring and fall, only to find out she has seasonal allergies. Most people know about hay fever. If they don't, they probably haven't watched the recent onslaught of TV ads for allergy medications!

When one suffers from yearlong allergies, the symptoms are not as clear-cut. The predominant symptoms include postnasal drip, persistent nasal congestion, and poor sleep. Because those symptoms are vaguer, people ignore them, compensate via an adaptive mechanism (e.g., mouth breathing instead of breathing through nose), or simply assume they have something else wrong with them ("I have always been congested; I don't think I have allergies").

Diagnosing Allergies

The diagnosis of allergic rhinitis is made by the patient and a health care professional. The patient supplies all the information that is needed; he or she undergoes taking of a detailed history and a medical exam. At this point, the health care specialist should be able to confirm the diagnosis by ordering and applying allergy tests identify the offending allergens.

Here are a few tips to keep in mind before you come into the office:

Try to recall possible triggering factors that precede your symptoms.

It is very important to note the time when symptoms began.

Try to identify allergens in your home, work, or school environment. If in doubt, take a picture with a cell phone or
a digital camera. Depending on circumstances, it may be
useful to keep a diary, as we often tend to forget many
important details.

Today, both skin testing and blood testing are widely used to
confirm allergic sensitivities. Both of those tests may be useful
for people whose symptoms are not well controlled with medications or in whom the offending allergen is not obvious.

Treatment

Treatment of allergic rhinitis includes reducing exposure to
allergens and other triggers, in combination with medication
therapy. In most people, these measures effectively control the
symptoms.

Reduction of exposure to allergens can often be difficult. Yet
a few simple measures can be used:

- Dust and dust mite avoidance: encase pillows, mattresses,
  and box springs in allergen control barriers. Remove heavy
  drapes, carpeting, and rugs, especially in bedrooms.
- Pet dander: the best avoidance would be to get rid of the
  pet, which is usually difficult to do. Pets are beloved com-
  panions and friends, and people prefer to take medications
  and suffer rather than get rid of their pets. There are special
  shampoos and pet wipes used to remove the allergens from
  the pet's pelt, coat, and hair. Limiting the pet to a certain
  part of the house (e.g., kitchen) can often be quite useful.
  Most importantly, don't allow your pet to share your bed.

- Pollen: keep windows closed during pollen season. Use a HEPA (high-efficiency particulate air) filter. Minimize early morning outdoor activity (5:00 A.M. to 10:00 A.M.), which is when the pollen counts are highest.

In summary, allergies of the upper respiratory tract are common, and not always recognized. Even in cases of infection, there may be an allergic component. Although there are many medications, both over-the-counter and prescription, for treating allergies, a methodical approach begins with identifying the allergens and then attempting to minimize contact, either by eliminating them from your home or avoiding places where those allergens are prevalent. Only after these two steps have been taken does it make sense to consider medical treatment, whether by the use of medications or by immunotherapy (desensitization).

5

Disorders of the Nose, Sinuses, and Throat: An Overview for Singers

ANTHONY F. JAHN, MD

The nose, sinuses, and pharynx form the upper part of the vocal tract, and therefore an important anatomic area for singers. A majority of singers seeking medical advice and treatment present with complaints localized to this area. This chapter describes some common disorders of the nose, sinuses, and pharynx, along with their management.

The structure of the nose is quite complex but can be broadly broken down into two major components: internal and external anatomy. Although the external anatomy of the nose plays a significant role in facial aesthetics, this chapter focuses on the internal nose, which plays a larger role in nasal function and dysfunction. The function of the nose is to inhale air, and in the process warm and humidify it. The second function is olfaction, or the sense of smell.

The nasal cavity is divided in the middle by a septum, consisting of bone in the back and cartilage in the front. The cartilage portion of the septum corresponds to the flexible part of the nose, whereas the bony part corresponds to the upper rigid part. Normally the septum is in the midline, although it may be somewhat curved or deviated. Depending on the degree of deviation, the septum may narrow one or both of the nasal cavities.

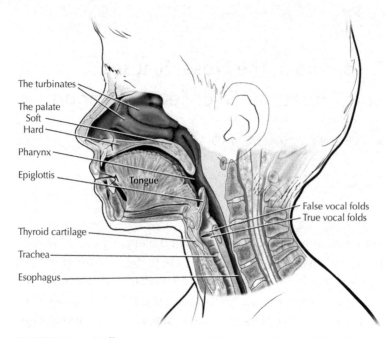

The turbinates
The palate
  Soft
  Hard
Pharynx
Epiglottis
Tongue
False vocal folds
True vocal folds
Thyroid cartilage
Trachea
Esophagus

FIGURE 5.1 Midline cross-section of the upper airway. ©2011 Carolyn R. Holmes, CMI

As air is inhaled, it travels to the back of the nose, where it enters the nasopharynx (Figure 5.1).

The nasopharynx is the uppermost portion of the pharynx, a tubelike structure that connects the nose, middle ear (via the Eustachian tube), oral cavity, larynx, and esophagus. The inhaled air travels down the pharynx through the larynx and then into the pulmonary system, where oxygen is absorbed and carbon dioxide is released.

The internal nose not only serves as a passageway for airflow but also cleans, warms, and humidifies that air. Several anatomic structures aid in this purpose, among them the nasal turbinates and possibly the paranasal sinuses (Figure 5.2).

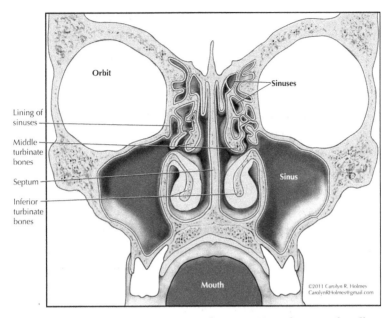

FIGURE 5.2 Cross section of nose and sinuses. Note the normal midline position of the nasal septum. The inferior turbinates project into the nasal passages, but do not obstruct air flow. ©2011 Carolyn R. Holmes, CMI

Turbinates are bony shelves covered by mucous membrane that project inward from the sides of the nose. Most people have three on each side, an inferior, middle, and superior turbinate. By increasing the surface area of the nasal mucosa, the turbinates aid in cleaning and humidifying air as it travels into the nasopharynx. The inferior turbinate is the largest and most important in the heating and humidification process. The role of the inferior turbinate is so significant in nasal physiology that, even if an overgrown inferior turbinate causes nasal obstruction, it should only be reduced, but not completely removed. Remarkably, in a short distance of three or four inches, cold and dry air is heated to body temperature and completely humidified.

The sinuses are mucous membrane lined cavities, outpouchings from the nasal cavity. There are four pairs of paranasal sinuses: the maxillary, ethmoid, frontal, and sphenoid. The maxillary sinuses are the largest of the four and lie in the cheeks, directly to the sides of the nose, above the upper jaw (or maxilla) and below the orbit. The ethmoid sinuses are between the eyes and above the maxillary sinuses, the frontal sinuses are in the forehead area, and the sphenoid sinuses are located in the middle of the head. The function of the paranasal sinuses is not entirely known, but most would agree that the open connection between the nasal cavity and the sinuses is important for good nasal health. The sinuses and the nasal cavities are all lined with mucous membrane, which secretes mucus and pushes it backward using tiny hairlike projections called cilia. The mucus blanket covering the mucous membrane catches environmental debris and pollutants and propels them out of the nose and into the nasopharynx. In this way, the inner lining of the nose is continuously cleaned as this blanket of mucus moves toward the back of the throat. In the course of a normal day, we swallow between a pint and a quart of mucus.

In singers, the nose and sinuses contribute to the quality of the voice. The air within the nose resonates during singing, amplifying and coloring the voice. In normal singing there is no direct connection between the air in the pharynx and air in the nose (since good technical singing involves raising the soft palate and separating these two compartments), but vibration is transmitted to the nasal cavities through the hard palate and the facial bones. The sinuses are also resonant cavities. Their contribution to the voice is less clear, although certainly the singer's perception of the voice "in the mask" is affected by resonance in these cavities. Swelling of the mucosal lining in the nose (and possibly the sinuses) might absorb some of the sound and muffle the voice.

The nose is also responsible for olfaction, or the sense of smell, which contributes considerably to our sense of taste. The nerve endings for olfaction are located at the apex of the nasal cavities, between the eyes. Whereas normal breathing lets air flow smoothly between the septum and the turbinates to the back of the throat, sniffing causes turbulent airflow around the turbinates, and eddies of odor-laden air swirl up to the olfactory area. When we are "stuffed up," which often occurs when there is allergic or infectious inflammation of the nasal mucosa, not only is our sense of smell decreased but we also tend to feel as if we can't really taste food as well as usual.

If the nasal and paranasal cavities become inflamed because of allergies or nasal infections, the mucus can build up in the sinuses and become infected, leading to a condition known as sinusitis. The causes of sinusitis are multiple. As mentioned earlier, allergies and nasal infections may lead to sinusitis, since both of these conditions cause swelling and inflammation of the nasal and paranasal sinus mucosa. If the mucous membrane becomes swollen, it can block off the small passages that connect the sinuses to the nasal cavity, and therefore the mucus in the sinuses can no longer get out. In these patients, the best way to prevent sinusitis is to adequately treat allergies and infections, which may involve both local (nasal spray) and systemic (pill) therapies.

Other people may develop frequent sinusitis because the passages that allow mucus to drain are abnormally narrow even in the absence of inflammation. These are patients who seemingly never have just a simple cold without getting sinusitis, which may last for weeks. In these patients, surgery may be the most effective way to open up their nasal and sinus drainage passages.

Infections of the nose are most commonly caused by the rhinovirus. This is what people refer to when they talk about the "common cold." We all are familiar with the symptoms of rhinovirus infection: stuffy or runny nose, feeling "under the weather," often accompanied by scratchy throat, red itchy eyes, or ear infection. There is no single cure-all for the common cold, and since it is caused by a virus and not bacteria antibiotics have absolutely no efficacy against it. In fact, taking antibiotics for the common cold can kill healthy bacteria in other parts of the body, leading to unwanted side effects such as vaginal yeast infections and diarrhea. However, a viral infection can damage the mucosa and leave it more susceptible to a secondary bacterial infection. If a cold has not gone away after a couple of days, or if the cold is accompanied by fever or the presence of particularly green mucus, this may be a sign of a secondary bacterial infection, and immediate medical attention should be sought.

When the nasal mucosa becomes inflamed it tends to secrete more mucus, which results in rhinitis, or "runny nose." Even if we blow our nose more frequently when we're having rhinitis, inevitably more mucus also escapes down the back of the nose into the nasopharynx. This is called postnasal drip. The mucus can then be coughed out through the mouth or swallowed into the esophagus. However, some of this excess mucus, along with any nasal bacteria or viruses we might be harboring, tends to find its way into the larynx and causes local irritation, also known as laryngitis. Along with irritation of the pharynx, soiling of the larynx by infected mucus can give the sensation of "scratchy throat" and can cause huskiness or hoarseness in the singer. If the infection continues unchecked, cough and bronchitis are the next symptoms.

In addition to blockage due to swollen mucosa, the holes that drain the sinuses can also be blocked by a deviated, or off-center, nasal septum. The deviated nasal septum is usually developmental: there may have been some slight deviation since birth, which may have worsened during the rapid growth phase of puberty. Septal deviation is often not obvious by looking at the outside of the nose alone, and thus it typically goes unnoticed for many

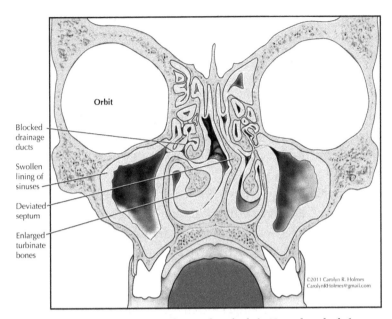

Orbit

Blocked
drainage
ducts

Swollen
lining of
sinuses

Deviated
septum

Enlarged
turbinate
bones

©2011 Carolyn R. Holmes
CarolynRHolmes@gmail.com

FIGURE 5.3 Nasal septum is deviated to the left. Note that the left maxillary sinus is obstructed, with swollen lining. The right inferior turbinate has overgrown to take up the extra room in the right nasal passage. The result is a nasal obstruction in both nasal passages. ©2011 Carolyn R. Holmes, CMI

years until it becomes symptomatic. Trauma to the nose can also result in a deviated septum. If the septum is off to one side, it leaves one side of the nasal cavity crowded and obstructed, and the other side empty and dry. When the mucosa becomes too dry, it is more likely to bleed. Interestingly, the turbinates attempt to compensate for this imbalance by hypertrophy, or increasing in size, on the side with the larger open space and shrinking on the more crowded side. The final result is often a bilateral obstruction: one side is blocked by the deviated septum, the other by the overgrown inferior turbinate (Figure 5.3).

Patients with a deviated nasal septum may complain of difficulty breathing, noisy breathing, recurrent nose bleeds on one side, snoring at night, or a history of recurrent sinusitis. These are the patients where a typical cold will often progress to sinusitis, rather than resolve normally. This problem can only truly be addressed surgically, although sinusitis can be staved off with antibiotics for the time being. Once the septum has been returned to its midline location, the surgeon may also decide to reduce the size of the inferior turbinates in order to improve airflow, through a procedure called turbinate reduction. As mentioned before, since the inferior turbinates are important for nasal humidification, they are usually not completely removed, just reduced. Surgery of the nasal septum and turbinates is fairly routine and does not take very long, but rare complications include perforation in the septum or septal hematoma (a collection of blood under the mucosa of the nasal septum), bleeding, and infection.

Sinusitis affects a large percentage of the general population and tends to respond well to oral antibiotics. Typical symptoms include blowing out green or white mucus, chronic infected postnasal drip, nasal obstruction, and headache concentrated around the cheeks, behind the eyes, or on the forehead, as well as decreased sense of smell and taste. Chronic sinusitis is also one of the most common causes of halitosis, or bad breath. When the doctor suspects sinusitis on the basis of the patient's symptoms and a physical examination, a CT scan of the sinuses is often ordered in order to confirm the diagnosis and determine the extent of the disease. The doctor takes many considerations into account in deciding whether or not to operate on the sinuses, most importantly how often the patient gets sinusitis and how well he or she has responded to nonsurgical treatment in the past. Ultimately, the risks and benefits of surgery should be carefully weighed before the doctor and patient decide how best to proceed.

Sinus surgery is usually done through the nostrils, using an endoscope similar to the orthopedist's arthroscope. A magnified image of the inside of the nose is shown on a television monitor, and the surgeon uses tiny instruments to open the sinuses and remove any obstructing tissue. In the case of nasal polyps (larger bits of inflamed tissue), greater amounts of mucous membrane may be removed, although in most cases only smaller pieces need to be excised to adequately open the passage between the inside of the nose and the adjacent sinus cavities. Sinus surgery can be very beneficial, but it can also carry potential complications. Again, the patient needs to discuss exactly what procedure is planned and understand expected benefits, alternative treatments, and potential complications. As with all elective surgical procedures, we encourage the singer to obtain multiple opinions before making a decision.

The impact of nasal and sinus disease on singers is significant. Difficulty breathing, decreased resonance, and difficulty placing the voice into the mask are some common complaints. Although "the mask" refers to bone-conducted resonance perceived over the cheeks and sinuses, the sinuses themselves play no role in the voice that emerges from the singer's mouth. In contrast, singers have commonly reported that, after undergoing appropriate septal and sinus surgery, they find it easier to place the voice into the mask, and the voice sounds larger. Interestingly, this change in sound is also reported by teachers who listen to their students, so it seems to be a real change, rather than just a change in internally perceived bone vibrations. This improvement in sound most likely reflects a change in the size of the internal nasal passages.

The oropharynx and mouth are an important part of the vocal tract. The size of the oral cavity is affected by the height of the palate and the position of the tongue, among other factors. The tonsils, if enlarged, may also play a role in the quality of the voice.

The tonsils are two almond-shaped structures that sit in the back of the mouth, on either side of the posterior tongue and the soft palate. Tonsils are made of lymphoid tissue, which plays an important role in how we acquire immunity during childhood. Similar tissue is found across the back of the tongue (lingual tonsils), in back of the pharynx (lateral pharyngeal bands), and in the nasopharynx (adenoids). Tonsils are very active in early childhood but serve no purpose after childhood. In most cases, they shrink and become insignificant in size. They persist, however, though rarely, and may be large enough to almost obstruct the back of the throat. Particularly at night, large tonsils can protrude into the airway, causing snoring and even sleep apnea. In other cases, the tonsils may be smaller but harbor a chronic low-grade infection that flares up repeatedly. In this situation, whenever the immune system becomes weak, whether from physical or emotional stress or concurrent illness, the patient develops tonsillitis. No amount of oral antibiotics can completely eradicate this infection, since the scarring within the tonsils prevents adequate tissue buildup of antibiotics. Less commonly, the tonsils can suddenly enlarge, from infectious mononucleosis or a tonsil abscess.

There is a common mistaken belief that singers should never have their tonsils operated on. In fact, in Damon Runyonesque lingo, a good singer used to be characterized as having "a great set of tonsils"! Certainly, medical therapy should always be tried before considering surgery, and the impact of chronically infected tonsils on the general well-being of the singer needs to be carefully considered. Still, if there is a valid clinical indication, tonsils can be removed. In singers this needs to be done with care, but it need not be avoided. If done with expertise and minimum trauma, singers should have no vocal difficulties following this procedure. On the positive side, a reduction in the number of sore throats, the opening of the posterior throat with cessation of snoring, and an even more open voice may be the benefits. One cause of a covered sounding voice is partial obstruction of the pharynx by enlarged tonsils; once they are removed, the voice will sound less muffled, and more forward.

In singers with upper airway obstruction during sleep (obstructive sleep apnea), removal of enlarged tonsils may give some relief, without the need to treat the soft palate.

In summary, the upper vocal tract is a vital aspect of voice production, and healthy open passages are important, not just vocally but also in more general terms of health and quality of life. Since these areas are open to the outside and are lined by mucous tissue, they share common diseases, involving viral and bacterial infections and allergies. Good hydration and saline irrigation of the nose are useful preventive measures. When inflammation does develop, it needs to be treated purposefully, whether with antibiotics, decongestants, or antihistamines. Once an infection or obstruction becomes indolent and fails to respond to medical management, appropriate surgery can be very helpful. The surgery should be performed by a surgeon who is familiar with the anatomy and physiology of singing. If surgery is being considered, the singer should seek a second, even a third, opinion before making a decision.

6

Hearing and Hearing Loss in Singers

ANTHONY F. JAHN, MD

MARSHALL CHASIN, AUD

An acute sense of hearing is an important part of singing. The singer constantly monitors his voice for intensity, pitch, and color. He simultaneously registers the sounds around him, whether piano, orchestra, or vocal ensemble. Most singers take their hearing for granted, but the sense of hearing is vulnerable on many levels, and its loss can be gradual, almost imperceptible.

Hearing testing is simple, and recommended to all singers who have difficulty with pitch or auditory discrimination.

The ear is a remarkable organ. It has evolved to perceive extremely soft sounds (*ppp*) and is able to tolerate very loud sounds (*fff*), and over a wide frequency range. The ear's sensitivity is so fine that, were the cochlea's hair cells (receptors) one order of magnitude more sensitive, we would actually hear the random (Brownian) movement of fluid molecules bumping into one another in the inner ear!

The frequency range in a newborn extends from 20 Hz (read as "Hertz," after the German scientist Heinrich Rudolf Hertz) to 20,000 Hz.[1] At the low-frequency end, this encompasses vibrations that are more felt than heard, lower than the lowest organ pedal. At the high-frequency end, it reaches dog-whistle frequencies, certainly higher than any musical instrument can go.

The ear is not equally sensitive at all frequencies, however. Hearing is most acute around 1,000 Hz. This is around the middle of the speech range (500 to 3,000 Hz), and maybe not coincidentally, it is around a tenor's high C. Within the speech range, vowels cluster around the lower end (starting from an octave below middle C), and consonants, especially high-frequency consonants (such as *s*, *sh*, *ts*, and *ch*) are at the higher frequency end, near the top note on the piano keyboard. There are no speech sounds that have frequencies on the left side of the piano keyboard (below 256 Hz), yet there are many low frequency musical notes that can be found here. Historically when hearing is tested, only the sounds on the right side of the piano keyboard are typically assessed. We can test for lower frequencies, but it is exceedingly difficult to say whether one "hears" the sound or "feels" it.

How We Hear

The ear has three main parts: the outer ear, the middle ear, and the inner ear. The outer ear is the part that can be seen when we look at another person, the part that we hang our glasses on. It also includes the ear canal, which is an inch-long tube, ending at the ear drum. The middle ear is an air-filled cavity behind the ear drum that contains the three smallest bones in our body: the malleus, incus, and stapes (or the hammer, the anvil, and the stirrup, if you remember your high school health classes).

The outer and middle ears both act to convey sound vibrations to the inner ear. Sound waves, which are vibrations of air molecules, arrive at the outer ear and are carried down the ear canal toward the eardrum. The eardrum divides the outer ear from the inner ear. The eardrum is a taut membrane, much like the drumhead on a snare drum. It is set into motion by the vibration of the air.

Embedded within the substance of the ear drum is a part of the malleus or hammer, the first of a chain of three tiny bones (or ossicles) that traverse the air-containing middle ear and connect the eardrum to the inner ear. As these tiny bones start to vibrate, air vibration is converted to mechanical oscillation. The hammer moves the anvil, and the anvil sets the innermost ossicle, the stirrup, into vibration. The footplate of the stirrup covers the oval window, an opening to the inner ear. The inner ear is filled with waterlike fluid, and the energy of the vibrating ossicles is passed into thee inner ear chambers, where it forms waves. Floating within this fluid bath are the receptors of the inner ears, called hair cells. As they start to vibrate, they generate an electrical signal, which stimulates the auditory nerve. The purpose of the hair cells is to transduce mechanical energy into electric energy. The electrical signal then travels through various relay stations into the central nervous system and eventually reaches the auditory cortex, where we consciously perceive sound. Figure 6.1 shows a schematic of this wonderful organ.

All of this is a tremendous simplification of the hearing process. It doesn't begin to explain how we can hear the individual instruments of a string quartet, or a Mahler symphony, or the one voice across the room at a noisy party that is calling our name (while filtering out that annoying person right next to us!). Many of these phenomena take place in the auditory portion of the brain rather than the ear, and we are only now beginning to understand how we perceive speech and music.

The explanation demonstrates that hearing has two components: conductive and sensorineural. The air vibrations that are sound are conducted down the ear canal, further conveyed as mechanical vibrations through the eardrum and the ossicles to the inner ear. The outer and middle ear are involved in the conductive part of hearing. In the inner ear, mechanical vibrations are changed to electric energy by the hair cells of the cochlea. The

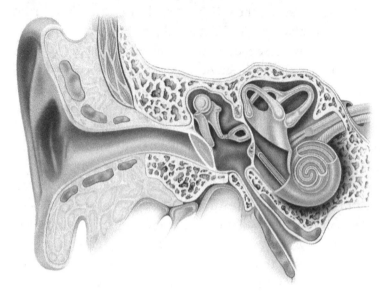

FIGURE 6.1 Schematic of the ear. Figure courtesy of Bernafon Canada. Used with permission.

electric impulse then travels up the brain. This is the sensorineural part of hearing.

It is evident from this that hearing loss can be conductive, sensorineural, or both. For example, conductive hearing loss occurs when the ear canal is occluded by wax, or there is fluid in the middle ear. Sensorineural loss occurs when the inner ear is damaged, or the higher auditory pathways are not working properly. It is also possible to have both problems: someone with noise damage to the inner ear could have wax in the ear canal as well. This is called a mixed hearing loss.

The inner ear (cochlea) receives sounds in two ways. One is through the ear canal, following the path described above. This is called air conduction. But sound can also be transmitted directly to the inner ear, though skull vibration. If you hold a tuning fork against your head, or your top teeth to the mouthpiece of a clarinet, the vibrations travel though the skull bones directly to the inner ear, bypassing the ear canal and middle ear. This is called bone conduction.

The singer hears simultaneously by both air and bone conduction. She hears the sounds around her, her own voice, the voices of others, the orchestra, through air conduction, via the ear canal. But she also hears her own voice through the bones of the skull, the vibrations of the facial bones and palate directly setting the cochlea into vibration. Although air-conducted hearing is normally dominant, there are circumstances where the singer relies on bone-conducted sound almost fully. In choral singing, the performer's ear canals are filled with the voices all around, and so the singer is flying "by instrument guidance only," i.e., monitoring the voice by bone-conducted sound and vibration.

If ambient sounds are distracting, one can increase the perception of bone-conducted sound by blocking the ear canal. Plugging the ear with your finger emphasizes bone-conducted sound to the ear, and actually directs the voice preferentially into the occluded ear. The cellist tuning in a noisy orchestra pit by putting the tuning peg of the instrument against the side of the head is another example of hearing by bone conduction. After Beethoven began to lose hearing, he was still able, for a while, to hear the piano using a "dentiphone," a stick held between the teeth, the other end touching the top of the instrument—again, taking advantage of bone conduction for hearing.

Common Causes of Hearing Loss

Practically speaking, there are two common causes of conductive hearing loss: earwax, and fluid in the middle ear. Wax is a normal secretion of the ear canal. Left untouched, it usually forms in the outer ear canal, and over time it falls out spontaneously. When it is manipulated using cotton swabs, it is not uncommon to push bits of wax into the deeper canal, and this may require removal. The best way to remove excessive wax is to loosen it over two or three days using eardrops or hydrogen peroxide, and then flush it out. You can use a rubber bulb, filled with lukewarm water and its tip placed into the outer part of the ear canal. Fairly vigorous flushing will dislodge the clump of wax without any damage. Then dry the ear using a rolled-up corner of a facial tissue to mop out any moisture. However if there has been previous damage to the ear (such as an eardrum perforation or hole), then wax should be removed only by your doctor.

The second common cause of conductive hearing loss, fluid accumulation in the middle ear, develops when the Eustachian tube is blocked. This can occur with a cold, with allergies, or after an airplane flight. Simple remedies include decongesting the nose with nose spray and then trying to pop the ears, or swallowing with the nose pinched shut. Oral decongestants can also help. Needless to say, if you are unable to relieve hearing loss, either from wax impaction or fluid accumulation, you need to see a doctor as soon as possible.

Sensorineural hearing loss (also called nerve loss or perceptive deafness) is usually more insidious. The most common cause—aging—results in a gradual loss of high frequencies, which progresses gradually over time into the speech frequencies. The initial loss is imperceptible. As it grows worse, you may be aware of difficulties listening to higher-pitched voices (women and children). Since high-frequency consonants provide speech clarity, you may also notice some difficulty in understanding speech, especially in noisy situations. As these frequencies are, at least initially, in the high range, you may have no difficulty with music. You may, however, note a difference in the color of the sound of instruments. Age-related hearing loss (sometimes referred to as presbycusis) can progress to the lower frequencies and cause significant impairment. Gabriel Fauré had a severe form of age-related hearing loss. A musicologist once reported, apparently with unintentional humor, that Fauré's hearing loss eventually became so great that he could no longer compose, so he became a music critic!

Aging of the ears usually causes a symmetrical sensorineural hearing loss. If the hearing loss is greater in one ear, the sufferer often loses a sense of sound direction. For good stereo sound localization, the thresholds in the two ears must be within 10 decibels of each other. If the difference is greater, the person cannot tell where the sound source is, although it may still be possible to hear the sound.

Noise Damage

A common and increasing problem in the pop music field is noise damage to the inner ear. The ears are meant to hear soft-to-medium sounds, and the cochlea saturates at intense noise levels. Loud noise damages the inner ear in several ways. Initially, the damage is usually temporary: several hours of decreased hearing, which recovers overnight. The hearing loss may be accompanied by a ringing or whooshing sound called tinnitus. If the loud sound exposure is persistent or repetitive, however, the damage becomes permanent and irreversible. Hearing loss occurs initially at higher frequencies near the top of the piano keyboard (4,000 to 6,000 Hz), but it can over time spread into the lower range and affect speech perception. Equally distressing, the tinnitus may become permanent. The likelihood of this occurrence varies with age, constitutional proclivity, and the type, intensity, and duration of the damaging noise.

Noise-induced hearing loss (which is further discussed in Chapter 7) and tinnitus are incurable, but also preventable. It is therefore extremely important to be aware of the duration of loud sound exposure and the sound levels involved. Occupational safety standards around the world currently mandate limiting industrial noise exposure to no more than 85 decibels of sound for an eight-hour day. This represents a reduction from previously acceptable limits, and it is very likely that the maximum permissible exposure will continue to go down as we become more aware of the insidious effects of chronic noise on the ear in the MP3 generation.

Testing Hearing

Hearing testing performed by an audiologist today is actually quite similar to the way it was performed in the 1960s. There are a few more tests that directly assess the function of the middle ear (such as to rule out ear infections) and some tests that are designed to obtain objective results without the person having to respond (such as otoacoustic emission testing). By far the most salient test, one that we may recall from the screenings performed by nurses in third grade, is that of pure tone testing. In this test, a series of tones or beeps at octave inervals (usually near the frequencies of the various C notes on the right side of a piano keyboard) are played through earphones in a sound-treated chamber. The tones are gradually made quieter until the person can no longer hear them. The threshold for each tone is then recorded on an audiogram (shown in Figure 6.2). In addition to the audiogram, the musical staff is written across the top, showing the correpondence between the letter notes used by musicians and the frequency numbers used on the audiogram.

A straight line across the top of the audiogram, in the range of 0 to 25 decibels, is considered normal hearing. If the quietest sounds a person can hear are greater than 25 dB, then this per-

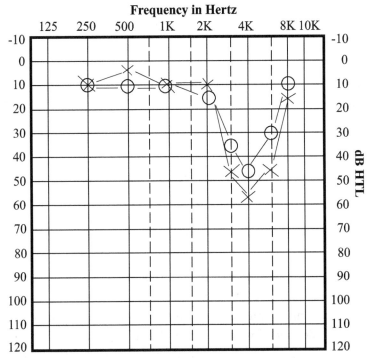

FIGURE 6.2 This shows a typical music induced hearing loss with the poorest hearing acuity at 4000 Hz (near the top end of the piano keyboard).

son has a hearing loss; the greater the decibel value needed before the sound can be heard, the greater the hearing loss. The degree of hearing loss can be further characterized as mild, moderate, severe, or profound.

In addition to "pure tone testing," there is "word recognition testing." This is a rather blunt test, and unless there is significant sensorineural hearing loss, word recognition testing does not typically provide much additional information. An audiologist may also perform acoustic immitance testing (also called acoustic impedance testing), where the mechanical function of the middle ear is indirectly assessed. Because the eardrum covers the opening to the middle ear like a curtain, the physician cannot always see the workings of the middle ear, so this test can be quite valuable.

Of the newer generation of audiological tests, otoacoustic emission testing (or OAE) has great promise for the musician. OAEs were first discovered in 1978 and were originally called "Kemp's echo" after the discoverer. In brief, Kemp found that when the ear is exposed to sounds, it can itself generate a sound in return! When any sound travels up from the ear, along the nerves to the brain, a part of it "loops" back around and returns to another part of the inner ear. This causes these different nerve endings or hair cells to vibrate, thereby setting up vibration in the fluid of the inner ear. But it does not stop here. This vibration causes the three bones in the middle ear to vibrate (like the tail wagging the dog), which in turn causes the eardrum to vibrate. Now the eardrum is acting like a loudspeaker rather than a microphone. This sound, the otoacoustic emission, is very quiet (on the order of only a few decibels), but it can be picked up in the ear canal with a specially designed computer. The presence of otoacoustic emissions usually indicates good hair cell function in the cochlea.

One important use of otoacoustic emissions is in the realm of hearing conservation. In the majority of cases (but not all), a change in the status of OAEs shows up long before one can measure an audiometic change in one's hearing levels, and before the patient is subjectively aware of hearing loss. This test can therefore be a sensitive and early indicator of cochlear damage. If our goal is hearing loss prevention, the use of OAEs shows great promise and indeed should be an integral part of any hearing assessment program for those in the performing arts.

In summary, the ability to hear clearly and through the full range of speech and music is essential to the singer, but it is often neglected during medical evaluations. Since the ears form the afferent loop of the singing process, monitoring the voice and the sounds of others on the stage or in the pit, we recommend that periodic hearing testing be part of every singer's health checkup.

Notes

1. For those readers over the age of sixty: you may recall the former name for Hertz as "cycles per second."

7

Hearing Conservation and Hearing Rehabilitation for Singers

MARSHALL CHASIN, AUD

DAVID GOLDFARB, MD

MARIS APPLEBAUM, AUD

Attention to hearing conservation is especially important for musical theater and other nonclassical genres, since sound is usually amplified to an unphysiologic and acoustically traumatic intensity, and the venue itself is often smaller and more reverberant. Furthermore, the singer often stands in front of the orchestra and the amplifiers, at the mercy of the man in charge of the soundboard. To heighten the excitement of the experience, sound levels are set well beyond the saturation level of the cochlea, where the music is felt rather than heard. Following two or three loud sets, a few hours of tinnitus and a temporary shift in auditory threshold is common. Permanent hearing loss can develop with repeated acoustic trauma, but it has been seen to occur after even a single explosive sound event. Although it is hard to conceive of the music of Mozart, Brahms, and the Beatles and the voice of Pavarotti as noise, repeated exposure to music at high intensity can cause noise-induced hearing loss in musicians. In some literature this is even referred to as music-induced hearing loss (distinct from noise-induced hearing loss), and it affects classical as well as rock musicians.

Prolonged exposure to loud music may initially cause a temporary threshold shift. This shift in hearing, also felt as a "fullness" or "feeling of dullness" in the ears, will usually resolve and return to the original threshold level after approximately sixteen to eighteen hours. Repeated exposure to high-intensity music may continue to cause shifts in hearing that can become permanent hearing loss over time. In addition to protecting one's hearing in practice and concert settings, one must also implement hearing conservation in general as all noise exposure is additive to hearing loss. It is best to minimize exposure to loud noise such as lawnmowers, motorcycles, personal stereo systems at loud volume, and firearms, to name a few. Noise-induced hearing loss can also be exacerbated by diabetes, cardiovascular disease, smoking, and ototoxic drugs.

The ability to perceive pitch and monitor one's own voice or music is crucial to the professional musician and singer. Noise-induced hearing loss causes tinnitus, hyperacusis (which is an abnormal sensitivity to loud sounds), and recruitment (an abnormal growth of sound loudness). It can also cause diplacusis, which is abnormal perception of a pure tone as off-pitch or double-pitch. Recruitment may make a small increase in sound seem as if it were a large increase in volume. Diplacusis may make a note sound flat, and hyperacusis may be so severe as to prevent the musician from playing at the correct level. All of these will make it difficult for the professional musician to monitor himself and the music around him.

Noise and Music-Induced Hearing Loss

Noise exposure and music exposure affect the ear in a similar manner. In most cases the only way to distinguish between noise exposure and music exposure is by the history. This is not really surprising because music is just made up of vibrations in the air, and factory noise, for instance, is also made up of vibrations in the air. A difference between noise and music is that music has a rich harmonic structure that has a well-defined relationship. For example, if a note has a harmonic that is twice the frequency of another (e.g., 880 Hz and 440 Hz) then they are one octave apart. In this example, both are called the same letter note, and in this case we are referring to the musical note A (sometimes written as A[440] and A[880]). There is rarely a time when successive overtones or higher frequencies on a factory floor have a well-defined relationship. Musicians (and most industrial workers) may refer to factory noise as dissonant. The complex differences between music and factory noise are primarily in the brain and not the ear. Yet since the ear is on the firing line for the mechanical air vibrations that are perceived as "sound," it is the ear that can suffer permanent hearing loss from prolonged exposure to loud music and loud noise alike.

When someone's hearing is tested, the results are recorded on an audiogram. An example of an audiogram is shown in Figure 7.1. The "Os" are for the right ear and the "Xs" are for the left ear. Across the top of the graph (the X axis) is frequency, much like a piano keyboard that goes from 250 Hz (close to middle C) to 8,000 Hz (about an octave above the top note on a piano keyboard). The frequency notes are spaced in a similar manner to that of the piano keyboard; each doubling of the frequency number (e.g., 500 Hz to 1,000 Hz) is one octave. The numbers along the vertical side of the audiogram represent decibels of sound. The sound threshold (a tone that is just barely heard) is identified for each frequency (plotted along the X axis), and its loudness (intensity) is plotted against the vertical scale (hearing threshold level, Y axis). The further down on the audiogram, the worse someone's hearing is. Normal hearing is a straight horizontal line near the top of the chart. It is difficult to test for the acuity of the really low sounds on the left side of the piano keyboard because it becomes very difficult to say whether one "hears" the sound or

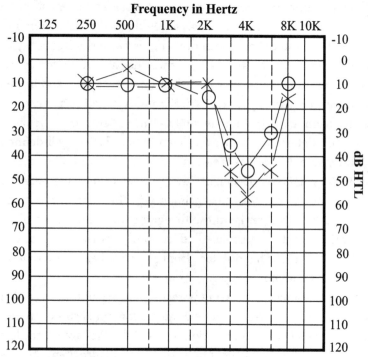

FIGURE 7.1 Audiogram showing a music or noise induced hearing loss in the higher frequency region (worse near the top note of the piano keyboard). This "notched" or V configuration is typical of long term music and noise exposure.

"feels" it. Any singer who has performed with a church organ is familiar with the sound of the low pedals, more of a physical throb thob than an actual tone.

The audiogram shows an interesting pattern or shape that is found in many cases of music and noise exposure. The audiogram shows excellent hearing acuity for the notes around the middle of the piano keyboard, but it falls off (poorer hearing acuity) for the notes near the top end of the piano keyboard (e.g., 4,000 Hz) and then recovers at 8,000 Hz. This local loss of hearing acuity in the 4,000 Hz region is typically seen in many cases of music exposure and is sometimes called "a noise induced notch." In almost all cases of industrial noise exposure, the right and left ears are rather similar. In some cases of music exposure there can be a difference or an asymmetry in the two ears. It is not uncommon for a violinist to have the left ear be slightly worse than the right simply because the instrumentalist holds a four-stringed noise generator closer to the left ear. If vocalists have asymmetrical hearing, it may be related to noisier musical instruments (such as the high hat of a drum kit) being closer to the left-rear side. We have also seen asymmetric hearing loss in voice teachers, whose right ear is closer to the singing student, an exposure repeated over decades of lessons. There are other causes of difference or asymmetry in the hearing, and if unexplained they should be investigated by an otolaryngologist.

Music Exposure for Those in the Performing Arts

Singers do not have themselves to blame for hearing loss. It is very rare for a vocalist to be able to generate and sustain a potentially damaging level of music. The human lungs are not designed to create sound at a damaging level. However, it is the orchestra or band backing up the singer that may be the culprit. And it may not be the musical performance (whether it is rock or opera) that is the sole cause. When we speak of music-induced hearing loss, it is exposure to a wide range of noise and music sources throughout the day and week that achieve a damaging "dose."

The term *dose* is not just a clever metaphor that conjures up an image of radiation workers in a nuclear facility being forced to take a vacation when their dose badge turns a certain color. The ear responds to loud music (and loud noise) according to the dose it receives, and dose is related to both the intensity and the duration of exposure. There is nothing wrong with a two-hour musical performance, but if this combines with six more shows in a week as well as rehearsals and teaching, the total exposure may be significant.

Specifically, one needs to be concerned with any prolonged sound levels in excess of 85 decibels (A-weighted), sometimes written as 85 dBA. The A-weighted scale corresponds to how the human ear receives sound. The vast majority of low-frequency energy generated by the bass notes on the left hand side of the piano keyboard bounce off the eardrum, but this is not the case for most of the higher-pitched sounds. The A-weighted decibel scale accounts for this. Sound level meters, which are small hand-held devices for measuring sound intensity, have a measurement setting for decibels in the A-weighted scale. Common sound levels of some musical instruments (in dBA) are shown in Table 7.1.

TABLE 7.1

Musical Instrument	Typical intensity range (dBA)
Normal piano playing	60–90
Loud piano playing	70–105
Violin	80–105
Symphonic music	86–102
Saxophone	75–110
Flute	92–105
Trombone	90–106
Tympani	74–94
Amplified rock music	102–108
Vocalist	70–90

Source: Adapted from Chasin (2006) shows typical intensity levels of a wide range of musical instruments measured from approximately 3 meters on the horizontal plane. Used with permission of Hearing Review.

The decibel scale is "logarithmic," meaning that every 3 decibels of increase in intensity (which is barely detectable) is double the potential damage. An 88 dBA sound is therefore twice as intense (and potentially twice as damaging) as an 85 dBA sound. However, there is an important correspondence between the sound level and how long one is exposed to it. A 90 dBA sound level for forty hours a week (as found in a factory, for example) is identical to a 93 dBA sound level for only twenty hours a week. This is also identical to potential damage from a 96 dBA sound (93 + 3) for only ten hours a week, and so on. A singer may not be exposed for forty hours a week but could be subjected to loud music for five or ten hours a week. The trick is to bring the exposure down to a point where there is no potential damage, e.g., 85 dBA for forty hours a week or 88 dbA for twenty hours a week, or even 100 dBA for one and a quarter hours a week. Recent research with the Canadian Opera Company found that opera singers were not at risk from music exposure since, given the number of hours they were exposed, the intensity level never exceeded a critical level.[1] It should also be pointed out that opera singers normally stand upstage from the orchestra, sing in large and relatively nonreverberant halls, and, apart from any special sound effects, are mostly exposed only to their own voices and the voices of other singers on the stage. However, these same opera singers should still take care when they mow the lawn and play the guitar.

The Need for Proper Hearing Protection

Prior to 1988, the only hearing protection available was industrial-strength earplugs, which tended to cause too much sound muffling for the performing artist. These old-style earplugs provided about 25–40 dB of attenuation (lessening of the music

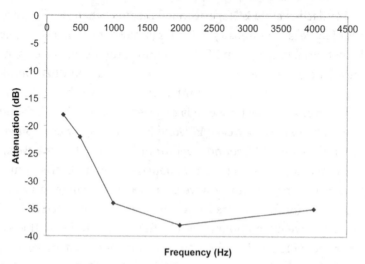

FIGURE 7.2 Industrial strength hearing protection which was the only option for musicians prior to 1988. These earplugs attenuate (or lessen) the lower frequencies only slightly but provides for significant higher frequency attenuation. When listening to music with these earplugs one would hear the fundamental energy but minimal higher frequency harmonic energy.

intensity). And they achieved differing amounts of sound attenuation depending on the frequency or pitch. Figure 7.2 shows how the attenuation varies as a function of frequency. In the figure, think of the horizontal axis (like the audiogram) as the piano keyboard and the vertical one as how much protection is afforded (with 0 dB meaning no change). Industrial-strength old-style plugs would result in a slight decrease in the fundamental energy and almost complete attenuation of the higher-frequency harmonics, but these harmonics are necessary for the beauty of music.

These old-style, industrial-strength earplugs not only treated the various sounds of music differently they caused an echo sensation by plugging up the ears. Also, with attenuation values up to about 40 dB, it was too much of a change for most musicians. Since the sound of many consonants in conversation are also in the higher-frequency range, these plugs limited the intelligibility of speech. Most important, the amount of sound attenuation was uncessarily too much.

Recall that for every 3 dB increase in sound level, the potential damage doubles. Stating this differently, for every 3 dB of attenuation (or lessening) of sound, the potential damage is cut in half. Consider a singer in front of a rock band, where the sound level has been measured at 100 dBA. Even if the singer were unprotected from this sound, she could still be safely in this environment for about fifteen minutes. Since a vocalist would be typically exposed for a longer period of time, and we know that it would be safe if only 85 dBA (or less) reached their ears, these musicians would require hearing protection having only about 15 dB of attenuation. Therefore, this 15 dB reduction (from 100 dBA to 85 dBA) is all the singer would need. Fifteen minutes exposure at 100 dBA is identical to eight hours at 85 dBA. A 15 dB attenuation hearing protector would minimize hearing damage in almost all musical venues, not just for singers but for other musicians sharing the stage as well.

In 1988, a new form of hearing protection became commercially available, called the ER-15. The ER stands for Etymotic Research (www.etymotic.com) and provides exactly 15 dB of attenuation for all sounds, regardless of pitch. This device uses a special attenuator element that fits into a silicon mold. This is a custom-made high-fidelity ear protector, which, unlike the attenuation pattern shown for industral-type ear protectors in Figure 7.2, attenuates all frequencies equally. The result is that the musician still hears all the music, but at a nondamaging level. Since all of the sounds of the music are treated equally (recall that industrial-type earplugs attenuate higher frequencies excessively),

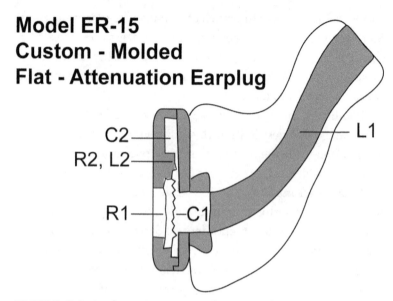

Model ER-15
Custom - Molded
Flat - Attenuation Earplug

FIGURE 7.3 A schematic cut away side view of the Musicians Earplugs (also called ER-15) which became available in 1988. These provide a uniform attenuation of all sound by exactly 15 decibels allowing the listener to hear music unaltered except that it is less damaging. Photo courtesy of Etymotic Research. Used with permission.

the bass still sounds like the bass, the treble like the treble, and so on. Since 1988 more than a hundred thousand pairs of the ER-15 uniform attenuation musician's earplugs have been fitted worldwide. A schematic cross-section drawing of the ER-15 is shown in Figure 7.3.

In 1992 it became apparent that a slightly stronger uniform attenuator musician's earplug was required for drummers and other percussionists, and the ER-25 earplug became available. As the name suggests, it offered exactly 25 dB of sound attenuation equally across the piano keyboard. A one-size-fits-all, non-custom version was also produced that has a uniform 20 dB attenuation of sound, and this is called the ER-20.

Ear Monitors

One cannot turn on any rock or pop video anymore without noticing "something" in the musicians' ears. These are called ear level monitors and are actually modifications of hearing aids. They are typically (but not always) custom-made like a hearing aid, and they have an amplifier, a loudspeaker (called a receiver), and a cable that forks down from the ear monitors to a body pack. The body pack uses an FM signal to receive (and transmit) the music and lyrics to the main instrument panel. The musician can get the mix of the music that he wants to hear without having to "compete" with the musician standing next to him. If this is done properly, a singer will be exposed to a sound level about 6 dB quieter than with the old-style wedge monitors that used to sit up on stage in front of the performers. A 6 dB quieter signal may not sound like a lot, but this is equivalent to a decrease of one-half of the normally acceptable sound exposure while still sufficiently loud for musicians because of the improved monitoring. Figure 7.4 shows a picture of a custom-made ear monitor (courtesy of Ultimate Ears, www.ultimateears.com).

And Let's Not Forget About Hearing Aids

There is no reason a hard-of-hearing vocalist (or any musician) should stop performing and enjoying his or her music. In many cases, someone who requires a hearing aid for listening to speech may not even require a hearing aid for music. Since music tends to be about 20–30 dB more intense than speech, a person with even mild to moderate hearing loss would be able to find music of all types enjoyable without a hearing aid. And for those people who still need a bit of boost for the singing or music, hearing aids have improved.

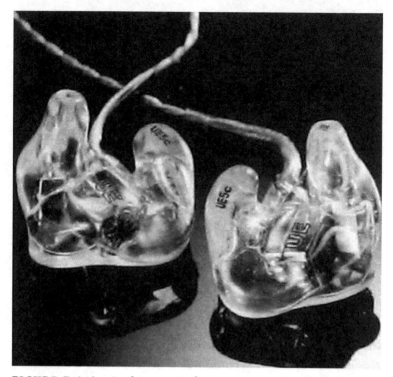

FIGURE 7.4 A pair of custom made ear monitors that allows the musician to hear the blend or mix of the music without having to have large on stage "wedge" monitors. With counselling musicians typically set the volume to about 6 decibels less intense while using ear monitors than with other types of on stage monitoring systems. Photo courtesy of Ultimate Ears. Used with permission.

The hearing aids of the 1980s and 1990s were actually excellent. The late 1980s saw the introduction of hearing aids with very wide bandwidths, meaing they were able to amplify a wide range of musical notes (in many cases up to two octaves above the top of the piano keyboard). These were called analog hearing aids. The late 1990s, however, saw a backslide in the ability of a hearing aid to amplify music with good fidelity. This corresponded to the introduction of digital hearing aids.

Although digital hearing aids had some great advantages over the older analog hearing aids, they had poorer ability to handle louder musical sounds. This isn't too bad for vocalists, since the loudest sound a singer can generate is typically well within the range of modern digital hearing aids. It is more of a problem for the intense instrumental sounds. Unfortunately, because of the specific way digital hearing aids process sounds, many (but not all) modern digital hearing aids tend to distort loud music. All digital hearing aids require a special component that converts the continuous sound of speech and music into "digits" that a computer can act on. This special component, called an "analog-to-digital converter," is the weak link in the vast majority of all modern hearing aids. Analog-to-digital converters work very well for speech and singing, but create a significant amount of distortion for louder music. The hearing aid industry is working feverishly to resolve this, and indeed, several ingenious methods have been found and are currently being developed. However, it may be some time before modern digital hearing aids catch up to the analog hearing aids of the late 1980s, at least for loud music.

Finally, a few words about the professional stigma of wearing a hearing aid. One of our patients, a professional opera singer with significant hearing loss, told us, "Walking out on stage with a hearing aid is tantamount to professional suicide." Nevertheless, the inability to hear, whether in a professional or a social situation, can also impair one's career advancement. If you are a singer who would benefit from hearing amplification, you have several options. You should try to use an aid that is the least visibly apparent but gives you the benefits you seek. Another option is to use the aid in social situations, but not during professional interactions or performance. Fitting a hearing aid into an ear canal that constantly changes in shape (as a singer opens and closes the mouth) is also a challenge, so be sure that the aids fit adequately, whether you are singing or not. Open fit aids or aids with soft molds may be an option to consider and discuss with your audiologist. Deep-insertion in-dwelling hearing aids are in their first generation, but as they are perfected they may offer yet another option for singers. These aids are deep in the ear canal, invisible, and past the hinge portion of the jaw, so they do not come loose or get dislodged with opening and closing the mouth.

A positive development is the increasing public recognition of hearing loss as a remediable condition. There is a growing epidemic of hearing loss and tinnitus among popular musicians, and with open advocacy on the part of well-known performers hearing loss is finally losing its social stigma and becoming just another impediment that can be overcome.

Notes

1. MacDonald, E., Behar, A., Wong, W., and Kunov, H. (2008). "Noise Exposure of Opera Musicians." *Canadian Acoustics*, 36(4): 11–16.

8

Sleep

The Art and Science

REBECCA J. SCOTT, PHD

As the old Irish proverb states, "A good laugh and a long sleep are the best cures in the doctor's book." Although we may not fully understand exactly why the world seems to look a little brighter after a good night's sleep, most of us can appreciate the sentiment behind such a statement. Indeed, as the mysteries of sleep have revealed themselves over the years, we now know that sleep (or lack thereof) affects all aspects of our physical, emotional, psychological health.

Think about it. We spend about one-third of our lives asleep. Every night, without much thought, we come home from a busy day; we take care of things around the house, tend to the children, and prepare for the following day. We might watch the latest reality TV show, surf the Internet, or read something before ultimately making a decision that is vital to our functioning: the decision to go to bed.

At first glance, sleep appears to be a quiet, passive state. In fact, some of my patients are fearful and resist sleep because they feel it is too similar to death. Nothing could be further from the truth. As we will review in this chapter, sleep is a very active state, one in which the body and mind recuperate. We will also review the two primary systems that regulate our sleep/wake cycle and that it is essential to understand in order to change and improve sleep. We will also explore some of the difficulties one can have with sleep, how to conquer those difficulties, and when to consult a sleep specialist.

Normal Sleep

You've all heard the statement "looks can be deceiving." This is especially true when observing someone sleep. What appears calm and steady on the surface can be very different from what is happening below that surface. Think of sleep as being like an ocean. On the surface, sleep has a peaceful appearance—so much so that it used to be thought that our mind and body switch off during sleep. However, like that ocean with its calm exterior, when we look below the surface we find all kinds of remarkable creatures, corals and plant life, all with a specific role in creating an entire ecosystem that exists unto itself. As technology has allowed us to look below the surface of sleep, we have found that we cycle between different stages of sleep, and that these stages are critical to our overall health.

Sleep is not a uniform state; it occurs in stages. When we close our eyes and start the transition into sleep, our limbs feels heavier, our breathing and heart rate slow, and our blood pressure drops. We might have strange and disconnected thoughts as we enter into a state of deep relaxation. For some, it may appear that this transition occurs quickly; however, the body prepares itself for sleep long before the transition actually takes place. In the healthy sleeper, it can take up to thirty minutes to fall asleep.

Figure 8.1 depicts a normal sleep pattern across an eight-hour night. There are two types of sleep: nonrapid-eye-movement sleep (non-REM), which consists of stages I, II, and III sleep; and rapid-eye-movement sleep (REM). Contrary to popular belief,

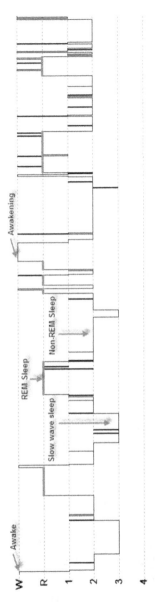

FIGURE 8.1 Plot of normal sleep across an 8-hour period. W = awake; R = rapid eye movement/ dream sleep; 1 = stage I sleep; 2 = stage II sleep; 3 = stage III sleep/slow wave sleep.

REM sleep is *not* the deepest stage of sleep but is synonymous with dream sleep. And even if we don't remember our dreams, we all dream every night.

We start off the night awake (W in Figure 8.1) and then progress through all the stages of non-REM sleep. Stage 1 sleep is the lightest stage of sleep, and we are only meant to spend about 2–8 percent of the night in this stage. Stage 1 sleep is so light that, if awakened during this stage, we feel certain we have not slept and will deny any accusations to the contrary. We then move into stage 2 sleep, which comprises about 45–55 percent of the night, before drifting into stage 3 sleep (or slow wave sleep). Stage 3 is the deepest stage of sleep and makes up about 10–20 percent of the night, with the majority occurring during the first third of the night. After about ninety minutes of non-REM sleep, we move into REM sleep. If awakened from REM sleep, we can typically recall, with great detail, having been in a dream. Approximately 20–25 percent of the night is spent in REM sleep, the majority occupying the final half of the night. On any given night, we repeat this cycle approximately four to six times.

In this day and age, it is increasingly difficult to dedicate sufficient time to sleep. There is so much to do, and those things usually get done at the expense of our sleep. There really are individual differences in sleep need, but the average person requires about seven or eight hours of sleep to feel well and function and perform at an optimal level. Despite knowing this intuitively, we sometimes find ourselves asking, "Do we really need all this sleep? What is the purpose"?

Well, going back to the ocean metaphor: the ocean has a purpose, helping to regulate our atmosphere and global temperature. There are processes occurring within the ocean that affect not only the inhabitants of those waters but life on land as well. This is the case with sleep too. It is not a trivial behavior we perform at the end of the day; it is a state that is critical for memory consolidation and information processing, and in which physical energy is repaired and muscle tissue restored. Without it, our state of wakefulness is dramatically altered. Everything is dulled. The boss who is barely tolerable to begin with becomes less so; a comment or critique that we can usually accept for what it is feels like an attack, and the antics of your child, which are normally so adorable, become as grating as nails down a chalk board. You get the point: we are irritable and lack energy, and our performance suffers; we have difficulty concentrating and experience memory lapses; our emotions are harder to regulate, and in some cases we might actually start falling asleep in inappropriate situations.

Additionally, sleep is also necessary for proper endocrine, metabolic, and immune functioning. For example, the common cold results from exposure to a viral infection; but how susceptible we are to developing those annoying cold symptoms and how long those symptoms last are mediated, in part, by sleep. Furthermore, obesity has also recently been linked to sleep. If we do not get enough sleep, we produce more ghrelin, a hormone secreted by the stomach that tells the brain, "Keep eating!" and less leptin, a hormone that tells the brain, "I'm full."

I'll let you in on a little secret. Though sleep can seem to be an elusive process, it is not as elusive as one might think. There are two separate systems that interact to consolidate sleep and promote alertness across the day. The first system, called process S, represents an internal sleep drive. Stated simply, the longer you've been awake, the greater your desire or drive to sleep. With every passing hour of wakefulness, this sleep drive builds and increases the likelihood of an easy transition into sleep. With the onset of sleep, this drive diminishes (which is why naps can interfere with our ability to sleep at night), and by the end of the night the sleep drive is very low. If process S were the only factor that affected sleep, we would all feel very alert in the morning and then struggle to remain alert as the day progressed.

But wait a minute. You're saying, "Why do I drag in the afternoon around 3:00 P.M. and then get a second wind in the evening?" Because there is a second process at play: Process C. This represents the internal circadian rhythm or "body clock" for sleep and wakefulness that occurs every twenty-four hours. As we have discovered, how sleepy or alert we feel is associated with the circadian rhythm of body temperature. When body temperature is highest (usually in the late morning and early evening) we feel most alert and vital. When body temperature drops (for a short period after lunch and then again at night), we feel tired and sleepy. Body temperature is generally lowest around 4:00 A.M. and then gradually rises across the morning hours.

By definition, circadian rhythms recur approximately every twenty-four hours, persist in the absence of any external cues, and help our bodies function in a manner that is consistent and in sync with the world around us; however, they are highly sensitive and can be "reset" by exposure to certain environmental stimuli. The strongest influence on the sleep rhythm is light; exposure to daylight in the morning hours helps organize our day while light at that same intensity in the evening can disrupt the sleep/wake cycle. Other factors, such as activity level, work schedule, social activity, and meals, can also affect the sleep rhythm.

The interaction of process C and process S explains why, if you've ever had to pull an all-nighter, it is possible to feel truly miserable and exhausted at the 3:00–4:00 A.M. hour (when your sleep drive is high and body temperature is low) and then feel better at 7:00–8:00 A.M. (when body temperature is rising) even though you have not slept. When these systems are working together, it is like a beautiful song in which two voices come together in perfect harmony; however, if they become disconnected, the song is lost and all we hear is noise.

Insomnia

Insomnia is defined as difficulty falling asleep or difficulty staying asleep, characterized by multiple brief awakenings, sustained awakenings, early morning awakenings and by the sense that one is not sleeping deeply. Insomnia has many causes, although poets and opera composers seem to favor a guilty conscience as the main one.[1]

Figure 8.2 depicts the sleep of someone with both sleep onset and maintenance insomnia.

Insomnia is a lonely, frustrating, and stressful experience that changes who you are and how you go about in the world. You lie awake at night thinking how you've "got to get some sleep" and that if you don't sleep you'll perform poorly, might get bad reviews, and won't be able to make it through the day. Anxious thoughts dominate, seeming to drive sleep even farther away. When you finally get through that next day, instead of spending an extra moment talking with friends or doing something else you enjoy, you feel the anxiety percolating. All you can think about is how you need to get into bed early tonight to "ensure" that you get at least some sleep. You can't understand how something you once did without much thought now seems impossible. To add insult to injury, your bed partner, almost as if mocking you, is sound asleep! You've lost all confidence in your ability to sleep and wonder if you'll ever feel that drowsy feeling again. What can you do?

Whether you have trouble falling asleep or staying asleep, the following suggestions will stabilize your sleep/wake cycle, strengthen your Process C and Process S, and begin restoring the healthy aspects of your sleep.

1. First and foremost (and I know how difficult this sounds), *stop trying*! Forget what your parents or coaches always told you

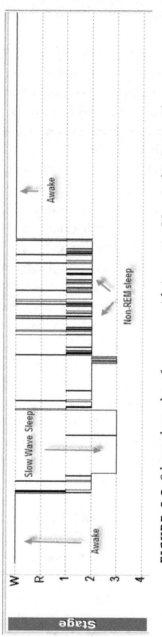

FIGURE 8.2 8-hour sleep plot of someone with insomnia. W = awake; R = rapid eye movement/dream sleep; 1 = stage I sleep; 2 = stage II sleep; 3 = stage III sleep/slow wave sleep.

about "trying harder." When it comes to sleep, the harder you try, the harder you'll fail; I assure you, you'll have better luck pinning Jell-O to the wall. You cannot force yourself to sleep; you can, however, set the stage to ensure that it makes its entrance.

2. Begin with a relaxing evening routine. Physiologically, the brain needs time to shift from a waking state to a sleep state. Think of your brain as a speeding car: you can't just hit the brakes and expect it to stop instantaneously. The alerting drive that has kept you active all day has to downshift, and the sleep drive then has to get in gear. To help this shift take place, spend the last hour of your day winding down, and do not go to bed until you have had this hour. Taking a warm bath, watching TV, reading a book, and practicing meditation or deep breathing are all methods of relaxation; however, the key is finding something that is relaxing to *you* and that does not interfere physiologically with the sleep process.

3. Dim the lights in your home one to two hours before going to bed. Remember that to get your best sleep you want process S and process C to work together in an organized manner. Bright overhead light interferes with melatonin production, a hormone in the body that promotes sleepiness and regulates the sleep/wake rhythm.

4. Stop late-night surfing. Turn off the computer for the hour before you go to bed. In addition to being mentally stimulating, the computer gives off light in the blue wavelength spectrum. Light in this spectrum suppresses melatonin and will interfere with sleep.

5. Do not go to bed on a full stomach. Although eating a light snack before bed can be a comforting ritual, a heavy meal just before bed can activate the digestive system and disturb sleep. The only system you want activated at night is the sleep system.

6. Limit caffeine in the evening. Caffeinated products (coffee, certain teas, and soda) early in the day can be helpful to counter-

act the consequences of a poor night of sleep; however, since the effects of caffeine can persist up to six to ten hours, caffeine in the evening can cause problems falling asleep and interfere with sleep quality.

7. Limit alcohol in the evening. Though having a drink can make it easier to fall asleep, the presence of alcohol in the system once one is asleep can lead to poor-quality sleep, nocturnal awakening, and early morning awakening.

8. Make sure your sleep environment is comfortable. Do not underestimate the importance of the sleeping environment. Comfortable bedding and a dark, quiet room that is neither too hot nor too cold are essential for good sleep.

9. Go to bed closer to the time when you're *actually* falling asleep rather than when you're *hoping* to fall asleep. This is especially true if you have trouble falling asleep. Though your first instinct might be to go to bed earlier in the evening to make up for sleep deprivation, restricting your time in bed (to six and a half or seven hours) for a short period actually helps to consolidate sleep and strengthen your body's natural "sleep drive."

10. If you awaken in the night and have trouble returning to sleep, don't panic. Reengage in whatever relaxing routine you were doing in the hour before you went to bed. The goal is to not let yourself lie awake in bed, feeling frustrated.

11. Get up at the same time every day. It may be tempting to sleep in after a night of poor sleep; however, no matter what your night was like, get up around the same time every morning. Variability in your sleep and wake times while you are going through a period of insomnia only serves to reinforce the insomnia.

12. Limit napping. If you are having trouble sleeping, you want to avoid taking naps. However, if a nap is unavoidable, nap as early in the day as possible and limit the nap to no longer than twenty to thirty minutes.

These are simple recommendations, but in my experience it can be difficult for patients to put them into practice. Expect that it may take you a few attempts to get it right, and that the first few nights tend to be the most difficult. Do not get overwhelmed and feel as if you have to do these things forever. They are critical during the initial stages of treatment, but once your sleep improves and you've gained some confidence in your sleep again, you will not have to be so regimented.

Jet Lag

Jet lag is of particular concern to singers, who frequently travel between engagements. It occurs after crossing several time zones and results when there is a mismatch between your naturally occurring rhythm for sleepiness and alertness and the socially accepted "daytime" and "nighttime" of the new city in which you've arrived. It is a temporary condition that resolves once your body clock adjusts to the new location. The severity of the jet lag depends on the number of times zones crossed as well as on the direction of travel, with eastbound travel being more difficult than flying west.

Although everyone responds to jet travel differently, the consequences of jet lag can be very similar to those of insomnia. If you are prone to jet lag, the best advice is to plan ahead! A couple of nights before your trip, start slowly shifting your sleep/wake time in the direction of the desired schedule at your new destination. Once you have arrived at your destination, force yourself into the locally appropriate sleep pattern as quickly as possible. Medications, exercise, caffeine, melatonin, and bright light therapy are all tools that can help speed the recovery from jet lag. If you are a frequent traveler or someone who has difficulty with jet lag, talk with your doctor or a sleep specialist to design a sleep program that will be most suitable to you and your needs.

Sleep Disordered Breathing and Sleep Apnea

When we sleep, our muscles relax. Snoring occurs because of relaxation of the tissues in the upper airway. Snoring can be smooth and regular, albeit loud, or it can be irregular and disrupt the quality of our sleep. Obstructive sleep apnea occurs when the tissues of the airway relax so much that the airway closes off and we stop breathing. When the airway is blocked, the oxygen in our blood drops until our brain steps in and "awakens" us with a loud snort and gasp. With this loud gasp, we awaken momentary and our breathing and blood oxygenation return to normal. This blockage of the airway can occur just a few times or up to several hundred times through the night.

Sleep apnea is a very serious disorder that requires evaluation and treatment. Even though the sleep of someone with sleep apnea is often highly disturbed, it is not uncommon for apnea sufferers to be unaware of their disorder. However, if you've ever shared a room or bed with someone suffering from apnea, the sound of the labored breathing, long breathing pauses followed by loud gasps, and the appearance of the apparent constant struggle to breathe are quite frightening. So frightening to watch, in fact, that is it is often the bed partner who urges the loved one to seek evaluation.

Other common symptoms of sleep apnea include daytime sleepiness and tiredness, low energy, difficulty concentrating, lack of focus, memory loss, weight gain, impotence or loss of sex drive, headaches, personality changes (such as increased irritability or depressed mood), dry or sore throat on awakening, restless sleep, and frequent awakening to urinate. Often these changes occur so gradually that we do not recognize the extent to which our lives, health, and overall functioning have been affected. However, if you experience any of these symptoms, or if someone has mentioned that your breathing in sleep sounds irregular, see a sleep specialist to review your symptoms and have a thorough evaluation. Untreated sleep apnea has very serious health consequences, such as high blood pressure, heart attack, stroke, cardiac arrhythmia, and change in glucose tolerance.

Once you speak to your doctor or consult a sleep specialist, an overnight sleep study (called a polysomnogram) is often recommended. This study is able to determine whether or not you have clinically significant sleep disordered breathing.

There are numerous treatment options for snoring and sleep apnea. Behavioral modification measures include sleeping on your side, sleeping with the head slightly elevated, weight loss, and avoiding alcohol and certain medications before bed. There are measures that open the obstructed airway, among them custom-made dental devices that move the bottom jaw forward in sleep, various upper airway surgeries to remove excess tissue in the airway and prevent airway collapse, and continuous positive airway pressure (CPAP) therapy.

Even though all of these treatments can be effective if you are a proper candidate (as determined by your sleep study and medical history), nasal CPAP is the most widely used treatment for moderate to severe sleep apnea. It works by blowing air into the back of the throat via a mask that is worn over the nose. CPAP is a highly effective treatment, but side effects, such as feelings of claustrophobia, nasal dryness and congestion, sneezing, and mask leakage, can interfere with your ability to successfully use this device. If you find that you have difficulty with treatment, first speak to your doctor to discuss all of your treatment options. Don't be afraid to speak to your doctor or a respiratory care company to make sure a mask is fitted properly. There are several styles of mask, so if you are not comfortable with one, try another. If you're having difficulty because of nasal dryness or cold-like symptoms, speak to your doctor about heated humidification, which typically resolves these side effects almost immediately.

For singers, management of obstructive sleep apnea may be particularly difficult, since some upper airway surgery may involve the soft palate, a vital part of the singer's anatomy. The drying and nasal-irritating aspects of a CPAP device can also be a problem. It is best to discuss these issues with your doctor, hopefully one that is familiar with treating vocal performers and their issues.

Seeing a Sleep Specialist

Too often, I sit with patients who have spent years suffering from the consequences of an untreated sleep disorder simply because they did not know they could get help, or they assumed that their poor sleep or tiredness was just a part of who they were. If you have difficulty sleeping or feel tired or sleepy and lack energy during the day, speak to your doctor or to a sleep disorder specialist. You can find a list of sleep specialists, cognitive-behavioral sleep specialists, and accredited sleep centers at the American Academy of Sleep Medicine's website (www.aasmnet.org). Take your sleep seriously, and don't let yourself feel out of control or victimized. Seek help, and see that the disorder is resolved!

Suggested Readings

Banks, S., and Dinges, D. "Behavioral and Physiological Consequences of Sleep Restriction." *Journal of Clinical Sleep Medicine* (Aug. 2007), 3(5): 519–528.

Castro, P., and Huber, M. "History of the Ocean." Rev. November 2008. http://marinebio.org/Oceans/History/.

Glovinsky, P., and Spielman, A. *The Insomnia Answer*. New York: Berkley, 2006.

Guillemets, T. "The Quote Garden." Rev. Nov. 7, 2006. http://www.quote garden.com.

Hauri, P., Jarman, M., and Linde, S. *No More Sleepless Nights*. New York: Wiley, 2001.

Jacobs, G. *Say Good Night to Insomnia*. New York: Holt, 1998.

Weaver, T. "Adherence to Positive Airway Pressure Therapy." *Current Opinions in Pulmonary Medicine* (Nov. 2006), 12(6): 409–413.

Notes

1. Witness Clytemnestra's plaintive "Ich habe keine gute Nächte!" in Act 1 of Strauss' *Elektra*.

9

Hormones and the Voice

JEAN ABITBOL, MD

Like a ship on the waves of the ocean, the voice travels through the ever-changing weatherscape of hormones and emotion. It changes through the voyage of the hormonal storm of our being. Its path, challenges and limitations, and emotional impact through reality is the voyage I propose to you.

Hormones represent a lifelong and intimate connection of the brain, via the hypothalamus, the pituitary gland, and the endocrine glands, to the muscles, cartilage, nerves, and covering cells of the larynx.

Why does puberty change the voice so much in humans? Why does a woman's voice change during her menstrual cycle? How can the vocal fold vibrations change at menopause, with a resulting deterioration of the voice? How does a cyclic pathology appear on a vocal fold, and why may the voice become impaired after the hormonal "earthquake" around the fifties?

The voice changes constantly, at the mercy of hormones, emotions, and many other subtle and invisible factors. To be effective in their therapy, physicians treating professional voice patients must accept the maxim that when artists complain of a vocal problem, most of the time they are right. This means that if we can't detect pathology of the vocal folds, it doesn't mean there isn't one; it simply means that we haven't found it.

How do hormones affect the voice?

Clearly, the larynx is a hormonal target. At puberty, it undergoes a host of changes These transformations are directed by our genetic makeup, but affected by our hormones. The impact of male hormones on the vocal folds is the key to the development of the male voice. Perhaps the most dramatic example is the castrato's voice, a child's voice that persists because he does not receive any testosterone (or more precisely, extremely little).

In addition to testosterone, a mighty hormonal factory goes into gear at puberty. Three masters manage it: the brain, the pituitary gland, and the hypothalamus. The first one directs: our brain, a neurological and emotional center, transmits information in the form of electrical impulses to the hypothalamus at the base of the encephalon. The hypothalamus relays this information to the pituitary gland. The pituitary then secretes its hormones and releases them into the bloodstream, where they migrate to the target organs as well as inform the hypothalamus and the pituitary gland that all is well, that the secretion rate is satisfactory. This feedback mechanism is remarkably precise and maintains our hormonal balance just as it should be, neither too high nor too low. If hormonal secretions are excessive, the hypothalamus and pituitary glands jointly diminish the stimulation of the gland concerned. Hormones therefore play an intermediary role between our brain and our various organs, including the larynx.

In certain respects, the hormone is like a cordless remote control, but its operating method is molecular rather than infrared. An infinitesimal amount suffices for a significant impact. Where vitamins are an indispensable element in our nutrition because the body does not produce them, hormones are produced by our cells but are just as indispensable to our survival. They accelerate, stabilize, or slow down their target organ.

The larynx is hormonally dependent, evolving with time and the sexual life of every individual. When you hear people speaking on the radio or on the telephone, you can identify their sex from the voice within a few tenths of a second. The voice is a secondary sexual characteristic. Of course, sex hormones influence it, but so do other hormones.

Timing has an important influence on hormonal activity. Certain hormones must be secreted at specific moments of our life: during our fetal development, at birth, or at puberty. The time window for optimal hormonal effect, especially for thyroid and growth hormones, is vital: before, and it's too soon; after, too late.

The thyroid hormones are a case in point. If they don't do their work in the first years of our life, this brings on irreversible physical and intellectual anomalies that can lead to cretinism, a form of physical and emotional retardation. Should one later try to palliate this hormonal deficiency with artificial substitutes, it would be to no avail: the damage will have been done. Nowadays, early diagnoses enable appropriate treatment to be prescribed in good time. The impact of our hormones dictates the need for a precise timetable.

Nowhere is the cyclic effect of hormones in the development and maintenance of normal function more evident than in a woman's monthly menstrual cycle, and the diurnal cycle present in both men and women. In our diurnal cycle, cortisone is naturally secreted by our body at the end of the day and in the early morning.

The Thyroid Gland

The role of the thyroid gland is to counter the aggressions of the outside world (the weather, cold, heat, stress). The thyroid is also indispensable to the evolution of the voice, and thyroid hormones play a determining role in our vocal register. Functionally, it can secrete an excess, or an inadequate, amount of thyroid hormone. Thyroid hormones have a profound effect on our metabolism. They act as do bellows on a fire, stimulating a majority of organs in our body and influencing our vocal timbre.

An inadequate level of thyroid hormone, however, can have a negative effect on voice quality. In a serious case of hypothyroidism, the voice becomes harsh, the vocal folds present a slight edema, and the vocal muscles grow congested. This well-known pathology regresses as soon as thyroid extracts are administered. The voice recovers its normal register and its natural harmonics.

Sex Hormones and the Voice

When thyroid function is normal, the essential elements that continuously dominate the quality of our voice are our sex hormones: estrogens, progesterone, and androgens.

What gives the voice its gender-specific characteristics? Our voice changes over the years, along with our life experience, our appearance, and our physique. It also changes as a function of our emotional environment. Where our fingerprint identifies a physical part of our anatomy that is unique to us, our voiceprint reveals our personality, our sensibility, and our sexuality. Let's try to follow the trail of the sexual voice. Let's retrace the steps of this miracle of life, from the embryo through to the adult and old age.

Puberty: A Hormonal Earthquake

The infant's voice has no sex. There is no way to identify a baby's cries as feminine and others as masculine. At puberty, the threshold between childhood and adulthood, our secondary sexual characteristics develop, and with them, the physical and psychological transformations specific to each sex.

Adolescence takes us down the path leading to sex-determined vocal frequencies. The male adolescent, now virile, slim, and athletic, is ill-served by his shrill, childlike falsetto. The adolescent female's voice also changes, beginning an odyssey of forty-plus years of hormonally determined vocal fluctuations. As a girl becomes a woman, she develops higher harmonics, as well as some lower ones that she previously lacked. In boys, the action of testosterone on the muscular and mucosal structure of the vocal cords favors the appearance of new low harmonics and the loss of some of the child's high harmonics.

The hormonal revolution is more impressive in men. The shape and covering of the vocal cords changes, thickens, grows, acquires more volume; but the thoracic cage, lungs, stature, and brain are also growing. In the West, men's left brain develops more than the right brain, whereas women maintain certain equilibrium between the rational brain and the emotional brain. The consequences of puberty for the voice may be more obvious in boys than in girls, but they exist in both sexes. It triggers emotional changes that are usually appropriate to the person's physical appearance. In women, the voice drops by a third of an octave compared to girls' voices; in men, the voice drops by an octave.

In male singers, a well-defined head voice and chest voice make their appearance after puberty. These two vocal techniques bring into play the ligaments and muscles located between the thyroid and the cricoid cartilages, which are more developed in men. They allow the larynx to rock (i.e., the thyroid cartilage to swivel back and forth on the cricoid), and significant enlargement of the laryngeal cartilages and lengthening of the vocal folds in men also makes it easier for them to sing in the head and chest registers.

In women, the changes to the larynx at puberty are less dramatic. The thyroid and cricoid cartilages hardly change. The vocal fold lengthens slightly and increases its muscle mass. The vocal fold remains very supple, with a fine mucous membrane. Small glandular cells keep the vocal folds lubricated and depend on feminine hormones (estrogens and progesterone). The ovaries enter their active period of reproduction. The first menstrual cycles appear, and they become progressively more regular. After a few months, the voice discovers new high-pitched and low-pitched harmonics. The periodicity of female hormone secretions gives rhythm to the adolescent girl's life cycles. The lunar cycle is orchestrated by the hypothalamo-pituitary axis, from the action of FSH and LH, two hormones that act directly on the ovaries to stimulate the secretion of estrogens and progesterone.

There are three hormones important for our sex life: androgens, estrogens, and progesterone. Even in women, some testosterone is secreted, although by the ovary. Each hormone triggers a modification of the mucous membranes, muscles, and bony tissues; therefore our laryngeal instrument, our voice, is also modified. It influences the cerebral cortex as well, thereby influencing the brain. This influence begins at puberty and persists for the rest of one's life.

Androgens give the strength and the desire to procreate. In women, the level of androgens must be around 150 µg/ml. If it is too low the libido fades away; if too high, masculinizing effects appear.

Estrogens have an impact on the voice timbre. The estrogens secreted by the ovaries have various implications for the larynx. They result in a slight thickening of the vocal fold mucous membrane, which creates greater vibratory amplitude. The voice acquires a good timbre. The desquamation of superficial cells is reduced, accompanied by a decrease in the need to clear one's throat and in the amount of laryngeal mucous fluid. The lipid cells under the vocal fold mucous membrane are stimulated. The voice becomes more supple (in the menstrual cycle, this is called the maturation phase, characterized by estrogen domination in the first two weeks of the cycle).

Regarding the cells of the genital and the vocal fold mucous membrane: Are they really different? The relationship and hormonal dependence of these two tissues was objectively confirmed by J. Abitbol et al. in 1986[1] and 1999[2] by comparative studies of smears taken from the vocal cords and the cervix of the uterus, during the same day of the menstrual cycle. The results were amazing; in both cases, the cellular characteristics were identical. There was a perfect correspondence between the smears taken from the cervix of the uterus and those taken from the vocal folds. This correspondence had long been suspected. Given that both have the same type of mucous membrane, it seemed logical they should demonstrate the same cyclical hormonal susceptibility. But now there was scientific, objective proof to support this. This is consistent with the observation that the voice can change with the menstrual cycle, or with hormonal treatment for endometriosis or menopause.

Actual hormonal receptors for estrogen and androgens were identified on the vocal folds by Voelter et al. (2008[3]), but not for progesterone. Androgen receptors were most frequently detected, especially in the basal and intermediate layer of the stratified epithelium and the lamina propria.

In addition to the effects on laryngeal mucous membranes discussed here, estrogens affect the metabolism of calcium, which influences the bony and cartilaginous structures of our larynx. Estrogens also improve the permeability of blood vessels and capillaries, which are quite numerous in the vocal cords, thereby increasing oxygenation. However, they have no effect on striated muscle.

Progesterone, found only in women, provokes a thickening of the vocal folds. As its name indicates, progesterone is a hormone that enables gestation to persist. It prepares the mucous membrane of the uterus for the implantation of the ovum. That is its primary role. With respect to the vocal folds, progesterone causes cells on the surface of the mucous membrane to desquamate. It thickens the secretions of the gland located below and above the vocal cords, causing, in 33 percent of our patients, during the four days preceding the menses dryness of the larynx, the need to clear one's throat, less agility when singing, and a narrowed vocal range. If the voice is strained during this phase, nodules or subepithelial hematoma may form. Progesterone also brings on a slight decrease in the muscle tone of the vocal cords, and it diminishes—and may even inhibit—the permeability of capillaries. This causes an accumulation of extravascular fluid, bringing on an edema of the vocal folds, which may remain swollen during the week prior to menses.

It is thanks to the estrogens that the intravascular fluid is transferred to the extravascular spaces in the surrounding tissues. When progesterone is then secreted, and if the balance between the two hormones is satisfactory, the interstitial fluid is be distributed, and edema of the vocal folds will be minimal. If, to the contrary, this is not the case, the progesterone will prevent the return of the interstitial fluid to the vessels, causing edema to form. The progesterone in this instance closes the door of the capillaries and prevents them from draining the tissues.

This imbalance between estrogens and progesterone causes a cyclical edema in the last week of the menstrual cycle, which is due to the accumulation of interstitial fluid in the vocal cords. A similar process causes some women to have swollen legs before their menses. A monophasic oral contraceptive pill avoids exaggeration of this phenomenon.

The Premenstrual Voice Syndrome

The premenstrual voice syndrome is characterized by voice fatigue, decreased range, loss of power in the singing voice, and fewer harmonics, caused by the dryness of the vocal tract and the resonance chambers. There is also an increased tendency toward laryngopharyngeal acid reflux. The syndrome starts four to six days before the menses (in women with no oral contraceptive pill) and continues for three days after the first day of the menses. We have seen this set of symptoms in a third of our female patients. Voice professionals are particularly sensitive to these problems, chiefly soprano and mezzo singers. Dynamic vocal imaging by videostroboscopy reveals congestion, microvaricosities (dilated tiny blood vessels), lack of vibratory amplitude at the vocal fold margins, edema, and cricoarytenoid inflammation owing to reflux.

The voice is more easily injured during the premenstrual phase than at other times in the menstrual cycle. The singer with a premenstrual vocal syndrome complains of tiredness, loss of *pianissimo*, an alteration in certain harmonics in the higher registers, a deficit in the power of the voice, and a veiled voice. The lubrication of the vocal folds is perturbed by the dryness of the atmosphere and the increasing effect of reflux. The examination often reveals microvaricosities on the vocal cord, a sign of venous fragility. The singer doesn't suffer from them; the folds vibrate normally. The danger they present stems from their fragility. Vigorous singing during this time may damage the vocal fold by causing a rupture in these fragile micro vessels. The microvaricose veins burst, but only under the submucosal layer. They burst under pressure during the very powerful vocalizations of a lyrical soprano in a high register. The result is hemorrhage and a hematoma, which can present as sudden though painless impairment of the voice.

There is no way to predict this accident. The treatment is simple: strict vocal rest combined with inhalations of Calyptol[4] (rosemary, thyme, essential oil of pine plants and eucalyptol), phlebotonics, minerals, and anti-inflammatory medicine.

Although the micropathology of premenstrual voice injury has become clear only relatively recently, this type of problem must have been known in earlier times. Since the nineteenth century, any female singer performing at La Scala Opera house in Milan can during the five days preceding her menses and during her menses cancel her performance and still receive her fees; the interval is called "the grace days."

General premenstrual changes are evident in all women, but only a third of these present a more noticeable edema of the vocal folds. Women on the biphasic pill can sometimes present these same symptoms. (A biphasic pill contains estrogens and a very small amount of progesterone on the first part of the cycle and estrogens and a strong dose of progesterone on the second part of the cycle; there is almost a reproduction of a natural cycle. A monophasic pill is taken for twenty-one days of the cycle; this pill releases the same amount of progesterone and estrogens every day.)

During this premenstrual period, formation of an edema can create or aggravate the formation of nodules on the vocal cords. This causes a hoarse voice for the six days prior to the menses and for the first two days of the menses. At first, the nodules are soft and vibrate adequately. From one cycle to another, this simple nodule hardens. Now the hoarseness is permanent.

This problem always requires speech therapy to enable the singer to rebalance the axis between her breathing and the vibration of the vocal fold. Sometimes microsurgery of the vocal folds is required. This intervention becomes necessary if the voice remains impaired between menses, as this can seriously handicap a singer's career. However, it's then more judicious to operate on these pathological vocal folds well clear of the week preceding the menses, thus allowing the organism to spontaneously reabsorb the edema of the vocal cords just described, which normally disappears between the third and twentieth days of the menstrual cycle.

Judicious use of medications may facilitate singing during the premenstrual phase. About two-thirds of singers do not need any hormonal treatment to avoid voice fatigue or voice vascular consequences. Instead, inhalation with Calyptol, vitamins (B5, B6, C), minerals (iron, calcium, magnesium; or copper, gold, silver), phlebotonics, anti-edema drugs (bromolein from pineapple extracts), and prostaglandin inhibitors (mefenamic acid such as Ponstyl). We always add anti-reflux treatment in the form of proton pump inhibitors such as omeprazole. Excellent clinical results are observed: the timing of the treatment is four days before the menses and four days after the first day of the menses every month for at least ten months.

In one-third of voice professionals, we may have to give a hormonal treatment with a monophasic oral contraceptive pill. Biphasic pills should be prescribed rarely, and only a gynecologist is the expert. The Voice Handicap Index is necessary to evaluate the patient. The type of pill depends on the individual and is prescribed by the gynecologist. A team approach is indispensable: the gynecologist, an otolaryngologist, and a voice therapist.

The Voice and Pregnancy

A professional singer can sing remarkably well while two to seven months pregnant. The vocal folds are then nicely plump and perfectly lubricated. The quality of the vibration is actually improved. The hormones that accompany a pregnancy confer a special warmth to the voice's harmonics; it is rounder, and it carries well. Pregnancy appears to beautify the voice. After the seventh month, breathing support is impaired—which is only normal. The sole problem that needs to be treated during pregnancy, in the context of our discussion, is gastric reflux.

The Voice and Menopause

During menopause, the menstrual cycle is progressively disrupted. But menopause, which today is of interest to us all, only relatively recently became topical.

In ancient Greek civilization (400 BC), the average life expectancy was twenty-three to twenty-seven years, and the menopausal woman didn't exist, or was an exception. Menopause still didn't exist in the Middle Ages, when life expectancy was twenty-three to forty years. Only in the twentieth century was menopause finally taken into consideration. Indeed, girls born in the 1980s can expect to live to the age of ninety-two! Menopause now corresponds to practically half a woman's life. By the end of the twentieth century, France accounted for nearly eight and a half million menopausal women. The continued importance of the singing voice, and of verbal communication and its effect on interpersonal relationships, all point to the essential problem that the voice and menopause are now beginning to pose.

Why do these changes in a woman's voice occur around this period of life?

During the peri-menopause, the progesterone level collapses, and very few estrogens remain. Equally, the secretion of male hormones also drops off considerably. But their presence, now that they're no longer counterbalanced by feminine hormones, can sometimes cause the voice to become more masculine.

The menopausal phase normally lasts from the age of forty-seven to fifty-five. The impact that the sex hormones had on their various target organs disappears, not without consequences. In the larynx, the vocal fold mucous membrane thickens. This is accompanied by lack of tonicity and loss of its contours. The voice becomes deeper and more masculine.

Management of the singing voice during and after menopause is a controversial subject. Should we use hormones or not?

These days, administration of substitute hormones enables the unpleasant consequences of this lack of sex hormones to be delayed to an increasingly later age, saving many women from a trying experience that is both mentally and physically hard to accept. In the 1950s, was this peri-menopause period not referred to as "the change of life," implying that an entire chapter in a woman's life was coming to a full stop? Our better understanding of our endocrinologic world has given the menopausal woman greater quality of life, on a daily basis.

But in some cases hormonal substitutes may be contraindicated. They are not recommended in cases notably of breast cancer, a high-risk family background, cardiovascular pathology, or cholesterol-related affliction. For this reason, a medical checkup is a prerequisite for women in their fifties who are considering their options. Thereafter, a regular checkup should be performed.

But the menopausal female voice doesn't necessarily become more masculine. Why is this? Observation of menopausal women has led us to categorize them into two vocal types. The first type, slim with very few fat cells, we will call the Modigliani type (as in Modigliani's paintings). The second, somewhat plumper, we'll call the Rubens type (as in Rubens paintings). Our clinical experience has shown us that the Rubens-type woman is less likely to suffer from voice deterioration at menopause. Why is this so?

Estrogen synthesis occurs on three levels: at the level of the ovaries (when they are functional), at the level of the brain (hypothalamus, tonsils, and hippocampus), and finally at the level of fat cells. These last are the ones that interest us here, because they are particularly active during the menopause. Since 1977, we have known that, in both men and women, fat cells can turn androgens into estrogens. The relationship between obesity and a higher secretion of estrones (estrogen derivatives) is also age-related, being higher in menopausal women. Thus, the lower need for hormone substitutes of our Rubens-type woman is because her fat cells transform her androgens into estrones. Meanwhile, our slim Modigliani woman is more likely to need hormone substitute therapy, prescribed, of course, with due respect to contra-indications.

Obese tenors have also been found to have a higher level of estrogens and a slightly lower level of testosterone than those found in baritones and bass singers. Indeed, these slim, deep bass singers with their bony figures have a higher level of androgens. They have no fat cells that could help the organism to metabolize testosterone into estrogens.

With age, muscle mass also diminishes; adipose mass increases, and cells are redistributed differently about the body. Corticosteroids encourage the increase of fat cells; therefore menopausal women need to be cautious about consuming them. A carefully considered hormone substitute therapy program, associated with vitamins and minerals, can bring considerable benefits to most female voice professionals if their body can tolerate it, which is far from being a given. I have noted that women thus treated are able to avoid developing a masculine voice as they age and are able to preserve a beautiful voice for significantly longer. I have been most impressed by certain sopranos who've kept the same tessitura until the age of sixty-five.

Male Hormones in Women

Women secrete androgens, but in small doses: via the adrenal glands just above the kidneys, and via the internal theca, a very specific part of the ovaries themselves. Indeed, the female sex requires a touch of testosterone to ensure a satisfactory level of libido and enough low-pitched harmonics in her voice to distinguish it from a child's voice. But the level of testosterone must be between 140 and 210 µg/dl. Too low, and the libido disappears; too high, and masculinity sets in and excess hirsutism can occur. This action is often irreversible, and aggravated by steroids.

I must insist that consumption of androgens leaves indelible marks in women. This is why voice professionals should check their medication carefully for the presence of androgenic anabolic derivatives. These elements may also be present in certain progesterone preparations and their molecular derivatives.

The Male Voice

The androgens secreted by the testes have a direct effect on the voice. They certainly act on muscles and bony tissues, but also on the brain. They increase aggressiveness; it is no accident that yelling is often an integral aspect of male expression in combat, both in men and in animals. This male hormone builds the laryngeal muscles, and it lends power to his call. The significant influence of androgens on his vocal print, on the power and frequencies of his call, without a doubt triggered the appearance of the secondary sexual attributes.

Androgens increase blood flow in the body and improve oxygenation and muscle performance. Note that cortisone can have an androgenic effect and act as a euphoriant. This induces some voice professionals to overdose on it, hoping to be at their best vocally. But doing so is dangerous, because it can have a rebound effect. When you come off cortisone, muscle tone decreases abruptly; tiredness, possibly even a light depression, may set in.

Conclusion: The Larynx Is an Emotional Target

We know that the larynx is a hormonal target. Pipitone and Gallup[5] showed the links among voice, seduction, and conception. They investigated ratings of female voice attractiveness as a function of menstrual cycle phase. Their results showed a significant increase in voice attractiveness ratings as the likelihood of conception increased across the menstrual cycle in naturally cycling women. There was no effect for women using hormonal contraceptives. It seems obvious that the impact of hormones on the larynx is the source of these changes.

Timbre and seduction are intimately connected. With both female voice and male voice, the ingredients are multiple. In our world, the seductiveness of a voice stems from its height, from its resonance, from the deep harmonics that ornament the higher pitches in a woman's voice, and equally from the rhythm of its silences. The feminine voice that seduces you owes its charm to deep overtones that are barely audible, and to the sensuous breadth of the vibratory emission. Sometimes the "sexy" quality is enhanced to an edema of the vocal cords, to a small nodule, or to a growth that's best left alone. This unusual frequency creates the landscape of these sensual feminine voices.

Our voice is one of the paths of the mind and imagination of every one of us. Like a scribe for our thoughts, it expresses our inner self, both in its immanence and in its transcendence.

Notes

1. Abitbol, J., et al. "Does a Hormonal Vocal Cord Cycle Exist in Women?" *J Voice*, 1989, 3: 157–162.

2. Abitbol, J., et al. "Sex Hormones and the Female Voice." *J Voice*, 1999, 13(3): 424–446.

3. Voelter, C., N. Kleinsasser, P. Joa, I. Nowack, R. Martínez, and R. Hagen. "Detection of Hormone Receptors in the Human Vocal Fold." *European Archives of Oto-Rhino-Laryngology*, October 2008, 265(10).

4. Calyptol, manufactured by Laboratoires Techni-Pharma, 7 Rue de l'industrie, Monaco.

5. Pipitone, R. N., and G. G. Gallup, Jr. "Women's Voice Attractiveness Varies Across the Menstrual Cycle." *Evolution and Human Behavior* 2008, 298: 268–274.

10

Pregnancy

A Primer for Singers

ANTHONY F. JAHN, MD

Until not so many years ago, the professional singer had to make an inevitable choice: career or baby? The choice, for many, was to sacrifice family for career. Happily, this is no longer the case; the typical female singer is able to combine both professions, mom and performer, and can succeed at both. This is due to many factors, including the ability to control and plan pregnancy and the more extensive social supports in place for the singer. Many singers indeed plan to have children, booking their gestation and concert schedules ahead of time.

For singers who are, or are planning to be, pregnant, there are numerous factors to consider. The purpose of this chapter is to take you through the various stages, from conception to the end of lactation, and discuss the effects that these major, albeit temporary, physical changes have on your singing. This is not primarily a general discussion of pregnancy; please keep in mind that the focus of this chapter is the voice, and it is written by a laryngologist, not an obstetrician.

Note: This chapter has been modified from a previously written article in *Classical Singer Magazine,* and is reproduced here with permission.

First, let me make a few general comments about infertility issues. If you are given hormones, either to induce ovulation or to facilitate implantation, these will have an effect on your voice. Most hormones, except for androgens, should cause only a temporary change in the voice, but the change may be persistent if you are making repeated or prolonged attempts at fertilization. Estrogen and progestins cause fluid retention. More importantly, synthetic progestins may break down into androgenlike compounds that can darken the voice. Lighter and higher voices are more at risk here. I can't comment on specific medications or specific cases; you really need to explore all of this with your fertility specialist, and then weigh the risks and benefits.

But let's assume you have become pregnant, perhaps the old-fashioned way. Pregnancy is a time of profound physical and emotional change; it is driven by hormones and affects every part of your body. Furthermore, as pregnancy progresses, these changes become more marked. Although delivery normally represents the end of pregnancy, the hormonal environment remains altered and doesn't return to normal until you have finished lactating and your periods have commenced again. So for singers who plan to breastfeed, these alterations may potentially last one to two years. Our bodies carry a remarkable variety of "as needed" information, reflexes, and capabilities that manifest only under very specific circumstances, perhaps just once or twice in a lifetime. Childbearing is a prime example of this. Consider the letdown reflex: a new mother may start lactating spontaneously, triggered by nothing more than the sound of a baby's cry.

From a greater perspective, singing during pregnancy is probably not as important for the survival of the species as making another human being. Nonetheless, many professional and amateur singers need to (or choose to) continue to sing during this time of great physical change. And in general, there is no reason you shouldn't—as long as you accept the limitations imposed on your vocal mechanism and lungs, your physical and emotional endurance, and what's going on below your diaphragm.

Let me preface everything that follows with one important disclaimer. Every woman is different! For many reasons, some can sing seemingly effortlessly (or with only mildly modified effort) through their entire pregnancy, stop right before delivery, and return to singing a few weeks later. Others are significantly vocally disabled for much of their pregnancy, and after delivery and weaning they get back to singing with great effort, only to find that their voice and technique have changed.

Looking at the hormones first, we see that when you become pregnant the normal cycling of estrogen and progesterone stops. Progesterone, or progestins, dominate the scene now. As the name implies, progestin promotes gestation: this allows the ovum to implant on the receptive surface of the uterine wall and for that attachment to continue as the baby grows. You will recall that progesterone is the dominant hormone during the week before your period, often a time of salt craving and fluid retention. This effect also occurs during pregnancy; there is a tendency to retain salt and for your tissues to swell. From the vocal point of view, hormonally driven fluid retention carries the same problems as singing during the premenstrual period: the voice may lose some sonority, and the high notes, especially with soft singing, may be unwieldy.

This is why pregnant women are encouraged to avoid salty foods, since the combination can lead to hypertension during pregnancy. Women who are prone to high blood pressure may develop a severe and dangerous form of hypertension during pregnancy, called preeclampsia or eclampsia.

The second hormonal issue pertains to low estrogen. Not only does progesterone dominate during pregnancy, but following delivery prolactin begins to increase. This hormone, as the name again suggests, supports lactation. But prolactin also suppresses estrogen, and in fact it suppresses normal menstruation. This built-in birth control is great, since it normally prevents the mother from becoming pregnant until she has stopped breastfeeding. On the other hand, the suppression of estrogen has a negative effect on the voice, almost like a temporary mini-menopause! So singing during breastfeeding may be unreliable. Not until the child is weaned, prolactin level drops, and the normal estrogen/progesterone cycle resumes will the voice return to its normal state.

For the sake of our discussion, the entire period can be divided into six parts: the three trimesters, the delivery, the postpartum period, and the period of lactation (which ends with the return of the menses).

The First Trimester

Each trimester of pregnancy carries its own signature as far as singing is concerned. During the first three months, you should have no significant difficulties, apart from morning sickness and the possible irritation to the throat that may come from vomiting. The effect of gastric contents coming up into the throat can cause irritation of the pharynx and elevation of the larynx. There are of course also hormonal changes, as discussed above, and you may need to more actively support the voice, especially at the top of your range. During the first trimester, the uterus is still below the pelvic rim and should not encumber your breathing or diaphragmatic movement, although pelvic floor sensation may be slightly altered.

The Second Trimester

In the second trimester, an expectant mother typically feels well, but the increasing distention of the abdomen can make support more difficult toward the end of the trimester. At the end of the sixth month, the top of the uterus is at the level of the navel, compressing the contents of the abdomen and resetting the "resting position" of the abdominal muscles. Interestingly, the mild stretch of these muscles can initially make contraction and support easier. All of these phenomena vary, depending on whether the expectant mom is slim or overweight, and they also vary with the size and shape of the pelvis. How you "carry" the baby (high or low) is also a factor, since carrying high will more quickly press up on the abdominal organs and the diaphragm.

Support is also compromised by the necessary adjustments in posture, as your center of balance shifts forward. The normal inward curve of the lumbar vertebrae (lumbar lordosis) is accentuated as the gravid uterus pulls the abdomen forward and downward. Support becomes more of a problem as the baby grows. The issue is not so much support in the conventional sense (although the muscles of the abdomen are stretched, they still work and are able to contract), but you will be unable to fill your lungs as fully, since descent of the diaphragm is impaired by the rising uterus. Long phrases become difficult—you may need to revise your breathing for certain types of music. Lower back pain is common, and contraction of the postural muscles of the back (like the psoas major) may sympathetically increase the muscle tone in your other muscles, such as in the pelvis.

There is another potential issue with the lower back that the late-second- and third-trimester mother should consider. One of the "as needed" contingencies in the pregnant woman is the synthesis of a hormone that loosens the ligaments and tendons. Appropriately named relaxin, this hormone can increase the possibility of dislocations and certainly worsen problems in the lower back. If you need to sing on stage, the angle of the stage's rake can become an important factor in your ability to perform, since your center of gravity has shifted, the curvature of the lower back is exaggerated, and the protective tendons and ligaments are looser than normal. Incidentally, relaxin is an amazing hormone: in rabbits, which give birth to multiple babies, relaxin actually dissolves the fibrous connection between the two pubic bones in front, allowing the rabbit pelvis to open like a book during delivery!

The Third Trimester

In the third trimester, all of the phenomena listed above become more encumbering. Around the seventh month, the top of the uterus is typically at the lower tip of the breastbone (xiphoid process). This is the highest point during pregnancy: in the eighth and ninth months, the uterus comes back down and protrudes forward. This is when the woman looks really pregnant and needs to rebalance her gait and standing posture. Fortunately, breathing becomes easier as the uterus moves away from the diaphragm.

GERD (gastroesophageal reflux disease) is a frequent accompanying feature of pregnancy and becomes an increasing problem as the enlarging uterus presses up on the stomach. Not only are the contents of the stomach (acid and enzymes) pushed up into the esophagus, but parts of the stomach itself may be pushed into the chest. The hiatus—a slit in the diaphragm through which the esophagus passes down to the stomach—may be stretched, allowing the lower esophagus and stomach, which normally belong in the abdomen, to slip up into the thorax, a condition known as a "hiatal hernia." If a singer develops this condition, it may or may not reverse completely after delivery, or it may recur if she puts on weight over time.

The effects of GERD on the voice are well known. Management of this problem includes measures such as elevating the head of the bed at night, using liquid antacids at bedtime, and generally controlling weight gain during pregnancy.

If your pregnancy was the successful outcome of in vitro fertilization, you may give birth to more than one baby, since several ova are typically implanted. This means, of course, that all of the comments regarding weight gain, reflux, postural changes, and breathing problems apply, but even more so!

One feature specific to the third trimester is increasing physical fatigue, which continues well into the postpartum period. Women need more rest. The quality of sleep changes; they may need to sleep in unaccustomed positions to accommodate the baby. Synthesizing a new human is hard work for your body, and you need to adjust your singing and performing to accommodate. Even if you have sung well during the first two trimesters, expect less endurance as you round the home stretch. As you change your technique, support, breathing, and laryngeal posturing to accommodate your (temporarily) new body, do this with conscious awareness, since you will have to unlearn this compensation after the baby is born.

Delivery

Delivery is a messy but magnificent event—one might say the *raison d'être* for our sexual existence. From the laryngeal point of view, it can be highly traumatic. Pushing for many hours can cause at least vocal fold edema, and in some cases vocal fold hemorrhage. Holding your breath and pushing raises the blood pressure in your head and can even cause some small blood vessels to rupture; it is not uncommon for women to develop facial edema or pinpoint bleeding (petechiae) in the skin of the face or over the sclera of the eyes.

A similar phenomenon happens to the vocal folds, which are contracted and forced together repeatedly and for prolonged periods during delivery. Vomiting is not uncommon. Much more rarely, stomach contents are aspirated into the larynx and trachea—a condition that carries the bizarrely musical name of Mendelssohn's Syndrome.

If delivery is by C-section, this is a decision that may be made emergently and after hours of attempts at pushing the baby out. Even if it is a planned C-section, the woman is usually intubated, so some intubation trauma to the larynx may occur.

For all of these reasons, you should consider not singing for at least two weeks after delivery. Though beneficial to the vocal folds, two weeks of such voice rest also allows the larynx to rise up in the neck into a position that is too high for optimal singing. So don't be surprised if your voice is below par. It will recover, once vocal fold edema or possible hemorrhage has resolved and your larynx is down where it should be.

Postpartum

In the postpartum period, two new issues are at play: vocal support and depression. Over the previous nine months, the abdominal muscles have gradually stretched out to accommodate the baby, and now they are loose. They have nothing to push against when you try to sing. The effect is similar (but even more dramatic) to what you might see with sudden severe weight loss. If you had a C-section, the abdominal muscles (recti abdominis) may have been further traumatized.

The muscles of the pelvic floor are also stretched and loose. If you had an episiotomy, pain in the perineal area is another burden. Over the ensuing few weeks, the abdominal and pelvic muscles will gradually tighten, but they may not go back to singing "trim" for several months. Kegel exercises are helpful to tone the pelvic floor muscles. You can also gently work the abdominal muscles, with advice from your obstetrician, but expect this to be a slow and gradual process.

Postpartum depression is common, and it may range from mild to severe. Expect to feel at least a bit down, since this also has an effect on your singing.

Breastfeeding Period

The prolactin issue has already been mentioned earlier. If you plan to breastfeed, expect a period of relative estrogen depletion, which can change your voice—less resonance, less color, less pliability to the vocal folds. This may continue into the sixth part of our discussion, when abdominal and pelvic tone have recovered, laryngeal edema from pushing and reflux has subsided, and laryngeal position is back to its vocally appropriate position—but the voice is still not right! Don't be impatient. Modify your singing schedule and repertoire to accommodate your temporary impairment. Things may not get back to normal until you have weaned the baby and your periods have resumed again.

Expect also to be chronically tired; your schedule now must mirror the baby's. This is the time that once was called the "period of confinement." You can certainly vocalize a bit, but spend your time sleeping as much as you can between feedings.

Although from the singing point of view choosing not to breastfeed may speed your vocal recovery, the physical and emotional advantages of breastfeeding to both you and the baby are so overwhelming that I would never advise this to any new mother, singer or not.

Summary

By way of general advice, I would suggest the following. Expect changes in your voice, your support, and your endurance, and accept these as part of the normal physiologic changes associated with pregnancy. Sing within your comfort zone. Every woman experiences pregnancy-associated vocal changes differently, depending on hormones, how much weight is gained, and how she carries the baby.

Singing can be continued as long as you are comfortable, depending on your fach, the role, your general physical condition, and the effect of pregnancy-related hormones on your voice. Stage performance, however, must take into account the increasing limits on your general endurance as your pregnancy continues. And consider the physical limitations of stance and posture. You are certainly less poised and "athletic" when pregnant.

Above all, don't be too hard on yourself and your vocal instrument; you are very busy making another human being! Pregnancy and childbearing are an incredible and unique adventure. This is a full-time job, but one that lasts only a few months. And you have the rest of your life to sing . . . perhaps beginning with a lullaby to your new baby.

11

Nutrition and Weight Management

SHARON ZARABI, RD, CDN, CPT

For years, singers have been struggling with managing excess weight. Obesity, defined as a body mass index (BMI) of 30 or above, can be calculated by dividing one's weight (in kilograms) by height (in meters squared). Excess weight has caused many performers to turn to various commercial crash diets and self-starvation as a means of achieving their weight loss goals. Although there are many abundant diet books out there, none is geared specifically for singers offering guidelines based on their specific needs and lifestyle.

The life of an opera singer is unique, and eating habits are reflected through daily regimen. An unbalanced, sporadic, erratic, unsteady job situation with specific demands is often reflected in irregular eating habits, a phenomenon that has led to the term "Diva Syndrome." This is defined by Angela Slover and Johanna Dwyer as "maladaptive eating behaviors and lifestyle characteristics that are prevalent among professional singers, predisposing them to obesity."[1] Such rituals are reinforced by a challenging life of traveling frequently for performances, late-night social gatherings leading to late-night eating, unpredictable work hours, fluctuating pay and resultant reliance on cheap fast food, overindulging at postperformance celebrations, bingeing patterns, and common taboo foods that may affect vocal delivery.

Singing professionals do not have a steady schedule. Sporadic hours of work lead to frequent snacking on readily available foods that are usually high in simple sugars, leading to an excessive intake of empty calories. Moreover, singers may be emotional eaters, leading to disordered, psychologically driven eating habits. They may base their self-esteem on the success of the performance and, if they are not living up to their own high expectations, use food as a coping mechanism for emotional comfort. Coaches, teachers, and instructors can be very critical, leading to more stress and disruptive bingeing incidents. In addition, loneliness, depression, as well as the emotional stress of an unstable lifestyle and financial dependence may contribute to bingeing patterns.

Bingeing is defined as an episode of eating marked by three particular features. First, the amount of food eaten is larger than most people would eat under normal circumstances. Second, the excessive eating occurs in a discrete period, usually less than two hours. And finally, the eating is accompanied by a subjective sense of loss of control.[2] Long hours without eating leading to starvation; even striving to avoid specific foods may also trigger bingeing episodes. If food intake is reduced, the thyroid responds by secreting fewer hormones, thus lowering the body's metabolism and conserving energy resources. This slowing of metabolism works against any dieter's goal, as less body fat is burned. Unfortunately, bingeing becomes a habitual lifestyle, where the feeling of being "stuffed" or eating beyond fullness becomes common and comes to signal the end of a meal. Like many obese individuals, they have desensitized the feeling of satiation, and the extra caloric intake leads to gradual but cumulative weight gain.

When singers are preparing to audition or perform, they often avoid specific foods and may even fast for several hours before stage time to control breathing and voice delivery. Singing on a full stomach, coupled with feelings of anxiety, stress, nervousness, and excitement, may initiate indigestion, nausea, vomiting, intestinal cramps, or loose stools.

Taboo foods that have been known to adversely affect vocal quality include chocolate, nuts, and dairy, which coat the throat. Caffeine, found in chocolate and of course coffee and sodas, dries out the vocal tract and also can cause what we all experience after a caffeine rush: the common "jitters." Carbonated beverages lead to gas, belching and increased reflux. By contrast, hot water with lemon and honey soothes the throat. Fruits, vegetables and high-fiber whole grains improve intestinal function.

Gastroesophageal reflux disease, also known as GERD, is a medical condition that can lead to serious vocal issues. Professor Rosalie Loeding comments that "75% of my voice rehab clients have reflux ranging from mild to severe."[3] Highly acidic foods, personal and physical stress and obesity variously contribute, by causing excessive abdominal pressure and acid production. Normal digestion begins with chewing, and then swallowing food that travels through the esophagus to be mixed with pancreatic enzyme and gastric juices, which are to be held down and led into the small and large intestines. A group of sphincters, including the cricopharyngeal sphincter, gastroesophageal sphincter and pyloric sphincter, ensure the downward flow of digested material. However, foods that are high in acid content, alcohol, chocolate, medications and cigarettes have been known to relax the sphincters, enabling gastric juices to push back through the esophagus, causing the feeling of heartburn (Tables 11.1a and 11.1b).

Communication regarding health and nutrition is often skewed and distorted, based on "what works for me." This is what leads to the latest fad diet and often to the yo-yo effect of losing weight and gaining almost double when coming off a diet. In these pages I avoid using the word *diet* in the sense of a regimen that deprives us of specific foods; I feel everything fits into a bal-

TABLE 11.1A High-acid foods.

- citrus fruits
- chocolate
- drinks with caffeine or alcohol
- fatty and fried foods
- garlic and onions
- mint flavorings
- spicy foods
- tomato-based foods, like spaghetti sauce, salsa, chili, and pizza

Source: http://digestive.niddk.nih.gov/ddiseases/pubs/gerd/

TABLE 11.1B Ways to prevent acid reflux.

Avoid eating 3 hours before bed
Take antacids (such as Tums® or Rolaids®) when symptoms flare
Eat larger meals earlier in the day
Avoid high fat foods, alcohol, and caffeine when appropriate

anced diet and can be eaten in moderation. Registered dietitians and health professionals can help singers in achieving an appropriate and healthy balanced diet, preventing further weight gain and treating the Diva Syndrome if the singers' lifestyle is understood. Nutritionists can play a major role in meal planning, as well as intervening in behavior modification. The role of a registered dietitian or nutritionist is to educate a singer on proper nutrition when an erratic lifestyle is evident, and to encourage healthy snacking to control blood sugars and prevent the feeling of hunger that leads one to binge.

Basic nutrition begins with understanding the six major nutrients and the effects they have on our bodies. Nutrients are elements of food that ensure maintenance of bodily functions and promote optimal performance. Calories, which provide the body with energy, are found in carbohydrates, protein, and fats. Good nutrition involves a balance of protein, carbohydrates, and fats (Exhibit 11.1) as well as vitamins, minerals, and water. The balance of these six macronutrients influences metabolism, which is the fuel for all of the body's functions. As mentioned before, any imbalance of calories (quantity and source) due to maladaptive eating patterns can disrupt the body's metabolism.

Carbohydrates

Carbohydrates can be categorized as simple or complex, depending on their molecular structure. Simple carbohydrates that are quickly metabolized include monosaccharides and disaccharides and are found in fruits, honey, sugar, corn syrup, and milk. Complex carbohydrates or polysaccharides are more difficult to break down, leading to longer transit time and a feeling of prolonged contentment in the GI tract. Since the breakdown and absorption takes longer, complex carbohydrates generate sugar more gradually, resulting in a slower and healthier release of insulin into the blood stream; there is no "sugar high" such as you might experience after eating a candy bar. Complex carbohydrates also tend to be associated with foods that have high fiber content. Wheat, corn, potatoes, barley, oats, beans, and vegetables are examples of high-fiber foods, containing a high proportion of the indigestible part of plants. Foods with high fiber content are good for our health, claiming to reduce cholesterol level, control blood sugars, and maintain colon and gut function.

An important function of carbohydrates is to provide fuel for the central nervous system and red blood cells. They help assist in fat breakdown. In the absence of carbohydrates, fats metabo-

EXHIBIT 11.1 Suggested portions and serving sizes.

STARCHES/ CARBOHYDRATE (1 serving = 80 cal, 15 gm carb)

Breads and Cereal
½ C cooked cereal
½ C grits

¾ C dry cereal
¼ C granola
¼ C grape nuts

1 light multigrain English muffin
2 slices light wheat bread
1 slice wheat, multigrain bread
¼ large deli bagel
½ bun
½ wheat pita bread
2 bread sticks

½ C pasta
½ C brown rice
½ C couscous
3 Tb cornmeal
1 corn tortilla 6″
1 flour tortilla 8″

Starchy Vegetables
½ C Idaho/Sweet potato
1 small potato
½ C dried or baked beans
½ C corn
½ C peas and carrots

Snack Foods
3 C popcorn
15 pretzels
15–20 fat free chips
1.5 sheets graham crackers
2 rice cakes
8 saltine crackers/animal crackers

Breads with Fat (125 calories)
1 biscuit, 2.5" diam
2" square cornbread
6 Ritz/clubhouse crackers
1 C croutons
2" square muffin
1 waffle, not belgian
1 pancake 4" diam
1 slice French toast
½ C stuffing
½ C Chinese noodles
1C croutons/crispy noodles
16 french fries

MILK (1 svg = 90 cal, 12 gm carb, 8 gm protein)
1 C milk, skim or 1%
1 C soymilk, lowfat
6 oz light/fat free yogurt

FRUIT (1 svg= 60 cal, 15 gm Carb, 0 protein)
1 C berries/cubed fruit
½ C fruit cup/canned fruit in
1 apple, orange, peach, pear
½ C applesauce
½ banana
12 Cherries
15 grapes
3 prunes/dried fruit
3 TB raisins
2 plums
¾ C pineapple
1 slice melon
1 kiwi
½ mango/papaya

continued

EXHIBIT 11.1 (continued)

VEGETABLES (1 svg= 25 cal, 5 gm carb, 2 gm pro)

½ cooked
1 C raw

Colorful, dark green, orange, red, leafy veggies:
Asparagus, green beans, broccoli, cauliflower, cabbage, Brussels
  sprouts, celery, cucumber, eggplant, leeks, okra, peppers,
  onions, mushrooms, collards, turnip greens, spinach, salad
  greens, tomatoes

FAT (1 svg= 45 cal, 5 gm fat)

Saturated Fat
  1 tsp butter
  1 slice bacon
  2 TB sour cream
  1 TB cream cheese
  2 TB coffee creamer
Polyunsaturated Fat
  1 tsp margarine
  1 TB mayonnaise
  1 tsp corn/ veg oil
  1 TB salad dressing
  1 TB low fat mayo
  1 TB sunflower/ pumpkin seeds
Monounsaturated fat
  1/8 avocado
  1 tsp olive/canola/peanut oil
  8–10 olives
  6–10 nuts
  2 tsp peanut butter
  2 tsp tahini paste (sesame)

PROTEIN 1 oz equivalents

Lean = 55 cal, 7 gm pro, 3 gm fat
   Beef: sirloin, round, flank, tenderloin, 98% fat free
   Poultry: chicken, turkey breast
   Fish: steaks, flaky, white, shellfish
      ½ can tuna in water, salmon
   Pork: ham, tenderloin, lean chop, Canadian bacon
   Cheese: 1% cottage cheese, light lauging cow cheese, alpine
   lace, 2TB parmesan cheese, 1 oz fat free cheese
   1 egg or ½ C egg substitute

High Fat Meat= 100 cal, 7 gm pro, 8 gm fat
   Cheese: swiss, Monterey jack, American, cheddar
   Pork: sausage, spare ribs, bacon, ground, bologna, hot dogs
   Fried and breaded: chicken, beef, pork, cheese

lize to ketones, which are highly acidic, causing bad breath and malnutrition (this is quite common among very low carbohydrate fad diets). Carbohydrates that are not used up are stored with water as glycogen, in the liver and muscle. This is an important fact to consider, since many dieters attribute weight gain to eating excessive fats; carbohydrates that are not metabolized are also stored and lead to weight gain. When following a very low carbohydrate diet such as Atkins or South Beach, it is easy for one to lose weight drastically because of loss of water. It is not fat loss but rather water weight that deceptively reduces the number on the scale.

Carbohydrates provide 4 calories per gram and according to the current recommendations of the U.S. Department of Agriculture should constitute 50 percent of our total caloric needs for the day.

Protein

Proteins are made up of individual units called amino acids. Each arrangement and pattern of amino acids forms a protein that is uniquely suited to various body functions. Proteins are necessary for building muscle and bone structure, fluid balance, synthesizing hormones, facilitating enzymatic reactions, regulating pH balance within the circulatory system, and contributing to the formation of antibodies to keep us healthy. Proteins are found in animal products such as chicken, beef, meat, dairy, and fish, as well as plant sources including legumes, beans, nuts, and soy products. Protein provides 4 calories per gram. The Recommended Daily Allowance of protein is 0.8 grams per kilogram of body weight, equating to 10–20 percent of total daily calorie needs.

Fats

Fats, also known as lipids, are essential for optimal heath and well-being. Since fats yield the highest number of calories per gram, they have acquired a bad reputation. In the early 1990s, low-fat diets were encouraged for weight loss, disregarding the important role they play as a fuel source for aerobic activity, providing a feeling of satiety, hormone regulation, and maintaining cell integrity. Fats are necessary to carry the fat-soluble vitamins as well (A, D, E, and K). Fats can be found in three forms. Saturated fats are solid at room temperature and are familiar to us as margarine, animal fats, coconut oil, palm oil, butter, and lard. These are the fats you want to limit, because of the adverse effects they have on our serum cholesterol and triglycerides. Monounsaturated fats, by contrast, are liquid at room temperature, and less likely to clog your arteries; examples are canola oil, olive oil, nuts, avocado, and sunflower oil. Polyunsaturated fats are the most beneficial and should ideally account for most of the fat in the diet. Polyunsaturated fats found in the omega3 form (EPA and DHA of fish, flax seed oil, and nuts) must be obtained in a 4:1 ratio with omega 6 fatty acids of corn oil, cottonseed oil, safflower oil, sunflower oil, and soybean oil. Fat provides 9 calories per gram and should comprise 10 percent of total daily calorie needs.

A Little Note on Alcohol

Alcohol contains 7 calories per gram and is considered a simple carbohydrate. Nonetheless, alcohol can fit into a balanced diet when considering calories throughout the day. Mixed drinks contain higher calories thanks to the addition of sweetened beverages to the highly caloric liquor. Table 11.2 lists common alcoholic beverages and calorie content. In any effort at weight loss, it is best to ask for low-calorie mixers or diet beverages when available; mix with club soda or a diet beverage. Like other simple carbs, alcohol lowers the blood sugar level, causing you to feel hungry. Additionally, intoxication leads to inhibition of your dieting resolve, which allows extra snacking to kick in without your even realizing it. Try to stay in control.

Energy Needs

Our bodies need a certain amount of calories (usually measured as kilocalories, kcal) to perform daily functions such as walking, breathing, blinking, thinking, etc. The ideal diet equation is simple: you should not take in any calories in excess of what you use up in the course of the day. However, in the fast-paced, supersize-me-portioned, generally sedentary lifestyle inhabited by

TABLE 11.2 Calories of alcoholic beverages

8 oz. beer (250 ml)	115kcal
1 shot of 80 proof liquor	approx 100 kcal
1 single measure of spirits	52kcal
1 bottle pf Hard Lemonade	285 kcal
1 small glass wine	80kcal
1 small glass sherry	68kcal
8 oz. Tonic Water	83 kcal
8 oz. Coca Cola	105 kcal
8 oz. Diet Cola	0 kcal
8 oz. Lemonade	60 kcal
8 oz. Orange Juice	72 kcal

References: http://www.weightlossresources.co.uk/logout/
news_features/alcohol.htm; http://www.calorieking.com

many opera singers, excessive calories quickly lead to an increase in weight. As an example, forty minutes of moderate exercise on the treadmill burns off about 400 calories, the equivalent of just one pastry from Starbucks! Even if you eat only one meal a day and are overweight, or claim that you don't eat meals and snack frequently throughout the day, gradual weight gain is evidence that you may be consuming in excess of your daily energy needs.

English BMR Formula

Women: BMR = 655 + (4.35 × weight in pounds) + (4.7 × height in inches) − (4.7 × age in years)

Men: BMR = 66 + (6.23 × weight in pounds) + (12.7 × height in inches) − (6.8 × age in years)

Harris Benedict Formula

To determine your total daily calorie needs, multiply your BMR by the appropriate activity factor, as follows:

If you are sedentary (little or no exercise) : Calorie calculation = BMR × 1.2

If you are lightly active (light exercise or sports 1–3 days/week) : Calorie calculation = BMR × 1.375

If you are moderately active (moderate exercise or sports 3–5 days/week) : Calorie calculation = BMR × 1.55

If you are very active (hard exercise or sports 6–7 days a week) : Calorie calculation = BMR × 1.725

If you are extra active (very hard exercise or sports plus physical job or training twice a week) : Calorie calculation = BMR × 1.9

Source: http://www.bmi-calculator.net/bmr-calculator/bmr-formula .php.

For every extra 3,500 calories ingested, one pound of fat is stored. Use the formulas in the box to calculate your daily caloric needs (BMR is basal metabolic rate).

Weight Loss

If an extra 3,500 calories is equivalent to one pound of excess body weight, then a 3,500 calorie deficit must equate to weight loss. Decreasing 500 calories per day (by consuming 300 calories less and using up 200 calories through moderate intensity exercise, e.g., 20 minutes of aerobic activity) for one week would initiate one pound of weight loss.

Dieting basically involves rebalancing your energy intake (food) and output (exercise) to achieve a balanced regimen that you can be comfortable with for a long time. The more gradual the weight loss, the longer it will last and the less effect it will have on voice quality. You can immediately eliminate 300 calories per day from your diet by avoiding sweetened beverages such as juice (even if it claims to be 100 percent fruit juice with no added sugars; it still contains excessive calories), soda, and smoothies. Such beverages contain as much as 300 calories in a 16 ounce serving and are made of simple sugar and water, with very little nutritional value. Reading food labels is also very important, looking for proper serving sizes and avoiding extra sugar. When reading labels, look for food items that have less than 10 grams of sugar per serving and more than than 3 grams of fiber per serving. And again, look at what constitutes a serving or portion; you may be surprised that it is often less than what you would normally consume.

The average individual will begin to lose weight by eating fewer than 1,500 calories per day. However very low calorie diets such as the Cambridge Diet, Liquid Protein shakes, Optifast/Medifast, and protein sparing modified fasts and detox diets can go as low as 500 calories per day. Many people who try such diets will find themselves overeating to compensate, and this may lead to a pattern of bingeing.

Repetition and Monotony

The North American menu is actually made up of various combinations of a small number of foods, usually wheat, beef, eggs, potatoes, and dairy products. A breakfast consisting of eggs, sausage, white toast, and hash browns is the same nutrient break-down as a lunch consisting of a hamburger, white bun, and fries; or a dinner of steak and potatoes or a bowl of white pasta. All are devoid of fruits and vegetables, and high in saturated fat and refined carbohydrates, which provide no fiber. In addition to the harmful health effects of these nutrients, eating such a monotonous diet can also produce allergies and food sensitivities. Among the most common food allergens are soy products, wheat products, dairy, and various nuts.

Getting the Most Bang for Your Buck

In addition to serving as a source of calories, nutrients play a vital role in regulating normal bodily functions. To eat well, you want to get the least amount of calories from the most nutritious sources and still feel full. Foods such as vegetables, whole grains, and beans that are dense in nutrients and fiber require more eating and chewing time and are absorbed more gradually, resulting in fewer calories consumed. Choosing a diet that is high in fiber and protein is therefore the key to healthy eating and weight control. Both protein and fiber nutrients take longer to digest, and they yield many health benefits. Here are examples of mix-and-match snacks, listed with proper serving sizes.

> Yogurt and chopped nuts
> > 4 oz. light yogurt topped with 1 tbsp. chopped nuts
> Apple and peanut butter
> > One medium apple and 1 tbsp. peanut butter
> Toasted cheese and tomato on wheat
> > Top one slice light whole wheat bread with 1 oz. reduced fat cheese and two or three slices of tomato. Toast in toaster oven.

Cottage cheese and berries

> 1 cup strawberries or blueberries and ½ cup low fat cottage cheese topped with 1 tsp. sunflower seeds. Sweeten with Splenda if desired.

Veggies with dip

> 1 cup raw baby carrots or broccoli florets and 1/3 cup reduced fat vegetable dip

Mexican tortilla wrap

> Top an 8-inch light whole wheat tortilla with ¼ cup fat free refried beans, ¼ cup shredded low fat cheese, and 1 tbsp. salsa. Microwave for 15–20 seconds and roll.

Celery and peanut butter

> 1 cup raw celery sticks and 1 tbsp. peanut butter

Breakfast sandwich

> One egg, 1 oz. reduced fat cheese on ½ light multigrain English muffin

Ricotta cheese dessert

> ½ cup part skim ricotta cheese mixed with one packet sugar substitute. Sprinkle with cinnamon and 1 tsp. almonds.

String cheese and reduced fat Triscuits

> 1 part skim mozzarella string cheese and five Triscuits

Tuna salad pita

> 1/2 whole wheat pita filled with ½ cup tuna, 1 tbsp. light mayo, and alfalfa sprouts

Peanut butter banana waffle

> Top one toasted low fat Nutri-grain or Kashi waffle with 1 tbsp. peanut butter and ½ small banana (sliced). Drizzle 1 tbsp. sugar-free maple syrup on top if desired.

Hummus and pita

> 2 oz. light whole wheat pita with 2 tbsp hummus

Supplements

In an effort to lose weight, many in our instant-gratification society turn to weight loss supplements as a quick means of weight loss. Before investing any money in such supplements, be sure to read the article "Foods, Drugs, or Frauds?" in the May 1985 issue of *Consumer Reports*, or check out www.nutrition.gov. Herbal supplements that claim to be "all natural," as well as vitamins and minerals, are not regulated by the Food and Drug Administration. This loophole allows companies to make false claims, so be sure to always read the fine print at the bottom of the label. In addition, there is never enough conclusive research to substantiate the potency of such supplements. There is no technical definition for the word *natural*. When they manufacture these supplements, how much of the active substance are they actually putting in before it is mixed with other fillers and extra ingredients? There is no supporting research on appetite stimulants or ergogenic aids such as the popular hoodia, phentarmine, ephedra, bitter orange extract, and guarana, just to name a few. Moreover, many of these products have been taken off the shelves for their potentially harmful side effects.

Common Stimulants

Ephedra (*Ephedra sinica*) claims to increase metabolic rate, restore thermogenic activity, and promote the release of the brain chemical neurotransmitter norepinephrine. Side effects include insomnia, dizziness, increased perspiration, and elevated blood pressure. Has been taken off shelves because of increased health risks and deaths.

Garlic (*Allium ativum*) claims to "boost thermogenesis." Comes in many forms of raw, dried, oil, or prepared commercial product.

Cayenne or red pepper (*Capsicum frutescens*) is a thermogenic food spice that claims to induce fat burning and help mobilize fat and sugar metabolism. Other pungent food spices such as cinnamon and ginger make the same claim, but there is little scientific evidence to verify such properties.

Ginseng (*Panax quinquefolius*) was used in ancient Chinese medicine to improve stamina during exercise, sharpen mental abilities, and relieve fatigue. Research indicates that ginseng may be able to raise basal metabolic rate as well. Side effects include headaches, skin problems, and other reactions.

Green tea (*Camellia sinensis*) claims to increase metabolic rate and stimulate thermogenesis thanks to caffeine content. It contains two related components not usually found in coffee—theophylline and theobromine—that boost thermogenic activity.

Yerba mate (*Ilex paraguariensis*) is another tea well known in South America, acting as a stimulant to boost thermogenesis. Stimulating effects come from a compound called mateine, which is a close relative to caffeine, plus small quantities of theophylline and theobromine. Mateine seems to have the stimulatory effects of caffeine without the side effects.

Hydroxycitric acid (HCA) is an extract from the fruit of a tree called *Garcinia cambogia,* found throughout India and Asia. Research indicates that HCA may promote fat burning indirectly by inhibiting the enzymes involved in the formation of fat; thus more fat is burned than stored. HCA also has been claimed to reduce appetite.

Carnitine is a nutrient found in meat and dairy products that can boost your metabolism by helping you burn fat more efficiently. No research has been conclusive.

DHEA (dehydroepiandrosterone), the most abundant hormone in the body, is naturally produced by the human adrenal glands and gonads and functions as an antioxidant and hormone regulator. Levels of this hormone tend to decrease with age. Animal studies seem to indicate that DHEA may promote thermogenic activity and decrease body fat; however, human studies have not proven this. Although for the general population no serious side effects have been reported, it should not be used by singers, since it is an androgenic (male sex) hormone, which may darken and masculinize the higher female voices.

Complementing Your Diet

Your best companion to a weight loss diet would be what you have always heard: exercise! Proper exercise increases the body's thermogenic response not only during the activity, but even long afterward. Once you have reset your body's energy consumption with regular exercise, the rate of metabolism will continue for some time, even in the absence of continued daily exercise. Of course, this doesn't last forever, but it does mean that skipping the occasional day of exercise will not harm your weight-maintenance routine. Why does exercise lead to higher metabolism? In addition to the calories you are burning at the time of your workout, regular and consistent exercise increases BMR. The more you use your muscles through light strength training, the more muscle fibers you build. Muscle is active tissue, and active tissue requires energy for function, hence expending calories. Think of your muscles as fat-burning machines. Strength training in addition to cardiovascular activity should be a part of your daily routine for sixty minutes at least three to four times a week. I promise you, the results will be evident!

Putting It All Together

Since balanced metabolism is the key to long-term successful weight loss, this chapter is less about dieting and more about regaining a state of improved health. The main problem of fad diets and weight loss programs is that even resolute dieters grow weary of the restrictions imposed by the Atkins, South Beach, Cabbage Soup, and Cookie Diets. Deprivation leads to frustration, and an eventual return to old eating habits. The best approach to weight loss is to take the information listed in this chapter and apply it to mindful eating skills. You really are what you eat, both in quality and quantity, and you need to scrutinize your meals with the same attention you use in looking at medications. There is no one diet that works for everyone, and particularly for singing performers, who need to battle daily obstacles that interfere with a consistent meal plan. The information listed here is to help you become more aware of poor eating habits and to *do something about them!* Knowing which foods are better for you than others (notice how I try to refrain from labeling foods as "good" or "bad") will not get you very far if you do not know how to apply it.

And what if you fall off the wagon? Having the occasional "cheat day" is part of life's little pleasures. Allow yourself the occasional dessert as a reward, without beating yourself up for lack of dietary resolution. What determines the overall quality of your diet is not the occasional treat, but what you eat the rest of the time, day in and day out. Try to avoid the "I'm on a diet" mindset, and instead envision your eating plan as a way of life. Until you change your eating behavior, modify old habits, and empower yourself, the road to success will only be a longer journey.

Successful Pointers

1. Keep a food journal of everything you eat. Include type of food or beverage, amount, time, and physical feeling of fullness or hunger.
2. Portion meals into three components, focusing on lean protein, vegetables and fruit, and whole grains. Wherever you see enriched bread, try to replace with 100 percent whole wheat or whole grain varieties.
3. Keep cut-up fruits and vegetables handy so you can snack on them at any time. Try to aim for two or three servings per day.
4. Avoid long hours without eating. Try to eat every four or five hours rather than "saving your appetite" for a huge meal. Grow more in tune with your feelings of hunger and fullness.
5. Avoid bringing trigger foods and junk food into the house. Make it a special trip to the store if you feel you "must" have it. Try to go shopping *after* a meal, never when you're hungry. Giving into temptation once in a while may prevent bingeing later in the day or week.
6. Choose calories you can chew rather than drink; this means drinking more water instead of juice, sports drinks, regular soda, alcohol, and specialty coffees.
7. Avoid mindless eating in front of the television or computer, or on the run. Put the fork down between bites. Savor the flavor. Make meal time enjoyable rather than a task. Sometimes you may make needing to snack or eat a meal into a habit, just because you are sitting in front of the television.
8. Plan ahead; know what you are going to order when at a restaurant or buffet so you are not tempted by high fat dishes.

9. Always include lean sources of protein at every meal to keep you satisfied: chicken, fish, shellfish, legumes, eggs, low fat dairy products, soy products, and lean meats.
10. Move your body; find an exercise that you like, whether it be dancing, walking, or aerobics, and stick to it.

Consistency is the key!

Conclusion

In order to operate at your peak, an appropriate balance between nutrition and weight control must be achieved. With the proper understanding, singers will gain greater control over their own health and their performance.

Further Reading and Links to Resources

www.usda.gov
www.nutrition.gov
www.eatright.org (to find a registered dietitian within your area)
www.healthfinder.gov
www.medlineplus.gov
www.mypyramid.gov

Personalized sites that help you track your weight goals, free of charge, with daily tips:

www.thedailyplate.com
www.sparkpeople.com
www.fitday.com

References

Borushek, Allan. *The Calorie King Calorie Fat and Carbohydrate Counter.* Costa Mesa, CA: Family Health Publications, 2008.

"Dietary Guidelines for Americans." 2005. U.S. Dept. of Health and Human Services. USDA. www.healthierus.gov/dietaryguidelines.

Kleiner, Susan, with Maggie Greenwood Robinson. *Power Eating*, 3rd ed. High Performance Nutrition. Champaign, IL: Human Kinetics, 2007.

U.S. Food and Drug Administration, Center for Food Safety and Applied Nutrition. "Overview of Dietary Supplements." http://www.health.gov.

Notes

1. Slover, A. N, and J. T. Dwyer. "Professional Singers with Obesity or Eating Related Problems." *Nutrition Today* (USA), June 1995, 30(3), pp. 123–127.

2. Mahan, K., and S. Escott-Stump. *Krause's Food, Nutrition, and Diet Therapy*, 11th ed. Philadelphia: Saunders, 2000, p. 594.

3. "Vocal Survival Techniques—Gastroesophageal Reflux." 1999. http://ent-consult.com/loedingger.html.

12

Little Black Dress, Part 1

Obesity and Bariatric Surgery for Singers

MITCHELL S. ROSLIN, MD

In some professions a large physique is considered beneficial and the norm. Certain athletes, such as sumo wrestlers, power weight lifters, and football linemen, are examples. Each of these activities requires an unusual accumulation of muscle and power. Within the performing arts, however, being excessively large is generally a disadvantage.

Historically, one major exception to this has been in opera. The stereotypical opera singer has a large body habitus. This has been accepted, since it was felt that the extra girth provided support for a powerful voice. Luciano Pavarotti, considered one of world's greatest tenors, was an obvious example. Prior to undergoing gastric bypass, soprano Debra Voigt was another. In fact, when she was told in London that she was too heavy to perform at Covent Gardens, the story made front-page news in the *New York Times*.

Although the overweight and buxom soprano is a caricature cliché, the saying "It ain't over until the fat lady sings" actually

Note: I would like to acknowledge the participation, in preparing this chapter, of Barrett Polan, who is a graduate of Hampton Sydney, is currently a medical student, and spent his summers as a research intern at Lenox Hill.

comes not from sports. In April 1978, a commentator at a professional basketball game coined the phrase. The expression referred to singer Kate Smith's performance, which often followed the conclusion of the game. Smith, a singer nationally known for her voice and her size, was instantly recognizable to generations of Americans (she also was famous for singing "Moon over the Mountain" to complete the broadcast day in the early days of television, and Irving Berlin wrote "God Bless America" for her). She entered the sports world when a public relations executive for the Philadelphia Flyers hockey team correlated the playing of the song and success for the team. Smith was then invited to sing "God Bless America" in person and became a regular guest at important games. The Flyers became champions, and Smith became a sports legend. Yogi Berra, the Hall of Fame catcher of the New York Yankees, is credited with saying "It ain't over till it's over," and the two events came together in San Antonio, when Smith was invited to sing "God Bless America," giving the world the now-famous saying "It ain't over until the fat lady sings." As this expression spread, so did the perception that opera singers should be large. In fact, for the majority of sports fans this cliché became the basis of their limited knowledge of opera.

For many other (and better) reasons, the overweight singer was accepted. Before the age of television, opera was, for most of America, an auditory rather than visual experience. Given the beauty of the music and the voice, the opera lover was willing to suspend disbelief, willing to accept that the obese soprano was ostensibly dying of consumption. It is, however, interesting that even in those early days a chubby Greek girl from Queens named Mary had to lose a lot of weight before she became Maria Callas, La Diva assoluta!

Times have changed. Opera is increasingly visual, the competition for roles is fierce, and the public expects to see believable drama and romance, whether in the theater, television, the movies. The question then becomes, Is there any vocal advantage to obesity?

Numerous theories have been developed to suggest that a large physique makes for a better singing voice. It has been suggested that fat in the area of the vocal cords provides an amplifying effect. More credibly, abdominal bulk was considered important for voice support, which involves contracting the abdominal muscles and pushing the abdominal contents up, toward the diaphragm. In less affluent times, when malnutrition and chronic illness was the norm for lower classes, obesity was considered a marker of prosperity and health. It was felt that if you were somewhat heavy, you had enough food to eat and therefore had the power to have a good voice.

The facts are different. In fact, the argument can be made that overweight singers sing well despite their body habitus, not because of it. Since the basis for a powerful voice is the ability to control respiration and a strong diaphragm, any impediment that interferes with respiratory function would have a negative impact. Obesity interferes with lung expansion. Most people with severe obesity have a restrictive disorder of their lungs. Simply stated, they cannot fully fill their lungs on inspiration. A large amount of fat in the midsection hinders motion of the diaphragm. Obesity also causes the pressure inside the abdomen to increase. This can lead to acid from the stomach refluxing up to the mouth and larynx and burning the vocal cords. This is called GERD, or gastroesophageal reflux disease. Other obesity-related factors that can have an impact on the voice include disturbed sleep patterns, increased risk for heart disease and stroke, and premature disability because of stress placed on the hip and knee joints. When obese vocalists sing well, it is because they have learned to compensate for the physiologic stress created by being overweight.

Obesity is generally becoming a significant problem in westernized cultures. Most epidemiologists believe this will be the first generation that will not outlive its predecessors. This is a startling fact when you consider the medical breakthroughs that have taken place. Despite efforts to detect deadly cancers, procedures such as cardiac stents, novel chemotherapeutic agents, and the money spent on health care research, people will not live longer. If you were born in the year 2000, there is a 50 percent chance that you will be treated for diabetes in your lifetime.

It is estimated that 60 percent of Americans are either overweight or obese. If it were just a size transition, it would not be concerning. We know we are getting taller, on average, and attribute this to the absence of malnutrition. However, the weight-to-height ratio is becoming disproportionately high, and with our larger waistlines come chronic diseases. These affect every system in our body. Best known are diabetes, hypertension, and hypercholesterolemia—together forming what is called "metabolic syndrome," related to obesity and poor dietary habits. All of these conditions make the occurrence of cardiovascular disease, heart attack, and stroke far more likely.

Recently it has been reported that obese teenagers have thickening of their carotid arteries. These findings highlight the fact that the atherosclerosis process starts early in life if you are obese. It is a disturbing thought to consider that future generations may have cardiac stents as well as open-heart surgery in their second or third decade of life.

Besides cardiac risk factors, obesity causes other problems. Obese people have disturbed sleeping patterns because of sleep apnea. Sleep apnea occurs when the soft palate drops down, obstructing the airway when sleeping. Modest weight loss is an effective treatment. Many are forced to sleep with machines that push air past the obstruction. As mentioned, obesity causes increased pressure in the abdomen. One of the consequences is reflux disease, pushing the acid of the stomach back up through the esophagus, and into the mouth. The increased pressure in the abdomen requires the heart to push harder to send blood through the body, resulting in hypertension. It also causes swelling of the legs because the blood in the veins of the legs has a more difficult time returning to the heart.

Other obesity-related conditions include severe degenerative joint disease and constant joint pain. There is a much greater impact on the joints when walking if you are overweight than if you are normal weight. As a result, there is a premature requirement for knee and hip replacement.

A lesser-known obesity-related disease, pseudotumor cerebri, leads to blindness. Again, probably because of the increased pressure throughout the body, fluid builds up in areas of the brain, especially around the eyes. This condition is commonly seen with tumors generating pressure, but in this condition there is no tumor. Although this is a rare occurrence, it is common to see young females who are overweight complain of migraine type headaches. Remarkably, these symptoms disappear with successful bariatric surgery and weight loss.

Obesity interferes with fertility. Men who are seriously obese have reduced testosterone and poor sperm production. Obese women have alteration of their female hormones, leading to irregular period, hair in unwanted places, and inability to ovulate. If they succeed in becoming pregnant, the pregnancy is far riskier. There is a higher early miscarriage rate. They have a greater chance of having a high-birthweight baby, secondary to gestational diabetes.

Obviously, it is imperative that we try to control our dietary intake. There is a thought process that states obesity is not causing these problems; instead, the culprit is poor diet containing excess fat and simple carbohydrates. Obesity is merely a marker for poor diet and sedentary lifestyle. In my opinion, this is really a difference in semantics. Very few people who have severe obesity have a physically active lifestyle or eat a healthy diet. There may be exceptions, but most are in denial about the amount of difficulty their weight causes in their performance.

What is perplexing is the source of the obesity epidemic. Why now? Why are we getting so heavy all of a sudden? Is this just a creation of the press and the numerous media outlets that need to put programming on television? Sadly, the truth is we are in fact getting larger. Ask any airline, look around the shopping malls, and go visit Disney World.

In 1996, there was not one state in the country that had an obesity rate greater than 20 percent. Fast-forward to the last Center for Disease Control Study in 2006: every state in the country with the exception of Colorado has an obesity rate (body mass index, or BMI > 30) greater than 20 percent. In fact, in four states than 30 percent of people are obese. BMI is a measurement that combines height and weight into one number that is then used to measure obesity. The number is calculated by taking your weight in kilograms and dividing by your height in meters squared. Although BMI is a handy convention for estimating obesity, it is still a calculated number, and there are people who have BMIs greater than 30 who do not have excess body fat. If you have a lot of muscle mass and are athletic, it is possible to have a BMI more than 30, but a low percentage of body fat. Since this occurs only rarely, BMI has become the accepted standard for determining obesity.

There are numerous popular theories to explain the obesity epidemic. Some authors point to our sedentary lifestyles. We drive more, and we are eating greater quantities of poor-quality food. Others have highlighted emotional factors. There is no clear consensus, but it is my belief that the obesity epidemic really began when America changed its farm policy.

From the time when Richard Nixon was president, the American farming industry has made corn the primary crop. A subsidy system was put in place so that there was a defined price for corn, eliminating the competitive free market. Since the government would guarantee paying for corn, there was no risk if there was excess supply. Therefore the only way to make more money was to grow more corn. This resulted in a surplus of corn. This surplus provided cheap (and unhealthy) feed for cattle. With cheap food and hormonal supplements, farmers raised cattle cheaper and faster. This trend continued, and the cheap fast food industry flourished. Corn syrup also gained prevalence as a sweetener and additive to other foods.

Numerous researchers have highlighted the contribution that cheap fast food has played in the obesity epidemic. Years ago it used to take five years of growth before cattle were market-ready. With the use of corn feed and additives, this time period has been significantly shortened. This rapid feeding has consequences. An old adage states, "You are what you eat." It stands to reason that a cow raised on grass would produce leaner and healthier steaks than one raised on corn and growth stimulants.

Another factor that we believe has received limited discussion is the unintended consequence of public health success in reducing cigarette smoking. Although it is certainly true that few things are more harmful to the human body than inhaling cigarette smoke, most ex-smokers will tell you that food often replaces cigarettes, with a resultant trend toward obesity.

There has also been a change in what we eat. Even though it looks as if there are more food choices at the supermarket, the truth is that many of our calories come from only two sources: corn and soy. As more of our calories are eaten outside the home, we delegate the responsibility for choosing healthy ingredients to strangers. We eat faster, and on the run. Instead of preparing fresh foods that are locally grown, we buy foods that have traveled a great distance and are adulterated with preservatives. In his two recent books, the food writer Michael Pollan (*The Omni-*

vore's Dilemma and *In Defense of Food*) has done an excellent job highlighting these issues.

Unfortunately, once people are obese there are very few treatment options that work. Also the faster somebody goes into treatment or begins to reassess lifestyle, and the earlier in the disease progression this occurs, the better the results. What this means is that diet and exercise therapy have a better chance to work with younger people who are less obese than it does with people as they advance in age and severity of condition. As a bariatric surgeon, I have for the last fifteen years reached several conclusions. One is that losing weight is very, very difficult. Two, once you become morbidly obese (that means a BMI more than 40, or being more than one hundred pounds overweight), losing weight and maintaining the weight loss are plain-out challenging ordeals without a surgical procedure. It can occasionally be done by people who live a very active lifestyle. However, once somebody has evinced irreversible changes from the wear and tear of obesity, the practicality of losing weight becomes exceedingly low, since they are unable to exercise enough to make a significant impact on their weight. In addition, once people progress to diabetes, especially those who are placed on insulin, the probability of maintaining weight loss without an aggressive surgical procedure is also low.

So, what constitutes a healthy diet? Years ago, people talked about just avoiding fat. The rationale for avoiding fat was that units of food contain differing amount of calories. The basic elements of food are protein, carbohydrates, and fats. Whereas protein and carbohydrates provide 4 calories per gram, fats are the most efficient source of energy and contain 9 calories per gram.

This appears to mean that if you eat 4 grams of fat you consume 36 calories, whereas if you eat 4 grams of a carbohydrate or a protein you eat approximately 16 calories. So logic dictates that if we avoid fats we will consume fewer calories and lose weight.

There is some truth to this, but there are also other factors to be considered. Size matters, and not only do larger portions of carbohydrates provide more calories in total but the excess calories are stored in the body as fat. As a result, the idea that you can eat as much of what you want and simply avoid fats is erroneous. It leads to people eating massive quantities of food and storing those excess calories as fat.

More recently, diet gurus have advocated eliminating all simple carbohydrates, and instead eating proteins, fats, and complex carbohydrates. The basis of these diets is that certain foods stimulate production of insulin. Insulin is the major anabolic hormone in the body, responsible not only for energy but also for clearing sugar from the blood and storing it as glycogen and fat. We all know that certain foods make us feel more full than others. With simple sugars and refined carbohydrates, we get a quick surge but, thanks to the blood-clearing effect of insulin, become hungry again shortly thereafter. This leads to eating more, and a vicious circle ensues. Thus it is thought that foods less stimulating of insulin will cause a less abrupt rise and fall in body sugar and keep you full for a longer time. The ease with which carbohydrates are broken down into simple "bad-for-you" sugars is measured by the glycemic index. The concept of a low glycemic index diet has been shown to be somewhat beneficial in a recent report by the Cochrane database review of all diet strategies.

Another approach is complete elimination of all carbohydrates, including complex fruits and vegetables. The idea is if the body cannot use carbohydrates, it has to use a different fuel, called ketones, to meet its energy needs. A process called ketolysis occurs, and there will be rapid weight loss. Numerous studies show that an "Atkins" type diet does not offer any advantage over a matched low-calorie diet with broader food choices. Additionally, consumption of foods high in cholesterol and fat such as bacon and cheese certainly makes cardiologists nervous.

So, what is the healthiest diet? From my perspective, we need to look at epidemiologic studies of the dietary habits of healthy subpopulations. On the basis of analysis of various populations such as Seventh Day Adventists and other groups that enjoy extended longevity, it would appear that they get most of their calories from things that grow in the ground. They eat fruits and vegetables and add in some low fat meats. Grains and carbohydrates are restricted to whole-grain varieties. When grains are refined, fiber is removed, which makes the grain easier to digest, and are broken down more rapidly into simple sugars, which is to say they have a higher glycemic index. What we preach is, if it grows in the ground, you can eat it; if your grandparents could eat it, you can eat it. Try to eat lean meats, and the lighter the color of the meat, the better; try as well to eat whole-grain pastas, whole-wheat breads, staying away from simple sugars or the things that turn into simple sugars. Do an experiment at your favorite bagel place: take a bite, leave the bagel in your mouth for a few minutes, and notice the sweet sensation. When you eat white bread or a big fluffy doughnut, it is similar to taking a spoon of sugar. And the nutritional value is similar to a package of Twizzlers.

Unfortunately, once people advance through the disease process and develop severe obesity (especially those with orthopedic limitations), there is very little that the patient can do to reverse the weight gain caused by poor diet. As a result, in the late 1990s there arose much interest in bariatric surgery. This happened for several reasons. To begin, there was increasing awareness of the dangers of obesity. Additionally, we came to realize that there were few alternatives offering the long-term success that surgery yields. At the same time, technical developments in abdominal surgery led to greatly decreased perioperative morbidity. We were now able to perform these operations through a laparoscope. This meant instead of large muscle-cutting incisions, we were able to perform these procedures, through small ports or trocars making small holes, using video imaging.

The purpose of bariatric surgery is to create an abnormality, to manipulate the stomach and intestine, to encourage people to eat less food. The expectation is that if you eat less food and lose weight, the whole body will get better, and this will more than compensate for the changes made in the digestive tract. People have to realize that bariatric surgery is a tradeoff. There is no way to do these procedures without changing the digestive tract and concomitantly generating surgery-related symptoms.

It is imperative when dealing with vocalists and performers to recognize the importance of avoiding trauma and damage to the vocal folds. Few substances can cause as much damage to the vocal folds as acid from the stomach. Unfortunately, the pressure on the abdomen or belly caused by obesity increases the possibility for this to occur. Additionally, care must be taken to recognize and minimize the risk of gastric reflux with any procedure being considered for bariatric surgery. Singers who are having a surgical procedure that requires intubation often request a small endotracheal tube with the idea that this will cause less vocal fold trauma. In our experience with performers, we advocate not a small tube but a properly sized one. Although a large tube may cause damage, a small tube might make airway exchange more difficult and permit greater movement of the tube during ventilation, also causing trauma. Thus, a properly sized tube is essential.

Similar to the general population, there is no ideal procedure for singers. All bariatric procedures have their advantages and disadvantages. Currently there are a variety of procedures being performed for weight loss, and many devices are in clinical development. They center on two objectives: either method to restrict the size of the stomach, or a way of getting the body to absorb fewer calories than are consumed.

The Lap Band

The laparoscopic adjustable gastric band was approved for clinical use in the United States in 2001. A circular band is placed around the stomach. Inside the band is a balloon that can be inflated by accessing a port placed under the skin with a needle and injecting fluid. The band is placed around the top of the stomach. The purpose of the band is to reduce the capacity of the stomach by placing an adjustable valve on the top part. This allows less food to cause the patient to feel full, and if this area remains filled for a period of time then the person will be less hungry between meals. Additionally, after the patient can eat more, the balloon can be further tightened.

The lap band has been a major advance for weight loss management. Recently, another product, the Realize band, has been approved for usage in the United States. It appears that the efficacy of both bands is similar. They can be placed through a laparoscopic procedure, which takes under one hour, and many low-risk (i.e., otherwise healthy) patients are having the procedure done on an outpatient basis. Bands are currently approved for the treatment of morbid obesity, meaning that patients have to have a BMI > 40 or 35. Studies are being completed to expand the indication to people with a BMI of 30. On average, recovery is rapid and most can return to work in less than one week. Obviously, recovery and results differ for those with permanent disabilities or impairment.

With a band, most people can lose half of their excess weight. This means if they are one hundred pounds overweight, on average they will lose fifty pounds. Although there is potential risk with any operation, the lap band procedure is considered safe; recent reports have highlighted a mortality rate for the procedure that is less than one in a thousand.

Despite these encouraging results, the band is not a perfect procedure. Approximately 20 percent of people are disappointed in their weight loss. For some, the band cannot be adjusted to find a zone where they are filled up with less food and feel satisfied. They continue to have adjustments until they develop severe symptoms. Then the band is loosened, and they regain weight.

An important fact for singers to understand is that a sign of a tight band is acid reflux and heartburn. If you experience these symptoms, the band needs to be loosened. If it cannot be tightened to provide adequate restriction, this may indicate the presence of a hernia and require surgical repositioning of the band and repair of the hiatal hernia.

In summary, band surgery has the lowest rate of serious complications in bariatric surgery. Weight loss is slower and is less overall than with stapling procedures. Band patients require frequent follow-up for adjustments and monitoring. A certain percentage will require revision procedures for issues arising from band placement. There is no change in the absorption of minerals, vitamins, and nutrients.

Stomach Stapling

In comparison to banding, stapling procedures require permanent alteration of the anatomy. The most prevalent stapling procedure is the laparoscopic gastric bypass (Roux-en-Y gastric bypass, or RYGB). With this procedure, a small portion of the existing stomach, called a pouch, is created with staplers. The size of this "new stomach" is around 15 to 20 ccs. The intestine is divided, a loop is brought up and attached to this new pouch, and the intestine is reattached. Food now passes from the mouth to the esophagus, into the small pouch, and then to the intestine. As a result, it bypasses most of the stomach and the first portion of the small intestine. Since the bypassed area is normally important for absorption of vitamins and minerals, this change in intestinal transit means that all bypass patients need to be put on lifetime vitamin and mineral supplementation.

With the Roux-en-Y gastric bypass procedure, patients can expect to lose 70 percent of their excess weight in the first year. Afterward, there is a degree of weight regain. Most studies show a 15 percent regain rate after three years. to prevent this, good habits need to be developed early. Bypass patients must avoid sugars or foods that are rapidly converted to sugars, such as refined grains.

Compared to laparoscopic adjustable gastric banding (LAGB), the stapling procedure offers both advantages and disadvantages. Fewer people are disappointed in their early weight loss with RYGB. Greater weight is lost. There is a higher chance of remission for diabetes, hypertension, and sleep apnea. However, rates of early mortality and serious complication are increased. Many recent reports show that the mortality rate with RYGB has been reduced to one in five hundred in top high-volume surgical centers, with a 3 percent serious complication rate.

Two other stapling procedures that are growing in popularity are the vertical sleeve gastrectomy and the duodenal switch. These procedures are related. A sleeve gastrectomy is a procedure where the area of the stomach that provides the major storage capacity is permanently removed. To perform a duodenal switch, the sleeve is constructed and then the first portion of the intestine, the duodenum, is divided. A bypass is then done to the duodenum. The sleeve gastrectomy is what is called a restrictive procedure, as its primary function is to reduce stomach capacity. The duodenal switch adds a malabsorptive element, meaning some of what is eaten is not properly digested and absorbed. The duodenal switch is the most successful bariatric procedure in terms of weight loss and prevention of relapse. On average, patients will lose 85 percent of their excess weight in three years, with minimal relapse. It is mandatory, however, that they take vitamins and supplements and have at least semiannual blood evaluation. With a sleeve gastrectomy, patients will lose around 60–70 percent of their excess weight over one year. Although long-term results are still being evaluated, it appears that properly done sleeves will have results two to three years out that will be similar to gastric bypass. It has become our practice preference to perform sleeve and duodenal switch on a larger number of patients. We contend that preserving the normal outlet valve of the stomach (called the pylorus) becomes an important aspect in obesity surgery.

So how can a singer figure out what to do? First, we have to realize that to perform to maximum capability, whether as an athlete or an entertainer, one needs to be healthy and physically fit. It is hard to be fit if overweight. Obesity has an impact on every organ system in the body and compromises breathing as well as diaphragmatic function,. Thus, eating right and being active has to be as important as vocal training and rehearsals.

Unfortunately, severe obesity is becoming a serious problem throughout the country. Once a person is severely obese, weight loss and fitness are difficult to regain. This is especially true as people become older and develop orthopedic impairment. For patients with severe obesity, treatment with surgery can be life-saving. There are now a variety of operations that can be safely performed, offer rapid recovery, and can assist in health management. The risk of intubation can be minimized. Bands or stapling procedures can be performed. If a band is selected, careful monitoring is necessary to reduce any risk of aspiration or reflux from a tight or slipped band.

In conclusion, singers are vocal athletes. As a result, overweight singers do not sing well because of obesity, but rather in spite of the negative impact that excess adiposity causes. It is imperative to prevent morbid or severe obesity in young entertainers, who are surrounded by food and beverage every night. Once severe obesity sets in, weight loss is quite complicated. Surgical procedures offer the best long-term control but need to be combined with dietary discretion and physical activity.

Control of obesity is a lifetime battle. Hopefully the health risks of obesity will be recognized by young performers, and people will realize that opera singers do not need to be fat. Opera singers and vocalists need not be heavy; rather, they need to be as healthy as they possibly can be.

13

Little Black Dress, Part 2

A Singer's Perspective on Bariatric Surgery

BY ORY BROWN

Why I Chose Bariatric Surgery

For almost as long as I can remember, I have been fighting obesity. I began "yo-yo" dieting in my early teens and over time lost and regained more than six hundred pounds. I am a classical singer (dramatic soprano), and quite apart from professional issues the years of carrying excess weight took their toll: I was in constant pain from overstressed joints, and I also had chronic acid reflux, which left my throat irritated and my larynx excessively elevated and out of position. I had high cholesterol and borderline high blood pressure and at the rate I was going was headed for a stroke or a heart attack within a few years. When performing, it was getting harder and harder for me to move gracefully onstage, and I was often short of breath and left with increasing difficulty sustaining the voice. The high larynx decreased the quality and power of my voice. Add to that the helplessness and low self-esteem I felt from years of failed dieting, and you can see why I was ready to have the surgery.

In October 2006, I had a laparoscopic Roux-en-Y gastric bypass procedure. This creates a permanent change in the stomach and is more drastic than gastric banding. The procedure went uneventfully. I was in the hospital for three days; I was quite sore for about a week but within the week was off all pain medications.

Initially my energy was somewhat sapped from the surgery, but I was able to go back to the gym within three weeks. I was back to light singing within ten days.

For the first month I was on liquids and pureed food but then progressed to eating more normal food. I was extremely careful to eat slowly and chew my food so that I didn't encounter problems with food getting stuck. I found out that eating too quickly can cause regurgitation. I also had to decrease my intake of sweet foods. In many patients, eating sugar after surgery causes what is known as "dumping syndrome," basically flooding the system with sugar: your heart races, you break out in a sweat, you feel very weak and are nauseated. This can last for up to an hour. It is not pleasant and for me was thus a good deterrent.

I didn't experience any hunger for about nine months and was able to lose 120 pounds, nearing my goal. At that time my hunger returned, and I entered the next phase of my new life.

I spent time getting used to my new way of eating. I learned to eat slowly, mindfully, not drinking and eating at the same time, getting in the necessary vitamins and grams of protein, and drinking eight glasses of water per day.

Although it is done laparoscopically, gastric bypass is major surgery, with significant consequences that affect your relationship to food for the rest of your life. I am pleased to say, however, that I have enjoyed many positive changes. Below I have listed some of the benefits of the gastric bypass surgery.

Since the surgery, I have lost more than 150 pounds. My joints are much less stressed, and I now have knee pain only occasionally (usually from running too hard at the gym!). My energy level is much improved, and some days I have energy to spare. My blood pressure and cholesterol are now normal. I still have occasional acid reflux, but it is much reduced. I also get fewer headaches, probably because I am eating healthier food.

Gastric bypass surgery also has some drawbacks, which should be weighed before considering undergoing this procedure.

First, there is a significant time commitment. In order for the surgery to be successful, I had to commit to some drastic and long-term alterations in my life—eating healthy food, taking vitamins, going to the gym—and this required my full attention. For me, this meant putting other things on the back burner, so to speak. Even though I am normal weight now, the issues with food haven't disappeared. I realize that if I don't continue this healthy lifestyle, I could gain the weight back.

Potential dehydration is a major concern. It is hard (especially during the first few months) to get enough fluid. I found that I could drink only a tiny bit at a time for many months. This meant I needed to take small sips all day long.

But the biggest issue for me has been getting used to my new body in terms of my singing voice. My support mechanism had to be reinvented. For my whole singing life, when I took in a breath the sheer weight of my lower abdomen assisted me in supporting the voice. I had the support of all that extra weight keeping the abdomen from collapsing during the exhalation. As my body changed I began to sing "off the voice" and had severe support issues. It is a challenge that can be overcome, but it is something that has to be dealt with.

For patients with significant obesity, a bariatric procedure is only the beginning of a lifelong commitment. I cannot stress enough the fact that the surgery enabled me to lose the weight, but in order for me to keep it off I have made several lifestyle changes. Here are some of the lifestyle changes required of me for the rest of my life to maintain my health.

I eat 75–100 grams of protein every day, along with vegetables and fruit. I take vitamins and nutritional supplements, and I avoid sugar and starches. I have yearly follow-up appointments with the bariatric surgeon and the nutritionist (this includes blood tests for protein, iron, calcium, and vitamins). I exercise three or four times a week for fifty minutes (cardio plus resistance training). I work with a therapist on stress-and-food issues, and I attend a support group for bariatric patients. A lot of work, and all in addition to my "real" life of auditioning, performing, and teaching!

From my experiences as a singer and bariatric surgery patient, here are some suggestions for other singers in my situation.

If you are considering bariatric surgery, it is important to be realistic about how your life will change and the sacrifices you will need to make for the procedure to be lastingly successful. First, I suggest that you do your research. There are many websites, but here are some I found helpful:

BariatricEdge.com
www.yourbariatricsurgeryguide.com
www.obesityhelp.com
www.nycbariatrics.com/default

Have (or gain) some insight into the psychological issues that result in overeating, and develop a sense of commitment to deal with them after surgery, and for the rest of your life.

Last but certainly not least, it is vital that you find a good bariatric surgeon, ideally one who has dealt with singers and understands the specific issues that affect what we do for a living.

I would say that although the first year after surgery had its challenges, this past year has been harder. The initial phase of weight loss was part of the postoperative period, and almost built into the procedure. It is only now that I am confronting my eating disorder on a daily basis, and learning to make healthier choices for myself regarding food, exercise, and lifestyle. Despite the difficulties, knowing what I know now, I would choose to have the surgery again in a heartbeat. It certainly was the right decision for me. The surgery changed my life, how I look at myself, and how I am regarded as a professional singer.

14

Skin Care for the Performing Artist

KAREN H. KIM, MD
PHILLIP C. SONG, MD

Having healthy skin is important for performing artists, who are often in the public eye. They are subjected to harsh lighting or camera close-ups that can magnify the slightest skin imperfections and signs of aging. There is therefore great pressure to remain healthy and youthful in appearance. Although aging is inevitable, aging of the skin is attributable not only to an individual's own genetic propensity (you can look at the older members of your family to get a clue as to how you will look at their age) but also the culmination of environmental factors that you are exposed to throughout your life. *The key to retaining healthy, youthful-appearing skin is prevention*, and avoidance of things known to harm the skin.

Without a doubt, smoking takes a heavy toll on the skin. It accelerates the aging process, causing wrinkles. Smoking reduces blood flow to the skin, which then restricts healthy nutrients from entering the skin. Smokers are not good candidates for surgery (including cosmetic surgery) because of their poor postoperative healing ability. Smokers have a tendency to develop characteristic vertical creases around the mouth ("smoker's lines") as well as creases around the eyes ("crow's feet"), likely due to the frequent repetitive muscle movements associated with smoking, and perhaps also as a direct effect of the heat of the cigarette smoke.

The sun emits ultraviolet radiation, which causes premature aging as well as skin cancers. Heavy sun exposure induces thinning of the superficial and deep layers of the skin. There is loss of collagen (the substance deep in the skin that gives it strength and support), leading to loose, flabbier skin. Sun-damaged skin also manifests as "age spots" or "sun spots," mottled discoloration, ruddiness, broken blood vessels, and wrinkles. You can also develop "actinic keratosis," small crusty spots or lesions, on sun-exposed skin, which, although benign, have the potential to develop into *squamous cell carcinoma*.

People who have had a lot of past sun exposure and those with a family history of skin cancer are at higher risk of developing skin cancer than those who do not. *Basal cell carcinoma* is the most common type of skin cancer and is easily treatable with surgery, electrodessication, and curettage or even a topical cream in some cases. Squamous cell carcinoma is the second most common type of skin cancer and, if treated early has excellent outcome. *Melanoma* is the most aggressive type of skin cancer and early diagnosis is crucial to its prognosis. A good rule of thumb to keep in mind is if any spot does not heal completely after a month, or if an irritated lesion heals and then recurs in the same area, it should be examined by a doctor. Also, if a mole changes in size, shape, or color, or if it becomes itchy or bleeds spontaneously, it should be evaluated immediately.

One of the most important measures for maintaining healthy skin is prevention of UV damage through sun protection. In general, the fairer your skin, the less inherent protection you have against the harmful ultraviolet rays of the sun. People with fair skin and light-colored eyes and hair have a higher chance of developing skin cancer than people with darker skin pigmentation.

However, anyone can develop skin cancer and therefore should make it a part of the daily routine to wear sunscreen. Application of sunscreen with an SPF of at least 15 is very important to maintaining healthy skin. Many moisturizers contain sunscreen, which is good for daily use. On days when you expect to be outdoors for an extended period of time, however, application of a separate sunscreen is recommended. There are numerous formulations available that are nongreasy and cosmetically acceptable. If you are outside for several hours, it is important to reapply sunscreen every three hours to maintain protection. Wearing a hat, sunglasses, and long sleeves is an additional way to protect yourself from the sun. In addition, there are excellent UV-protection garments widely available for people who spend a lot of time outdoors.

Cosmeceuticals

If you look in any drugstore or department store, you will see myriad lotions and potions that promise youth and vitality to your skin. Be aware that many of these products contain ingredients whose efficacy has not been scientifically proven. Amid the range of items and price tags, the best products are not necessarily the most expensive.

People love to ask what special cleanser they should use. I stress that the most important aspect about a cleanser is that it should not strip away the skin's natural oils and be gentle enough to be tolerated well by all skin types. Two examples are Cetaphil cleanser or CeraVe cleanser. They are noncomedogenic (they don't cause acne) and gentle for those with sensitive skin.

Topical retinoids are a mainstay in skin rejuvenation. Retinoids are vitamin A derivatives that stimulate collagen growth and have antioxidant properties. Over-the-counter formulations contain retinol, a precursor to retinoic acid, the biologically active form of Vitamin A. Prescription-strength retinoids are available as tazarotene and tretinoin in varying concentrations. Retinoids improve fine lines and lighten dark spots and should be incorporated into everyone's healthy skin maintenance program. Applied to the skin, retinoids promote new collagen (the substance in the skin that is responsible for its firmness and resilience). Applied consistently, topical retinoids have been shown to soften fine lines and improve skin texture and skin discoloration. It should be pointed out that oral retinoids, such as isotretinoin (i.e., Accutane), which are often recommended for severe acne, may be drying not only to the skin but also to the vocal tract of the singer.

Vitamin C is a natural compound with potent anti-inflammatory and antioxidant properties. It can also stimulate collagen growth and reduce hyperpigmentation (skin discoloration). Topical Vitamin C is useful in fighting signs of aging and is also helpful for skin cancer prevention.

Vitamin E applied topically helps to restore natural Vitamin E that is lost as a result of oxidative stress from either the sun or the environment. Like Vitamin C, Vitamin E is a potent antioxidant that protects the skin against the harmful free radical damage that occurs from the sun and environment. By restoring the depleted vitamins, Vitamin E has been shown to be effective in protecting the skin from ultraviolet radiation. Vitamin C and E together may have synergistic effects, and their antioxidant effects may be boosted. Therefore, you may find topical Vitamin C and Vitamin E available as a combination serum.

Niacinamide and nicotinic acid (known as Vitamin B_3) have skin-lightening and anti-inflammatory properties. They can also reduce oil production in the skin. Clinical studies have shown that niacinamide can improve acne and rosacea, and it may be helpful in protecting irritated skin from injury.

Polyphenols are found in white, green, and black tea and have very strong anti-inflammatory and antioxidant capabilities. They show strong anticancer properties as well. Topical application of green tea has been shown to reduce skin redness and signs of sun damage.

Other topical compounds known to have potent anti-inflammatory and antioxidant effects are coffee berry, soy, feverfew, and mushroom extracts.

Chemical Peels

For skin that has begun to show signs of aging or environmental damage, the patient seeking help has access to a variety of rejuvenation procedures. The general principle common to many of them is to remove the damaged layers of the skin and allow the deeper layers to regenerate, leading to a smoother and tighter skin appearance.

There are a variety of chemical peels ranging from very superficial peels with hardly any recovery time to more extensive chemical peels with longer "downtime" to restore skin texture and wrinkles. Glycolic acid, salicylic acid, and Jessner peels exfoliate the skin at varying depths. They are all corrosive to some extent, and care must be taken during application. With any of the treatments, there is a risk of scarring, pigmentary problems, and infection. These are potent medical therapies and should be performed under the supervision of a physician. In particular, people with a history of herpetic infections should notify the physician before undertaking any of these treatments, as herpetic outbreaks ("cold sores" or "fever blisters") can occur after treatment.

Glycolic acid peels of less than 70 percent concentration, trichloroacetic (TCA) acid peels up to 20 percent, and a combination peel with resorcinol, salicylic acid, lactic acid, and ethanol (called Jessner's solution) are superficial peels that act on the uppermost surface of the skin. These are commonly known as "lunchtime peels" and are helpful when performed as a series of treatments. They improve dark spots and acne, and make the skin feel softer and smoother.

Medium-depth peels penetrate to slightly deeper layers of the skin (the upper reticular dermis). They are produced by TCA peels of 35–40 percent, along with Jessner's peels or 70 percent glycolic acid peels. Scars and wrinkles, along with precancerous lesions called actinic keratosis, can be treated with these medium-depth peels. They have a longer recovery time than superficial peels, signified by crusting and redness, which can last a few days or longer.

Deep chemical peels affect the midreticular dermis and improve deep wrinkles and scars. Baker's formula (combination of phenol, croton oil, septisol, and distilled water) is a common deep chemical peel. It has fallen out of favor because of the risk of cardiac arrhythmia and liver and kidney abnormalities. Deep chemical peels have a long recovery time that requires good, vigilant aftercare. There is also a higher risk of infection, scarring, and skin lightening associated with deep chemical.

Lasers and Light Sources

With recent technological innovations, lasers have emerged as a useful and popular way of improving skin and reversing signs of aging and sun damage. *Laser* is an acronym that stands for light amplification by stimulated emission of radiation; it consists of a monochromatic beam of light, usually in the visible or infrared range. Because the light beam has synchronized waves of the same wavelength, a laser conveys more physical energy than conventional light and can be used to physically alter tissue. Lasers are useful in treating specific conditions in the skin based, on the idea of "selective photothermolysis": specific components in the skin will absorb certain wavelengths of energy and can be destroyed such that other structures in the skin are spared and not damaged. This can be especially helpful when you have isolated spots or areas that you want to focus on.

Intense pulsed light therapy (IPL) is also helpful for treating signs of skin aging. IPLs are devices that project multiple wavelengths of light simultaneously onto the skin, to treat a number of skin targets at the same time. So for example, someone with numerous brown spots and broken blood vessels may benefit from treatments with an IPL, since some of the wavelengths are absorbed by the blood vessels, and others by the pigmented skin areas.

Common skin conditions that are treated with lasers and pulsed light devices are redness, broken blood vessels, and brown spots (solar lentigines). Skin redness and broken blood vessels can be effectively treated with the pulsed dye laser, KTP laser, diode laser, and alexandrite laser and IPL. The recovery period is typically just a few hours, although occasionally some crusting occurs, which clears after a few days. For very stubborn spots, you may experience mild bruising, which typically lasts five to seven days after treatment.

Brown spots, or sun spots (solar lentigo), can be eliminated with a Q-switched ruby or alexandrite laser or pulsed light therapy. For brown spots on the face, there is crusting that appears after treatment, which lasts for five to seven days. On the body, the scabs can last up to two weeks.

Laser therapy is also an excellent treatment for unwanted facial or body hair. For men prone to ingrown hairs along the beard area or for women who have been experiencing new or increased facial hair growth, laser hair removal is an excellent long-term treatment to eradicate the problem. People who, by contrast, pluck can end up with more ingrown hairs or inflammation around the hair follicle. They may also develop telltale dark spots where the hair has been plucked, which can be difficult to disguise. With lasers, which can be successfully used on dark and fair skin, unwanted dark hair is easily eliminated.

For fine lines and wrinkles, injectable materials such as hyaluronic acids (Restylane, Perlane, Juvederm Ultra, UltraPlus), collagen (Cosmoderm, Cosmoplast, Evolence), and botulinum toxin A (Botox, Reloxin) can be used. Some of these fillers are discussed in greater detail in the next chapter.

Laser treatments are helpful as adjuncts to fillers, or as an alternative option for people who do not want injectable agents. The most aggressive and impressive outcome can be achieved with laser resurfacing using a carbon dioxide laser or erbium laser. These destroy the superficial layers of the skin and allow new skin and new collagen to grow. As a result, there is visible skin tightening and smoother texture. Shallow and deep wrinkles can be dramatically improved. This procedure, which gained popularity about ten years ago, is currently not in high demand because of the long postoperative recovery and higher risk of complications. Excellent and vigilant wound care is critical. There is a significant amount of crusting, which can last for one or two weeks after the procedure, as well as redness that can linger for several months afterward. Higher risk of scarring, infection, and skin discoloration is associated with this procedure compared to less invasive laser procedures.

In light of the demand for skin rejuvenation and laser treatments with minimal recovery time, the concept of "fractionated resurfacing" was introduced in 2004. New skin and collagen can now be produced without the weeks of crusting, oozing, and extensive wound aftercare. This is accomplished with a new generation of lasers that create microscopic holes in the skin (invisible to the naked eye) that are then filled in quickly with new skin and collagen growth. Wrinkles, acne scars, skin discoloration, and enlarged pores can be improved with only two days of redness and no open wounds or sores after treatment. A series of treatments are usually necessary for best results (typically three to six treatments delivered at three- or four-week intervals). There are multiple devices that deliver fractionated resurfacing currently available, among them Fraxel Re:Store and Re:pair (Reliant Technologies), Affirm (Cynosure), Pearl Cutera, Active FX and Deep FX (Lumenis) as well as Palomar's Lux1540 nm Laser.

In addition to resurfacing techniques, a variety of skin-tightening procedures are also available for the face and the body. ThermaCool by Thermage is the original device that delivers radio-frequency energy to the deep collagen layer of the skin (dermis) and stimulates breakdown of the existing, loose collagen and production of new, thicker collagen. The formation of this new collagen is thought to be responsible for the skin-tightening effect. Individuals with mild facial laxity, especially around the jowls, are good candidates for this treatment. This device has since been modified to allow deeper penetration to thicker skin, so that it can be used on other parts of the body such as the arms, abdomen, and legs.

Cutera Titan is a broadband light device that has also been used for skin tightening. Instead of radio frequency energy, broadband light energy is applied to the skin to promote new collagen formation and consequently tighten skin. The advantages to these devices is the minimal recovery period (people may experience mild redness lasting a few hours) and the absence of a surgical scar compared to facelift or abdominoplasty. The disadvantages are that the results are quite variable, ranging from very subtle changes to moderate tightening. Such noninvasive skin tightening procedures are not suitable for those with extensive skin laxity. In those cases, surgery is the best option.

Today, adults are generally looking to maintain a healthy and youthful vitality, beginning at a younger age. Even when there are no career-impacting or financial considerations, the goal for many people, performers or otherwise, is to look healthier and more rested rather than alter their appearance dramatically. We are fortunate that we have made great strides in understanding the skin aging process and to have technological innovations that enable us to improve our skin and keep us looking healthy. From the most fundamental steps of topical skin care and sun protection to more sophisticated tools such as lasers and light devices, the modern-age performer has a great multitude of options to look the best she or he can.

15

Minimally Invasive Cosmetic Techniques

ANDREW BLITZER, MD, DDS

Facial aging is accepted by some as the inevitable consequence of aging. Others feel that any treatment that will make them look young and vigorous is an advantage in a competitive world. It has long been said that men get better with age, while women just get older. This clearly is not true, and an increasing number of men are now also seeking procedures to rejuvenate their appearance.

For singers and other professional performers, the constant scrutiny of a critical audience, as well as the competitive nature of their profession, adds to the general desire to maintain a youthful appearance. These performers are always in the public eye, whether on stage, on interview shows, or in magazines. A fine voice no longer compensates for an appearance that may suggest fatigue and aging. Since artists are often hired not on the basis of stage performance but from audition (therefore without the benefit of stage makeup), their facial appearance must naturally suggest youth and vitality.

In an era when time is of the essence, many people have decided that minimally invasive procedures are better than those requiring significant downtime. A variety of minor in-office procedures are now readily available for facial rejuvenation. These procedures restore lost tissue volume to the face and minimize facial lines, creating a face that is more refreshed and relaxed and may be more youthful in appearance.

Although in-office facial rejuvenation techniques are effective, they should be used judiciously, clearly these procedures need to be included in a program of healthy eating, cessation of smoking, exercise, and minimizing sun exposure. A careful discussion of exactly what the singer would like to change, and why, should take place. Only after this discussion can a clear treatment plan be made to meet realistic expectations. Patients with unrealistic expectations or a body-dysmorphic disorder will never be happy and may need psychological intervention.

Botox

Botox (Botulinum neurotoxin A) is a bacterial product that decreases the chemical released by nerves that causes muscles to contract. Botulinum toxin extract was first used as an investigational drug by Dr. Alan Scott in the late 1970s for eye muscle conditions. In the early 1980s we began using the toxin to treat neurologic problems affecting the face and neck, such as twitching of the eyelids and face. We soon realized that some of the patients receiving the toxin for a medical condition (muscle spasms) also noted a cosmetic benefit, relaxation and smoothing of their "aging" lines. In 1989, when Botox was approved by the FDA for eye conditions and facial spasms, we began to treat patients with this medication in an off-label fashion, for cosmetic reasons only, and saw profound benefits in creating a more relaxed and youthful appearance. In 2001, Botox was approved by the FDA as safe and effective for treatment of frown lines, and this application spread through the medical cosmetic community. Since that time, many thousands of people have been treated around the world with dramatic results and virtually no adverse effects. In fact, Botox therapy has become the most popular cosmetic procedure performed by doctors worldwide.

How does Botox work? Frown lines, as well as some wrinkles, result from the contraction of facial mimetic muscles, which corrugate the overlying skin. By relaxing these muscles, the overlying skin smoothes out, and the wrinkles disappear. Examples include horizontal lines over the forehead produced by raising the eyebrows ("surprise" expression) and the shorter vertical lines between the eyebrows above the top of the nose produced by the "frowning" expression.

But not all facial lines are a result of excessive muscle contraction. Many people have aging or damaged skin, with lines related to excessive sun exposure and smoking. These noxious elements can cause breakdown of elastic fibers and collagen in the skin, with loss of skin tone. This results in fine etched lines and an "alligator skin" appearance. These finer lines are not benefited by Botox injections, since they are not caused by muscle contractions but loss of tissue elements within the skin itself. The treatment of such fine wrinkles requires good skin care and moisturizers, retinoic acid products, and in some cases chemical "peels" or laser resurfacing. More detailed information about these products and treatments can be found elsewhere in this book.

Some normally occurring facial lines and contours, such as nasolabial lines (between the cheeks and mouth), normally deepen with age as a result of loss of tissue volume (reduction of fat and collagen). These are generally deeper lines that are present at rest and worsen with facial gestures. These types of volume reduction lines and depressions are best managed with injections of "filler" agents such as collagen and hyaluronic acid gels (Restylane, Juviderm, etc.). Filler agents used to replenish lost volume are made of biocompatible materials that recontour the facial area being treated. There are other agents that are more viscous and are used to augment bony contours underlying the skin and soft tissues. All of these products used for volumizing cheeks, lips, and lines last about four months. After that time, they are gradually absorbed into the body, and the injections need to be repeated. In some instances, fat from another part of the body can by harvested and reinjected into the facial tissues as a volumizing agent. Although this is a person's own tissue, it is no more permanent than extraneous filler materials, and additionally it creates the possibility of having complications and pain at the donor site.

Collagen products were the first injectable materials commercially available for facial augmentation. The first was a bovine (cow) collagen. This required a skin test one month prior to augmentation to identify those who might have allergies or skin reactions to the protein. Since then, we have developed a porcine (pig) collagen with fewer sensitivities, and a human collagen that is nearly sensitivity-free.

The first injectable hyaluronic gels (polypeptides normally found in skin) were derived from rooster combs, which are particularly rich in this substance. There were patients who developed sensitivity reactions to this avian material, and therefore we now use bioengineered hyaluronic acid gels, such as Restylane and Juviderm. These materials are virtually free of sensitivity reactions and last four to six months.

One of the newer materials used for volumizing and recontouring of the bony structures is Radiesse, a powdered form of calcium hydroxylapatite (the dominant mineral substance found in human bone, therefore biocompatible) in a pastelike vehicle. Since this material tends to be rigid, it cannot be placed superficially in the skin. Hydroxyapatite paste can create significant volumizing of the cheeks, fill defects in the nose and chin, and even recontour the jaw bone line. This material lasts nine to twelve months.

Yet another new product that has been approved for deep volumizing (particularly in patients who develop lipodystrophy, where fat disappears from the face) is Sculptra (injectable poly-L-lactic acid). This material must also be placed at a deeper level, but it can create a volumizing effect which lasts for a year or more.

For patients who require still larger volumes or who want more permanent volume results, surgically placed implants are available, particularly for the chin, cheeks, jaw line, and nose.

An older and more permanent but somewhat controversial injectable material is silicone. This had been injected for years and was removed from the market by the FDA because of many sensitivity reactions, granuloma formation, infections, and scarring. Although much of the literature on silicone complications comes from a study of breast implants and may not apply elsewhere, the material has acquired notoriety. Liquid silicone is available only for some severe eye conditions, and its use as a cosmetic agent is even illegal in a number of states.

Optimal management of some facial lines requires a reduction of muscle function with Botox, followed by the addition of a "filler" or volumizing material. This two-pronged approach is particularly good for deep frown lines, deep "crow's feet" lines, "lip stick" or "smokers lip" lines, "marionette" lower facial lines, and chin creases.

Minimally Invasive Approaches

Here is an outline of minimally invasive approaches to specific areas of the face:

Glabellar or "frown" lines: These vertical lines between the brows are caused by contraction of the corrugator muscle used during

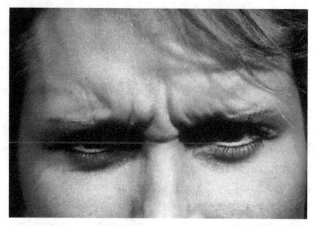

FIGURE 15.1 Frown lines, before cosmetic procedure.

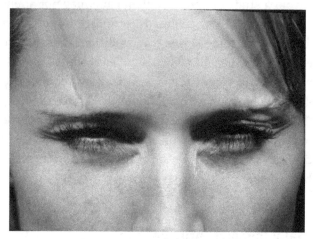

FIGURE 15.2 Frown lines, after cosmetic procedure.

a worried, angry or frowning appearance. This is the most common site for cosmetic injection. With reduction of the contraction of this muscle, the lines minimize. For people with very deep furrows, it may be necessary to add a filler material under the deep fold (Figures 15.1 and 15.2).

Horizontal forehead lines: These lines are produced by the underlying frontalis muscle, which contracts the skin and causes a horizontal pleating. These lines are easily diminished with weakening of the frontalis muscle using Botox. Too much weakness, however, leaves a motionless forehead, an appearance that has been caricatured in many cartoons about Botox. It is much better to leave some vertical movement for gesturing, and yet limiting the amount of wrinkling that occurs. This point is of particular significance to singers and other performers, who need to use the face to convey expression or signal intention during performance.

Eyebrow position: The position of the eyebrows is directly related to the muscle pull upward (frontalis muscle), downward (orbicularis oculi, eyelid muscle), and inward (corrugator muscle). By changing the balance of these muscles, one can change the shape and position of the brow.

"Bunny scrunch" lines: These oblique lines along the nose on smiling or laughing are a result of overcontraction of the nasalis muscle and can be reduced with Botox (Figure 15.3).

"Crow's feet" or lateral canthal lines: These are a result of contraction of the orbicularis oculi (eyelid) muscles during a laugh or squint. An overactive muscle produces large folds in the outer corners of the eyes. These can be reduced with Botox, or if they are deep they may require a filler as well.

Nasolabial lines or furrows can be best handled with a filling agent. Occasionally, a small amount of Botox high up in the line will eliminate the upper part of the line and minimize the "gummy" smile.

"Lipstick" lines or smokers' lines in the upper and lower lips are from contraction of the orbicularis oris. They come from puckering of the lips, which pleats the skin. Since the muscle responsible for these lines also closes the lips, these are difficult to eradicate completely with toxin without causing oral incompe-

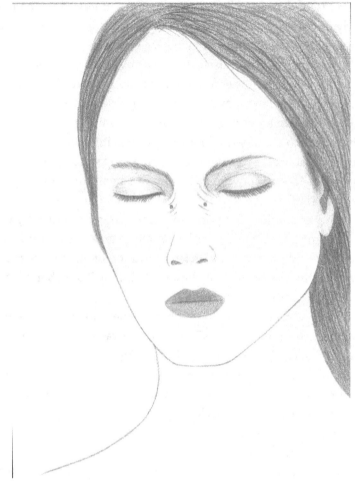

FIGURE 15.3 "Bunny Scrunch" lines

tence and drooling or speech difficulties. Therefore these lines are best treated with a small amount of toxin, fillers, and sometimes skin resurfacing (Figure 15.4).

"Marionette" lines: These come from active contraction of the depressor anguli oris muscle and its attachment to other facial

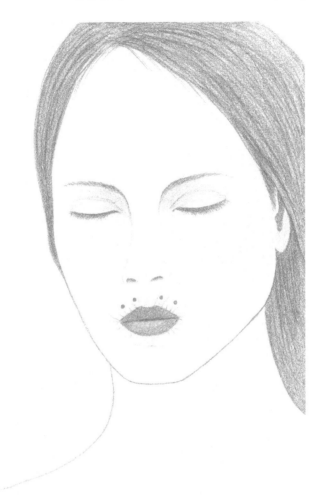

FIGURE 15.4 "Lipstick" lines or smokers' lines

mimetic muscles. A small amount of toxin injected into the muscle as well as a filling agent manages this line very well.

"Popply" chin or "Peau d'orange" chin: This is caused by over-contraction of the mentalis muscle and is easily corrected with Botox injection into these muscles (Figure 15.5).

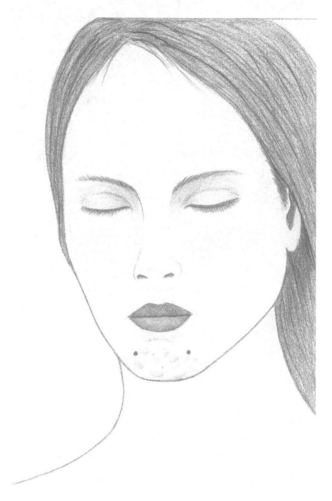

FIGURE 15.5 "Popply" chin or "Peau d'orange" chin

Neck bands: These bands are caused by an enlarged or more visible edge of the platysma muscle. Injections of these bands with Botox can reduce the amount of the band showing. The appearance of neck bands is sometimes exaggerated after weight loss or face lift surgery (Figures 15.6 and 15.7).

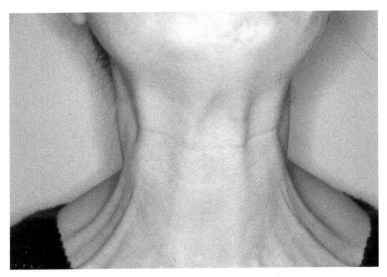

FIGURE 15.6 "Neck bands", before cosmetic procedure.

In addition to treating wrinkles of furrows that result from aging or tissue loss, Botox may also be used for other applications, which may be of relevance to the performing vocal artist.

Excessive facial sweating (hyperhidrosis): Many people have over-active sweat glands, particularly under stress. Botox has been very successfully used to treat underarm sweating and "sweaty palms." Performers who are under hot lights and must deal with stage stress may have excessive facial sweating. Injections into the skin in the area block the neurotransmitter to the sweat glands and thereby allow shrinking and decreased function (atrophy) of the glands for a time. This can markedly decrease the quantity of sweat and makes performing under these extreme conditions much easier.

Facial weakness and asymmetry: A number of studies on what constitutes an attractive face have shown that facial symmetry is perceived as healthy and desirable. Conversely, even minor de-

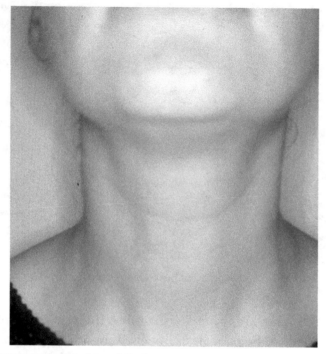

FIGURE 15.7 "Neck bands", after cosmetic procedure.

grees of asymmetry may be perceived as unhealthy and unattractive. Patients who have had facial nerve injuries, who might have had incomplete recovery from a "Bell's" palsy, or who have developmental facial asymmetry can also have their appearance balanced with Botox. This is done by slightly reducing muscle contraction in the more actively contracting side of the face. To most eyes, it is this asymmetry that is noticeable, and not the reduced function. Subtly weakening the stronger side and occasionally using some fillers can greatly improve facial symmetry, and improve appearance.

Cosmetic enhancement has become a staple in our health-conscious, energetic, and fit population. Vocal performers in particular are under intense visual scrutiny, whether on stage, in magazines, or on HD televised performances. Minimally invasive in-office facial rejuvenation techniques have emerged and allow changes in appearance with minimal side effects. Consultation with an experienced facial esthetic physician and surgeon can provide a realistic assessment for every individual.

16

Anesthesia for Singers

ANTHONY F. JAHN, MD

Although we all agree singers are special people, in at least one way they are like everyone else: at some time or other, they will likely undergo surgery. This surgical procedure may be a simple wisdom tooth extraction, a tonsillectomy, perhaps a Caesarian section, or an orthopedic operation. The procedure may take minutes or many hours, and it may be elective or life-saving. Without doubt, anesthesia will be required.

In medical history, the story of surgery prior to anaesthesia was long, complicated, and painful. When general anaesthesia, in the form of chloroform, was discovered in 1847, its appearance was hailed and blessed by all. Dr. James Simpson, a Scottish obstetrician, was the first to use chloroform to eliminate the pain of childbirth, and his patient named her daughter Anaesthesia as a sign of gratitude.

Until a generation ago, anesthesia usually meant one of two things: either a complete general anesthetic, which renders the patient unconscious, or simple local injection of the surgical area with a local anesthetic, as a dentist does before pulling a tooth.

Note: Some of the material in this chapter has appeared previously, in *Classical Singer Magazine*, and the NATS (National Association of Teachers of Singing) *Journal*.

For singers, general anesthesia has raised concerns: it usually involves inserting an endotracheal tube, which is made of rather stiff plastic, through the back of the throat, passing between the vocal folds and into the windpipe. This allows the anesthetist to administer oxygen and anesthetic gases during the procedure directly to the lungs, while at the same time protecting the airway and preventing aspiration of fluids from the throat.

In the singing community, there is trepidation about general anesthesia. Stories of prolonged hoarseness, even of permanent change to the voice, abound. The concern centers on intubation, and the possible damage caused by the endotracheal tube, which sits between the vocal folds for the duration of the surgical procedure. In fact, fear of anesthesia is at times greater than fear of surgery! However, surgery is quite common nowadays. In addition to the treatment of serious conditions, many singers undergo cosmetic procedures to maintain youthful appearance. There are numerous anesthesia options for such situations, options that either completely avoid touching the larynx or do so in a safer and more controlled way. Some of these are outlined here.

Anesthetists often prefer general anesthesia with intubation, since this is a safe and predictable way of controlling and monitoring the patient's cardiac and pulmonary function during surgery. It turns out, however, that there are techniques to avoid having to do this, while still allowing a safe and painless surgical procedure.

Most minor procedures that do not involve the airway can be performed using intravenous sedation and local anesthesia. For example, a sinus procedure, excision of lumps and bumps anywhere on the body, and even most cosmetic surgery in the facial area (such as eyelids or a rhinoplasty) may be carried out using intravenous injection of sedating medication. This means the patient is rendered sleepy but not unconscious, which is often called "twilight sleep." While in this state, the surgeon infiltrates a local anesthetic into the tissues (the famous "mosquito bite"), and the procedure is performed painlessly. If the surgery is on a limb (such as a carpal tunnel release), a regional block can also be used: the nerves going to the surgical site are numbed, in combination with intravenous sedation. During the procedure, the patient is drowsy or lightly sleepy, but rousable, and able to respond to the surgeon. In addition to local injection of anesthetic in the surgical area, any discomfort can also be controlled by the anesthetist through the IV.

Local (or regional) anesthesia with IV sedation has two potential advantages for a singer: it does not require that a tube be placed into (and pulled out of) the larynx, and since the patient is awake though sleepy, the chance for aspiration of stomach contents into the windpipe is minimized. In addition to having no pain, patients usually also have little recollection of the procedure with adequate intravenous sedation; just ask anyone who has had a colonoscopy!

If general anesthesia is required for a procedure that does not involve the mouth or throat, another good option is laryngeal mask anesthesia. The laryngeal mask is like a small oxygen mask inserted through the mouth. During the procedure, the laryngeal mask is positioned in the back of the pharynx. Rather than going between the vocal folds, it sits tightly on top of the larynx, like a cap. All of the usual inhalational agents can be given through the laryngeal mask, and the mask protects the larynx, preventing acid reflux during the operation. It is ideal for shorter procedures that require general anesthesia, or for patients who turn squeamish at the thought of being awake during surgery. As a singer, you should always discuss the laryngeal mask with your anesthetist; it is not always appropriate, but in many cases it is the ideal compromise between local anesthesia with IV sedation and a full intubational general anesthetic. Although laryngeal mask anesthesia is a good option in experienced hands, it is also not without potential complications. For this reason, the singer should not insist on this method if the anesthesiologist is more experienced with conventional intubation, and particularly if in his or her judgment intubation is the safer course.

So far, we have been speaking of anesthesia as if there were always a choice. This of course is not always so: it does not take into account emergency operations, major procedures, or serious illnesses. So-called crash intubation, which is done to save a life, e.g., after a car accident or in another imminently life-threatening situation, is rare but might be necessary. In cases of persistent unconsciousness or major illness, a patient may need to remain intubated (usually in the ICU) for assisted breathing, often for a prolonged period of time. In elective surgery, which involves the mouth or pharynx (as with a tonsillectomy), and in surgery of the vocal folds an endotracheal tube is typically used, to give the doctor access (the laryngeal mask is somewhat bulky and obstructs the surgeon's vision) while protecting the patient's airway. Although you should be aware of all options, you need naturally to defer to the doctor's experience: your life and well-being take precedence over a temporary encumbrance to your voice.

So, if intubational general anesthetic is the only choice, what can be done to minimize trauma to the larynx? First, tell the anesthetist that you are a professional singer! She needs to understand that your livelihood and your well-being (professional and emotional) depend on your voice. If possible, meet the anesthesiologist before the procedure. This meeting may be brief, and just before the surgery, but take advantage of it. If you have any recommendations from other singers or your laryngologist for a specific voice-friendly anesthetist, make use of the knowledge.

When I speak with an anesthesiologist before operating on a singer, I make a number of requests. I ask them to intubate and extubate personally. This is potentially important in a teaching hospital, where less-experienced physicians-in-training may be involved in your care. I ask them to use the smallest caliber tube that they feel can safely provide anesthesia. I ask them that, if possible, the patient be completely relaxed during the insertion and removal of the tube, as well as during the case. This prevents inadvertent movement of the vocal folds during the procedure. At the end of the procedure, we make sure to suction out any stomach acid to prevent reflux during reversal of anaesthesia.

What should you personally do to minimize any complications to your larynx? First, be sure your stomach is empty at the time of surgery; hospitals usually tell you to not take anything by mouth for six hours before the procedure. This includes all solids (remember, milk curdles and is considered a solid), and even clear fluids. If you are prone to acid reflux (GERD), check with your internist about your anti-reflux medications, and do take them the day before surgery. Additionally, a tablespoon of your favorite liquid antacid (my preference is Gaviscon) should be taken as you go to bed the night before your operation.

Immediately after surgery, you should be on complete voice rest. This is equally important, whether you had laryngeal surgery or an appendectomy. Breathe through your nose in the recovery room, and be sure you are breathing humidified air (or oxygen), which the recovery room nurses can provide. My personal recommendation is that you not use your voice at all for forty-eight hours. After that time, you can start to speak softly, with minimal pressure to the larynx.[1] As you begin to vocalize, don't push beyond where you are vocally and proprioceptively comfortable. Your high notes (especially singing *p* or *pp*) may take up to a week to return. These recommendations are based on personal preference and clinical experience; your own laryngologist may recommend a different postoperative schedule.

In order to minimize reflux during convalescence, as you begin eating after surgery have frequent smaller meals that are easily digestible rather than a large one, and strictly avoid foods that cause heartburn. And don't forget your GERD medications, if you take these normally. Keep in mind that when you put the voice at rest (even for twenty-four to forty-eight hours), there is a tendency for the larynx to rise in the neck. As you vocalize, concentrate on lowering the larynx to its trained singing position, and avoid excessive tension in the muscles of the neck and the floor of the mouth. Rarely, the lungs may take a couple of days to fully re-inflate. This, along with muscle splinting in cases of abdominal or thoracic surgery, may temporarily change your breathing and support mechanism. Many pain medications contain codeine, which is constipating. Straining on the toilet involves tightening the larynx and pushing the vocal folds together. For this reason, make sure that your bowels are working well after surgery. This involves drinking lots of water, and possibly taking a mild laxative.

If after a week you are still hoarse, see your laryngologist for an examination. Though there are occasional incidents of significant trauma to the larynx, in most elective surgery situations they are rare. A visit is important, then, for documentation and (usually) reassurance. It is not uncommon to be slightly husky after anesthesia; if you are severely hoarse, you should be examined as soon as possible. This will help to identify any possible damage, and allow expeditious treatment.

If you follow these suggestions, you should have a great anesthetic experience. And then in turn you can sing the praises of your anesthesiologist to the next patient!

Notes

1. This is for surgery that did not involve the larynx. After laryngeal surgery, I usually recommend a full week of vocal rest.

17

Facial Plastic Surgery

MAURICE M. KHOSH, MD, FACS

Cosmetic facial plastic surgery is increasingly popular in the United States and worldwide. Popular culture's embrace of plastic surgery has led to broader acceptance of cosmetic surgery as an option for improving one's appearance.

Stage performers in particular often carry the burden of being scrutinized not only in their performance but also in their appearance. The desire to look better on a personal level, as well as the desire to be more attractive on stage or to the camera, entices many performers to seek facial plastic surgery.

Advances in medical and surgical knowledge, instrumentation, and medications have made cosmetic surgery safer and more reliable, and recovery shorter and more comfortable. A range of options are now available for patients who seek enhanced facial appearance, varying from minor procedures to produce subtle changes to more comprehensive treatment for significant facial rejuvenation.

Surgical procedures may need to be modified to suit singers or other professional performers. In general, techniques that allow faster healing and a shorter recovery are preferred. Currently, there are nonsurgical, office-based procedures that can help rejuvenate facial appearance. Those options, using injections, lasers, and topical treatments, are discussed elsewhere in this book. This chapter focuses on surgical treatments.

Specific discussion of facial plastic surgery procedures is preceded by a discussion of preoperative considerations, including nutrition, medications, and nonprescription supplements. We will then cover several facial cosmetic procedures: rhinoplasty (cosmetic nasal surgery), facial rejuvenation, facial implants, and fat grafting to the face. For each procedure, the indications, postoperative expectations, and potential complications are briefly discussed.

Preoperative Considerations

Cosmetic surgery is elective; it therefore behooves the surgeon and the patient to ensure that every procedure is performed with the utmost safety. The process begins with choosing the right surgeon. Board certification, a review of the surgeon's qualifications, and assessment of the surgical volume are broad measures of a surgeon's competency. Review of pre- and postsurgical results and conversations with former patients can help instill confidence with regard to your surgeon's abilities. Most cosmetic surgical procedures require sedation or general anesthesia, which is best carried out in a certified operating room or surgical facility. There are particular anesthetic considerations that pertain to singers and vocal performers (as discussed in Chapter 16). If endotracheal intubation (placement of breathing tube through the vocal folds and into the trachea) is necessary, the anesthesiologist should use the smallest-sized tube that is safe to use. This minimizes vocal fold trauma and postoperative swelling. Another mode of general anesthesia, laryngeal mask airway (LMA), uses a mask that fits over the larynx and avoids traumatizing the vocal folds. This mode of delivering anesthesia cannot be employed with every patient, and it must be discussed with the surgeon and the anesthesiologist.

A patient's overall health status is very important in assessing his or her suitability to undergo surgery. Health issues such as high blood pressure, cardiac problems, respiratory issues (such as asthma), bleeding disorders, and obesity need to be evaluated. In certain cases, surgery may need to be deferred until the specific medical problems are addressed. Such decisions should be made in consultation with your internist or medical doctor and your surgeon.

Singers and vocal performers are quite aware of the detrimental effects of smoking. Aside from affecting the larynx and vocal abilities, smoking causes premature facial aging by producing skin wrinkles that are due to loss of skin elasticity. Smoking has also been associated with poor skin healing after surgery. Wound infections, poor scarring, and bleeding from surgical incisions have been attributed to smoking. In patients who smoke, cosmetic surgery should be deferred until the patient can commit to not smoking for two weeks prior to surgery, and at least weeks afterward.

Nonprescription nutritional supplements and vitamins are widely used. Some of these supplements can be helpful in recovery from surgery, while others can be harmful. You should discuss all your medications with your surgeon, including herbal and vitamin supplements. Our current medical knowledge indicates that the commonly used "G" herbal supplements (garlic, ginko, ginseng, and ginger) can lead to increased risk of bleeding. Fish oil and glucosamine can similarly raise the risk of bleeding. There are potential cardiac side effects from the use of kava, St. John's wort, ephedra, echinacea, licorice root, and goldenseal. It is recommended that most herbal supplements be stopped two weeks before surgery. On the plus side, arnica montana may impart some benefit in reducing postoperative bruising and swelling. You should discuss its use with your surgeon.

Cosmetic Surgical Procedures

Rhinoplasty

Rhinoplasty refers to alterations in the external appearance of the nose. Septoplasty, or repair of a deviated septum, refers to straightening of the midline wall inside the nose to improve breathing. Typically, septoplasty alone has no impact on the shape of the nose. Septoplasty is commonly combined with rhinoplasty to enhance breathing while improving the cosmetic appearance of the nose. Most patients equate rhinoplasty with reducing the size of the nose. However, rhinoplasty can also increase the size of the nose either in projection or in length. This form of surgery, known as augmentation rhinoplasty, is most often sought by Asian and African American patients who have a flat or inadequately projected nose, or as a revision operation for patients who had overly aggressive reduction in the size of the nose.

Rhinoplasty can enhance the onstage or on-camera appearance of performers by improving the most prominent feature on the face, and increasing overall facial symmetry and proportionality. Singers, though, need to be acutely aware of the breathing and phonating effects of the surgery. Any reduction in the size of the nose must be in consideration of its potential effect on the physiology of the nose. The nose must be evaluated internally to diagnose any obstruction that could be due to a deviated septum or nasal congestion. If an obstruction is found, it should be addressed at the time of surgery. During the rhinoplasty procedure, excessive reduction of the dorsum (nasal bridge) and overnarrowing of the tip should be strictly avoided. Overly aggressive surgery in this area will not only result in an unnatural "operated" look to the nose but also result in a dysfunctional nose in terms of breathing and resonance.

Since facial proportionality plays an important role in our perception of nasal shape, it is important to assess the projection of the chin and its relation to the nose. A small or underprojected chin may give the false illusion that the nose is too large. In such cases, improving chin projection through placement of a chin implant can enhance the appearance of the nose, and minimize the need for reducing the size of the nose.

Cosmetic surgery of the nose can affect the nasal tip, the nasal dorsum, or both. The patient and the surgeon must discuss the desired effects from the surgery. Computer-generated imaging during the consultation can help the patient and surgeon communicate better in regard to realistic expectations from surgery.

The surgical approach for rhinoplasty is classified as open or closed. In the closed approach, all incisions are hidden within the nose. In the open approach, there is a small and normally imperceptible incision in the columella (the middle strut separating the nostrils) skin. Each approach has its own advantages and disadvantages. The closed approach is faster, and there is typically less swelling in the postoperative phase. The open approach is more precise, as there is better visualization of the nasal anatomy during the course of surgery. The open approach is especially useful during revision surgery, and when there is asymmetry in the tip region. Either approach will allow the surgeon to manipulate the nasal bones and cartilages (Figures 17.1 through 17.4).

A detailed discussion of rhinoplasty techniques is beyond the scope of this chapter. However, in broad terms, reducing the dorsum involves shaving the nasal bones and cartilages. Alternatively, the dorsum may be augmented by placement of cartilage grafts or synthetic implants in this area. Releasing the nasal bones and placing them closer to the midline allows narrowing of

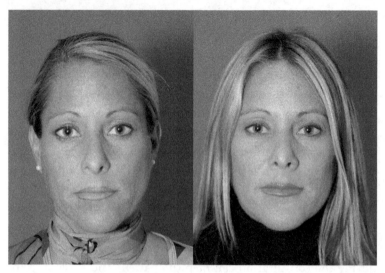

FIGURE 17.1 Rhinoplasty in this 41 year-old patient allowed subtle improvement of her nasal appearance. This operation was performed via an internal approach.

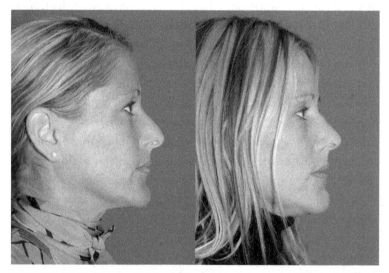

FIGURE 17.2 The profile view demonstrated removal of the dorsal hump and refinement of the nasal tip.

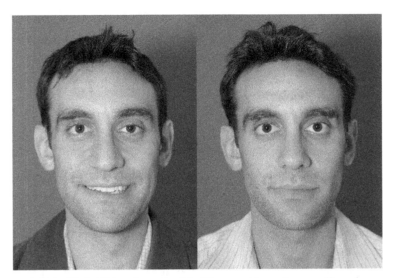

FIGURE 17.3 Rhinoplasty in this 38 year-old gentleman allowed correction of a large dorsal nasal hump and a droopy nasal tip. An external approach was used in performing the rhinoplasty.

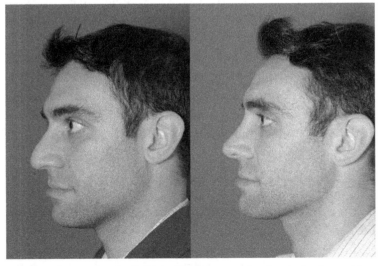

FIGURE 17.4 The profile view demonstrates the change in the position of the nasal tip, and appearance of the dorsum of the nose.

the nose. Removing a small wedge of skin from the corners of the nostrils can reduce the nostril width. Shaving the nasal tip cartilages and binding them with sutures narrows and refines the tip. More sophisticated procedures involve placement of cartilage grafts in the nasal tip region.

At the conclusion of surgery, tape and a small cast are commonly applied to the nose. In the past, the nose would be packed with gauze for one or two days. Currently, few surgeons pack the nose, as it is quite uncomfortable for patients. Patients are discharged home from the recovery room. The nose tends to ooze some bloody discharge for one or two days. Mild to moderate bruising for a week is commonly seen over the nasal bridge and around the eyes, especially if the nasal bones have been narrowed. Pain is usually well controlled by oral medication, and narcotic pain medication is often not necessary past the third day. Once the cast is removed, patients may apply makeup to hide bruising. The initial nasal stuffiness is often resolved after two weeks. Although the final cosmetic results of rhinoplasty may take up to six months to manifest, most singers or performers return to their activities within two to four weeks.

From the vocal point of view, temporary nasal stuffiness can impair the sensation of the voice, particularly in the mask, and nasal obstruction may also have a negative effect on breathing and support. These issues, however, are temporary, and resolve as the nasal swelling (both internal and external) disappears.

Upper Face Rejuvenation: Brow Lift and Eyelid Surgery

Sagging of the brow, droopiness, redundancy of the upper eyelids, and a puffy appearance to the lower eyelids are early but telling facial manifestations of aging. In the upper eyelid, descent of the brow can exacerbate the droopy appearance of the eyelid. These anatomic changes can impart a fatigued or sad look to the

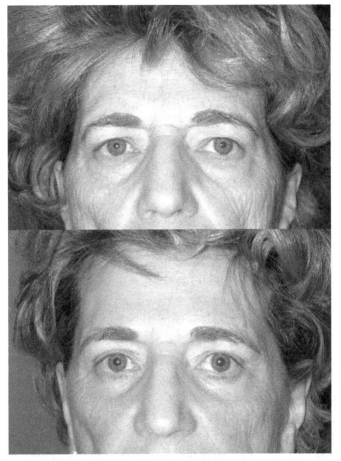

FIGURE 17.5 In this 69 year-old woman, upper and lower blepharo-plasty was used to rejuvenate the appearance of her eyes, while skin laser resurfacing helped improve the facial wrinkles.

patient. Brow lifting and eyelid surgery can be very effective in reversing the aging look of the upper face, giving the patient a refreshed and rested look (Figure 17.5).

Although upper eyelid surgery can be comfortably performed under local anesthesia alone, brow lifting and lower eyelid surgery requires sedation or general anesthesia. Oftentimes, upper face rejuvenation procedures are combined with facelift surgery or fat grafting for total facial rejuvenation.

Brow lift surgery has benefited greatly from advances in surgical technology. Currently, the procedure is performed with a minimally invasive endoscope, using small, hidden incisions. This avoids a long scar in the hairline, and the loss of sensation in the upper scalp, unpleasant side effects of the older open surgical techniques.

Through several small incisions in the hairline, small endoscopic cameras, and thin instruments are passed. The surgical field is visualized on a television monitor. Forehead tissues are elevated upward, and held in place by attachment to the bone of the forehead. When both brow lift and upper eyelid surgery are deemed appropriate, the brow lift is performed first. Elevation of the brow often minimizes the need for skin removal from the upper eyelids.

In upper eyelid surgery, an ellipse of redundant eyelid skin is removed. Puffiness of the corner of the eyelid near the nose may be present from herniation of fatty tissue. The puffiness can be eliminated by careful excision of the excessive fat; the eyelid incision is then closed with fine sutures.

Lower eyelid surgery can be performed through one of two approaches: on the eyelid skin (transcutaneous approach) or hidden just inside the eyelid (transconjunctival approach). The transcutaneous approach is used if there is significant skin redundancy of the lower eyelid, typically found in older patients. The transconjunctival approach is better suited to younger patients who have puffy lower eyelids without significant skin redundancy.

In the transcutaneous approach, an incision is made just below the eyelashes. The thin eyelid muscle is then divided, and the orbital fat below is identified. The fat is trimmed as necessary, and the redundant eyelid skin is trimmed prior to closure. In older patients with droopy ("hound dog") lower lids, the eyelid can be further tightened through a procedure known as canthoplasty.

In the transconjunctival approach, the incision is made inside the eyelid (conjunctival membrane). An instrument is used to retract the eyelid skin and allow visualization. The orbital fat can thus be reached without incising the eyelid muscle. This approach avoids the risk of causing lid margin retraction; however, lower eyelid skin redundancy cannot be addressed thorough this approach.

Our advancing knowledge of eyelid aging has taught us that in addressing eyelid puffiness fat removal should be done very conservatively. Past experience has shown that patients who have significant amounts of fat removed from the lower eyelid develop a skeletonized and hollow-appearing eye socket, a problem that can be difficult to correct. A hollowed eye socket is quite counterproductive to the patient's desire for a younger and healthier look. A more natural and youthful eyelid has some degree of fullness, as can be seen in pictures of young models in glamour magazines.

The puffiness that is seen in the lower eyelids of older patients is partly an optical illusion. The apparent fullness of the lower eyelid is exacerbated by descent of fat just below the orbital rim (midface fat). Descent of midface fat leads to creation of a hollow between the lower lid and the cheek, also known as a tear trough deformity. In the past, disruption of the smooth transition from the eyelid to the cheek was interpreted as excess fat accumulation in the lower eyelid. In an effort to recreate a smooth contour, surgeons would remove fat from the orbit. A more appropriate rejuvenation would entail restoration of midface fullness through fat grafting, midface suspension, or place-

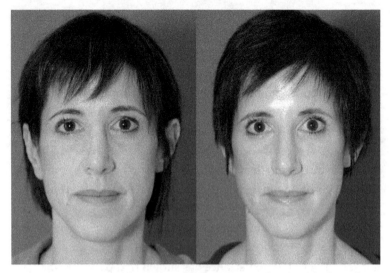

FIGURE 17.6 A combination of fat grafting and upper blepharoplasty helped rejuvenate the facial features of this 45 year-old patient.

ment of an implant in the area. In my opinion, the fat grafting approach can achieve the most natural result with diminished risk (Figure 17.6).

All upper face rejuvenation procedures discussed here can be performed as outpatient surgery. Following upper facial rejuvenation, patients may expect bruising and swelling, which will subside within two weeks. Most patients are able to resume their daily work activities after two weeks. The final cosmetic benefits of the surgery will be manifest in three to six months. These treatments carry a very low risk of complications such as bleeding or infection. Risk of injury to vision during eyelid surgery is extraordinarily low. Brow lift surgery carries a very low risk of injuring the sensory nerves in the forehead. A more realistic risk from surgery would be the possibility of bleeding or slight asymmetry.

Lower Face Rejuvenation: Facelift, Neck Liposuction, Fat Grafting

In a series of self-portraits, Rembrandt tellingly demonstrated the effects of facial aging: formation of jowls in the lower jaw, accumulation of fat in the neck, redundancy of neck skin and loss of definition in the neck line, downturn of corners of the mouth, and creation of folds from the corners of the nose to the mouth. A volumetric assessment of the aging face shows a transition from a heart-shaped frame to a rectangular contour to the face. The anatomic correlate to these findings is descent of mid-face fat, accumulation of fat in the neck, elongation of ligaments and muscles in the neck, and loss of skin elasticity. Lower face rejuvenation surgery aims to reverse these signs of aging.

Lower facial rejuvenation must be performed with the goal of creating a natural and attractive result. Younger patients in their late fifties or early sixties who retain good skin elasticity can expect the best results from a facelift operation. Patients with well-developed bony structure can also expect better results. Singers or vocal performers who plan to have facial rejuvenation should ask their surgeon to avoid excess tightening of the neck. A very tight neck will have an impact on the position and excursion of the larynx, which can affect the voice quality of a professional performer. The pulled-back, windswept look of a "tight facelift" should also be avoided; it can be a source of distraction to the audience.

Facelift surgery is the ultimate rejuvenation procedure for the lower face and neck. In 1974, Dr. Tord Skoog described a major innovation in the facelift operation; his technique continues to be the most commonly practiced method for the facelift operation. Prior to Skoog, facelift operation involved excision only of extra skin. Skoog espoused tightening of the SMAS[1] fascia, the tissue layer below the skin, which covers the facial muscles. The fascia-tightening step renders the facelift results longer-lasting. In a variation of the SMAS fascia facelift, known as the deep plane facelift, the fascia flap elevation is carried further toward the corners of the mouth in an effort to achieve better rejuvenation in the fold of tissue between the nose and the corner of the mouth.

During the facelift operation, the skin incision begins in front of the ear, extends slightly into the ear canal, and curves around the base of the ear lobule unto the back of the ear. The incision ends in the hair-bearing scalp next to the ear. Because the incisions are hidden in skin folds and behind the ear, the final scar is not noticeable.

Next, a flap of skin is elevated toward the midcheek. The SMAS fascia is then incised and dissected toward the midcheek as a flap. The SMAS fascia flap is pulled back toward the ear, and elevated superiorly. This maneuver tightens the muscles in the neck and eliminates the sagging folds of the face. The SMAS fascia is then sutured in its elevated and retracted position. Any extra skin in the face is now removed while avoiding excess tension on the wound edges. All incisions are then closed (Figures 17.7 and 17.8).

Neck liposuction is a common component of a facelift operation, and usually performed as the first surgical step. Through a small incision in the midline of the upper neck, a cannula is inserted below the skin to vacuum the excess fat deposits. If there is a separation of the neck muscles in the midline, the muscle edges can be reapproximated at this time. In younger patients with fullness in the neck, liposuction alone can enhance the neck appearance without a facelift operation. However, when significant skin redundancy is present, a facelift operation is necessary to reposition the excess neck skin. Placement of a chin implant can further enhance a facelift operation by increasing the chin projection and giving more definition to the neck. The chin im-

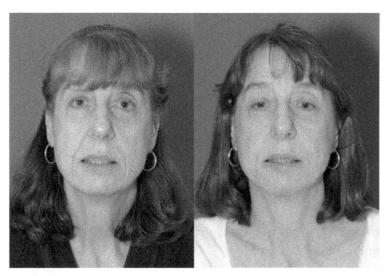

FIGURE 17.7 In this 68 year-old patient, a SMAS facelift was used to rejuvenate the face, highlighting the cheeks and changing the facial contour from rectangular to heart shaped.

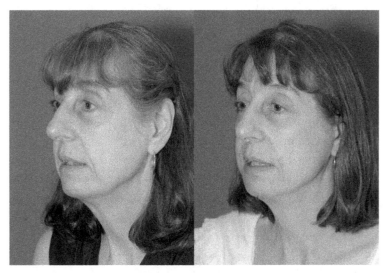

FIGURE 17.8 The oblique view demonstrated the improvement in the jowl region.

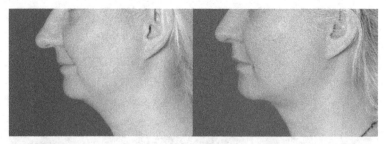

FIGURE 17.9 In this 35 year-old patient, the neck-line was enhanced via neck liposuction and placement of a small chin implant, while her over projected nose was corrected with rhinoplasty.

plant can be inserted through the same incision used for neck liposuction (Figure 17.9).

As discussed in the upper face rejuvenation section, fat grafting is used to restore volume loss in the face secondary to gravity and aging. Fat grafting can be especially useful in enhancing the cheek projection, rejuvenating the contour of the medial cheek, and effacing the fold between the corners of the nose and the mouth.

Recovery from lower face rejuvenation is surprising for its minimal postsurgical pain. Although patients may stay in a hospital overnight, most are discharged home after the procedure. Depending on the preference of the surgeon, small drains can be placed under the skin flaps to drain any blood, and a bulky soft pressure dressing is applied. Drains or pressure dressings are removed after one day; sutures are removed after seven to ten days. Patients can expect moderate swelling of the face and bruising of the lower face and neck, which can last up to two weeks. Although the final results may not be manifest until six months, most performers may return to work after four weeks.

Serious complications from lower face rejuvenation are exceedingly rare. Minor complications such as blood accumulation under the skin flaps or noticeable scars can occur, albeit very infrequently. These complications can be rectified easily during an office visit. Adverse cosmetic results such as excessively "pulled" appearance, or ear lobe malposition, are more difficult to resolve.

Conclusion

In singers and performers, cosmetic facial surgery can improve self-confidence and may help boost a professional career. Choosing the appropriate surgeon carries added importance for performers, since agents, critics, and audiences will scrutinize not just the patient's performance but the cosmetic results also. The ideal outcome of cosmetic facial surgery should be natural and fitting for the patient. It is important for the performer to have a frank and thorough consultation with the surgeon to discuss the feasibility of a desired outcome. Computer-generated imaging and a review of pre- and postoperative results in previous patients can aid in making an informed decision regarding surgery.

Finally, it is paramount for any patient undergoing cosmetic facial surgery to realize that recovery from surgery involves not only physical healing but also psychological mending. It is not uncommon for patients to feel sad, depressed, or unhappy in the postoperative period. A supportive family and peer group will aid the patient in facing the emotional challenges of recovering from plastic surgery. Conversely, patients with signs of depression or anxiety should postpone cosmetic facial surgery until such psychological factors are resolved.

Notes

1. Superficial musculoaponeurotic system.

18

Advances in Laryngeal Surgery for Singers

STEVEN M. ZEITELS, MD, FACS

Transoral mirror-guided resection of lesions on the vocal-fold edge in singers and performing artists has been done since the nineteenth century, after Manuel Garcia,[1] the renowned opera teacher, popularized mirror laryngoscopy. The critical pathway for decision making that faced the patient and surgeon then remains unchanged today. Cooperatively, the patient and surgeon must carefully assess whether the lesion(s) are of greater liability to the vocal instrument and career than the operation to excise the lesion(s). This judgment requires detailed communication and *mutual responsibility* for the chosen management course.[2]

Surgery typically strikes a chord of fear in most performing artists, especially the notion of undergoing a procedure on the vocal folds. Much of the fear, which is rooted in apprehension concerning the unknown, can usually be reduced with knowledge. This chapter gives the singer and voice teacher vital information to assuage the natural fears that are attendant with prospective phonomicrosurgery (endoscopic microsurgery of the vocal folds that is designed to preserve or improve the voice). Furthermore, this knowledge should offer individuals the fundamentals to develop an individualized coherent approach to the surgical decision-making process as well as to the preoperative and postoperative management.

Most commonly, singers require laryngeal surgery to correct benign structural abnormalities of the vocal folds, including nodules, polyps, cysts, ectasias, and varices. Less frequently, they develop dysplasia and cancer.[3] Today, phonomicrosurgery is done under general anesthesia through the mouth by means of a direct laryngoscope, which is a lighted tube (speculum) that provides visualization of the vocal folds. A surgical microscope is used to enhance the precision of the procedure by magnifying the vocal-fold surgical view. Phonomicrosurgical procedures strive to microscopically remove any abnormal tissue from the vocal folds, while maximally preserving the normal phonatory tissue. This leads to improved vibration (enhanced oscillation) of the vocal folds, which results in superior quality.

Phonomicrosurgery in performing artists has historically been associated with controversy because of variable results as well as divergent opinions about the pathogenesis of lesions and the potential for nonsurgical reversibility. Furthermore, the tremendous societal visibility of performers leads to significant publicity both in and out of the entertainment industry if suboptimal surgical outcomes occur. Paradoxically, excellent results are often obscured by the artists' desire to conceal the injury and reconstruction for fear it will imply that their singing technique is flawed, which could have a career-damaging affect. It is not uncommon, and understandable, for singers to not make their surgery public knowledge.

Surgical intervention in performing artists presents the laryngologist with a unique set of circumstances. The patient population is typically outgoing, often quite sophisticated from prior laryngological problems, and frequently outspoken about previous care. A "reticent performer" is almost an oxymoron. Singers are vocal athletes and therefore should be managed at a level of precision and sophistication commensurate with their needs. The indication for phonomicrosurgical intervention is rarely due to a general health problem for the patient; phonomicrosurgery is typically done because there is a functional performing deficit accompanied by a lesion that can be attributed as a major etiological factor.

There is no exact formula for which patients should undergo surgical intervention or how long any patient should undergo voice therapy prior to surgery. The timing of surgery and the extent of preoperative voice therapy should be individualized on the basis of lesion characteristics as well as concomitant inflammation from vocal abuse, reflux, infection, menstrual swelling, and smoking. Furthermore, preference of the patient, voice therapist, and surgeon are interdependent influences in the decision-making process. Finally, performance, recording, and traveling schedules frequently delineate the window of opportunity for comprehensive intervention.

Patient bias about management strategies from previous experiences of their performing colleagues is an extremely important consideration. The surgeon should generally avoid persuading a performer to undergo surgery. Furthermore, surgeons must discuss the possibility that the voice can be made worse by a procedure. This approach engenders a mutual responsibility for the decision of pursuing the elective procedure. Finally, surgeons should generally relate their personal experience with the particular problem, not quoted literature, especially if the patient inquires. Singers readily share their experiences within their professional circles, and unfavorable results will often become widespread information owing to collegial networking among performing artists.

Patients should not be unduly fearful of surgery since many of them are performing with injured vocal folds and a procedure will often be an opportunity for significant skill advancement.

Many performers have been masking the lesion-induced vocal aberration by expending tremendous compensatory effort. In addition to acoustical vocal improvement, patients should understand that effort of phonation may decrease and stamina may improve, which are a reflection of enhanced aerodynamic function.

The management of performing artists requires a collaborative team approach, in and out of the operating room. The speech pathologist or singing therapist is an especially critical member of the team.

Symptoms and the Visit to the Laryngologist

If a vocalist has persistent dysphonia, a visual examination of the vocal folds by a well-trained laryngologist is necessary. Voice teachers' sensitivity to subtle acoustic changes in their students' voice quality is essential for the diagnosis of many vocal-fold lesions. Alternatively, it is not unusual for a vocalist to sound normal to others, but he or she may notice the need for greater aerodynamic support to achieve the same acoustical outcome. This may be associated with decreased stamina and increased recovery time after extensive voice use. Other symptoms include loss of range, especially in the upper register, and difficulty with precise onset of selected notes. Finally the passagio may become unstable, especially when done softly.

The performer should speak to colleagues as to which regional laryngologists are familiar and skilled with the special needs of the vocalist. Laryngeal stroboscopy is necessary to adequately assess any structural abnormalities of the vocal folds. A stroboscope, which provides a slow-motion video analysis of vocal-fold vibration, should be available in the office of any laryngologist managing vocalists. From a number factors, such as overuse and inflammation from infection or reflux, the stroboscopic examination may need to be repeated to accurately determine whether changes of the vocal-fold tissue are reversible or irreversible.

Lesions such as bilateral nodules (on both vocal folds) that are observed by stroboscopy may not resolve with appropriate medical management (e.g., reflux) or vocal therapy rehabilitation. The decision to undergo phonomicrosurgical resection is primarily based on the issue that the vocalist is not meeting his or her vocal needs, along with the fact that the nodules have not resolved with appropriate management. The lack of regression of the nodules suggests permanent changes within the layered microstructure of the vocal-fold tissue. Unilateral (one-sided) vocal-fold lesions such as polyps or cysts almost always reflect permanent tissue changes that require excision (removal) to improve the voice. However, in occasional situations, either type of lesions may regress spontaneously.

If a performer has decided that vocal-fold surgery is necessary to restore the voice, a number of issues must be addressed. Many individuals will seek the assistance of family members, as well as knowledgeable teachers, coaches, and colleagues. It is of paramount importance that the vocalist have complete confidence in (1) the decision to proceed with removal of the lesion, and (2) the surgeon. In some instances, this leads to a second opinion regarding the decision. However, he or she should avoid seeking a multiplicity of opinions, which eventually leads to confusion and impairs the ability to develop a healthy doctor-patient relationship. It is imperative the vocalist-patient trust the surgeon who is to perform the procedure.

Perioperative Surgical Issues

It is common for anxiety and fear to develop as the plan for surgery materializes. The most effective means to neutralize natural fear and apprehension about the upcoming surgery is knowledge and thoughtful consideration of the impending issues. Realistic goals and expectations for the operation must be carefully discussed with the surgeon. Although unlikely, the vocalist should understand that any vocal-fold procedure can result in a worse voice. This may be for a number of reasons, the most common being postoperative scarring. Although scarring may be the result of nonoptimal surgical practices, unavoidable scarring can occur despite excellent technique. This is more likely to happen in patients with a rheumatologic disorder such as arthritis or lupus. Phonatory mucosal scarring may also occur spontaneously, be secondary to uncontrolled reflux, or result from inappropriate voice use after the procedure. Undetectable and unexpected vocal fold pathology at the time of surgery may also lead to an unexpected vocal outcome. The singer should understand that the stroboscopic exam in the clinic is not as accurate as a microscopic exam under general anesthesia.

There are a number of considerations related to the timing of a vocal-fold procedure. The urgency of a procedure relates to the exact nature of the lesion and the vocal needs of the patient. Ideally, there should be only modified voice use during the week prior to the operation so that there is no risk of an acute hemorrhage, which would complicate the operation. Women should try to avoid voice procedures during the premenstrual and menstrual period for reasons of possible swelling of the lesions and the vocal-fold tissue. Since all patients require some combination of voice rest and modified voice use postoperatively, great care should be taken to schedule the surgery at an appropriate time with regard to future singing obligations. Additionally, most singers will require some vocal rehabilitation subsequent to the procedure to reduce stylistic compensatory strategies that frequently develop while they are singing with the vocal-fold pathology. Important engagements should be avoided for at least six weeks after the operation so that there is no undue pressure during the rehabilitation period.

It is important for patients undergoing surgery not to be taking aspirin or other nonsteroidal anti-inflammatory agents such as ibuprofen, because these medications can result in excessive bleeding, which can complicate a procedure. Normal coagulation (clotting) is critical during phonomicrosurgery.

It is understandable that reflux is common in singers because they have strong abdominal musculature, and increased intraabdominal pressure lends the aerodynamic support of the voice. Many surgeons will recommend use of anti-reflux medications during the perioperative period. There is a growing body of literature to suggest that a majority of vocal-fold lesions occur in patients with reflux laryngopharyngitis. It is believed that the reflux creates a change in tissues that renders them susceptible to injury, which leads to the genesis of vocal-fold lesions.

Technical Aspects of Phonomicrosurgery

There have been significant technical improvements in phonomicrosurgical techniques and instrumentation during the past fifteen years.[4] In the 1990s, the carbon dioxide (CO_2) laser was abandoned by many surgeons from concerns about imprecise heat administration to phonatory mucosa. This led to a trend toward the exclusive use of cold instruments instead of the CO_2 laser during phonomicrosurgery.[5] The introduction of subepithelial infusion[6] of saline and adrenaline greatly enhanced surgeons' ability to optimally preserve the pliability and delicate layered microstructure of phonatory membranes. It became clear that in removing polyps, nodules, and cysts, preserving the overlying vocal membranes was critical for obtaining optimal vocal outcome in singers. The recent introduction of 532nm pulsed-KTP (potassium titanyl phosphate) angiolytic laser several years ago has greatly enhanced surgeons' ability to treat delicate vascular lesions such as ectasias and varices.

The technical aspects of excising vocal nodules are partially responsible for the controversy regarding the appropriateness of surgical resection. Until the aforementioned microsurgical developments, most surgeons, voice teachers, and speech pathologists were proponents of conservative management of vocal-fold nodules with exclusive use of voice therapy. There has been a paradigmatic shift toward surgical resection of refractory vocal nodules in recent years. The rationale for more liberal use of surgery in the treatment of vocal nodules is twofold. First, here is an increasing body of knowledge that has substantiated the anatomical persistence of the nodules despite adequate voice therapy. It has been observed that patients' voice quality and singing improves with such conservative management, but there is a plateau in that improvement. Examination of the removed tissues indicates permanent tissue changes. Second, there have been significant improvements in both the techniques for excision and microsurgical instrumentation.

There are relatively few complications related to phonomicrosurgery apart from dysphonia (hoarseness, or an abnormal voice). The most common temporary problem following microsurgery of the vocal folds is mild oral trauma from the metal laryngoscope speculum. It is not unusual to sustain temporary changes such as mild cuts and abrasions of the membranes and numbness of the tongue from pressure. Occasionally, there is permanent dental trauma such as chips or dislodgement of teeth.

Final Comments

Phonomicrosurgery to improve voice quality does not need to be a frightening experience. There are a number of vocalists who are in fact quite relieved to be undergoing an operation that can potentially restore an injured voice, or potentiate future professional and technical development and growth. There is almost always some microscopic scarring, with any procedure. Phonomicrosurgery is indicated when the deleterious effect on singing by lesion(s) in the vocal fold(s) is greater than the unavoidable surgically induced microscopic scarring. The enhanced technical sophistication of current phonomicrosurgical procedures has made many individuals surgical candidates in a way that was not so even a decade ago. This is very encouraging for a multitude of performers because many professionals are able to reestablish faltering careers and many students are able to maximize their conservatory experience.

Notes

1. Garcia, M. "Observations on the Human Voice." *Proceedings of the Royal Society of London*, 1855, 7: 397–410.

2. Zeitels, S. M., Hillman, R. E., Desloge, R. B., Mauri, M., and Doyle, P. B. "Phonomicrosurgery in Singers and Performing Artists: Treatment Outcomes, Management Theories, and Future Directions." *Annals of Otology, Rhinology, and Laryngology*, 2002, 111(Supplement 190): 21–40.

3. Zeitels, S. M., and Sataloff, R. T. "Dysplasia and Cancer of the Vocal Fold: Considerations for the Performing Artist and Voice Teacher." *Journal of Singing*, 1999, 55: 35–38.

4. Zeitels et al. "Phonomicrosurgery in Singers and Performing Artists"; Zeitels, S. M. *Atlas of Phonomicrosurgery and Other Endolaryngeal Procedures for Benign and Malignant Disease.* San Diego: Singular, 2001; Zeitels, S. M., Akst, L., Burns, J. A., Hillman, R. E., Broadhurst, M. S., and Anderson, R. R. "Pulsed Angiolytic Laser Treatment of Ectasias and Varices in Singers." *Ann Otol Rhinol Laryngol*, 2006, 115: 571–580.

5. Zeitels, S. M. "Laser Versus Cold Instruments for Microlaryngoscopic Surgery." *Laryngoscope*, 1996, 106: 545–552.

6. Zeitels, S. M., and Vaughan, C. W. "A Submucosal Vocal Fold Infusion Needle." *Otolaryngology: Head and Neck Surgery*, 1991, 105: 478–479; Kass, E. S., Hillman, R. E., and Zeitels, S. M. "The Submucosal Infusion Technique in Phonomicrosurgery." *Annals of Otology, Rhinology, and Laryngology*, 1996, 105: 341–347.

19

Home Remedies

ANTHONY F. JAHN, MD

Home remedies are a time-honored tradition in the singing community. Although vocal disorders are often transient and self-limiting, for singers there is an urgency to getting better, and many illnesses having a vocal impact respond well to commonsense home treatment. There may not be a need, or indeed even a benefit, to rushing to prescription medications: it is important also to remember that good singing has been around for a long time and precedes the discovery of antibiotics and steroids by many centuries.

There is a mythology surrounding home remedies, special throat sprays, and gargles that enhances their therapeutic effect. Placebo forms an important part of most treatments, and so also with home remedies: it reinforces the body's natural ability to overcome injury, fatigue, and most infections. Nonetheless, many remedies do in fact help to speed recovery, are readily available, and can avoid the cost of medical visits and medications.

It is not possible to list every folk remedy here, but certain principles are common to many treatments, and you should choose your remedy according to these guidelines.

Management of Oversinging Injury

An injury of the vocal tract may come from oversinging, caus-ing strain to the soft tissues of the larynx. One result of excess trauma is edema: the blood vessels become more porous and allow leakage of fluid into the tissues. The temporary effect is swelling and a degree of immobility. The vocal folds become somewhat stiff, and the voice becomes hoarse. There is a reason for this edema: it is your body's way of telling you to put the structure at rest, so it can recover! The hoarseness may be minor, affecting the high notes only, or it can be more severe, leaving the singer with almost no voice. Swelling also exerts pressure on nerve receptors in the vocal tissues and muscles, causing an ache or pain. Persistent oversinging can also strain the muscles of the neck, making them tight and tender.

The remedy for this sort of injury is simple: voice rest. In cases where hoarseness or discomfort clearly follows oversing-ing, immediate voice rest is the best treatment. If possible, you should impose complete silence on yourself, extending not only to singing but also conversational speech, and even whispering. Avoid noisy environments if possible, since merely hearing loud sounds can cause an involuntary tensing of the vocal muscles. Listening to music that you know may have a similar effect, as your brain tells your larynx to position itself ready to sing along. Massage to the neck and shoulders as well as gentle Yoga-type stretching are good adjuncts to voice rest.

If you look at a conventional athletic injury—say, a wrenched knee—immobilization is the first measure, followed by an ice pack to reduce swelling, and later gentle massage and mobiliza-tion. Massage keeps the blood circulating and helps to get rid of lactic acid in the muscles. You can not apply an ice pack to your larynx; you can, however, massage the vocal folds. This is done naturally, by breathing. As you breathe in and out through your nose, the vocal folds adduct and abduct gently. The muscles also contract with swallowing and open with yawning. The larynx therefore is never completely at rest but is gently moving. Some speech therapists even advocate controlled low-pitched gentle phonation or "warming down" after vocal overuse. Over time, the inflammation from trauma resolves, and the swelling recedes as tissue fluids return to the blood vessels.

One word of caution about voice rest. If you keep silent for more than a day or two, expect the larynx to rise in the neck. It simply begins to assume its pretrained, normally higher position. As you begin to vocalize, you need to bring it down again, which expands the resonant spaces of the pharynx. Resuming vocal activity after prolonged voice rest without attention to this phenomenon may leave you singing with a high larynx and excess muscle tension.

Management of Infectious Inflammation

Infection of the vocal tract is most commonly viral, less frequently bacterial or fungal. The local inflammatory mechanism on the tissue level is somewhat similar to trauma, as the blood vessels again become leaky, and tissue edema develops. There is a critical difference, however: lots of open, leaky blood vessels are important to allow antibodies and white blood cells to come out of the vessels and accumulate in the area in order to get rid of the infection. The strategy with infections, therefore, is to increase local circulation. This is why tissue infection responds to heat, while swelling from trauma responds to cooling.

Many singers use gargles or inhalers to address afflictions of the throat and to try to improve the voice. The purpose of these maneuvers is to bring a solution into direct contact with inflamed areas in the upper respiratory tract, and they can be very effective if properly used. For gargles and inhalers to work, they must reach the affected areas of the vocal tract. There are specific indications for rinsing, gargling, and inhaling solutions, and they are not interchangeable.

Oral rinses or mouthwashes have no benefit specific to the singer. They stay in the anterior two-thirds of the mouth cavity and are useful for dental problems or infections affecting the mouth (such as a yeast infection of the gums or palate).

Commercial mouthwashes, if used excessively, can actually do more harm than good. They do temporarily reduce the bacterial count in the mouth, but they can also damage the mucous membranes. The remaining bacteria reproduce rapidly, and within a short time they are back in full force. The end result is a full complement of bacteria, which are now free to act on mucous membranes that may have been damaged by the mouthwash. An unpublished study by Dr. Michael Hawke in Toronto revealed a large variety of bacteria and yeast cultured from the mouth of patients who used commercial mouthwashes regularly. If you use mouthwashes, they should be saline or peroxide-based, or medically prescribed. Good dental care will do more for bad breath than commercial mouthwashes.

Sore throat (pharyngitis and tonsillitis) responds well to gargles. Gargling involves holding a quantity of solution in the back of the throat while blowing air out. This causes the solution to bubble and percolate, soothing the mucous membranes it contacts. The best gargle is a solution of warm water and salt or baking soda. The heat helps to increase circulation to the infected part of the throat; the salt (which makes the gargle hypertonic in comparison to normal tissue fluids) draws edema fluid from the tissues and reduces swelling and pain. The classic British actor's gargle— port wine—probably had more effect after it was swallowed.

How far back does the gargle go? Radiologic studies by Dr. Bob Feder in Los Angeles have shown that the gargled solution does not go past the posterior tonsillar pillars (the back of the oropharynx). Gargles are therefore of no benefit for hoarseness or any other laryngeal condition. Since the gargled liquid doesn't descend into the hypopharynx, a voiced gargle is no more beneficial than an unvoiced one.

To get a solution farther down the respiratory tract, it must be either a vapor or in aerosol form. Vapor is the gas form of liquids, while aerosol is a fog of tiny, mechanically fragmented droplets of a liquid (in medical use, usually a saline solution), which can be generated by a nebulizer. The most common vapor is steam (water vapor), although certain volatile oils may also be carried with steam into the throat. A drop or two of eucalyptus oil in boiling water makes a soothing inhaler, taking advantage of both the heat of the steam and the medicinal effects of the volatile oil. This is the main advantage of steam, in that it carries both moisture and heat to the involved areas.

Since steam is usually inhaled from a pot or through a mask, the warming and moisturizing helps the nose and nasopharynx, as well as the pharynx and larynx. Steam can travel as far as the upper trachea, but inhaled water vapor cools rapidly and precipitates, normally creating a watery coating no farther down than the lower pharynx and upper part of the larynx. To get steam farther down involves inhaling it, whether at a higher temperature, more rapidly, or closer to the source. This creates the risk of a burn and should be avoided. If you are using a vaporizer to humidify your bedroom, there is no benefit to hot versus cold. Either way, by the time the water droplets reach your respiratory tract, they will be cool—or at most, at body temperature.

Aerosols are mixtures of air and finely dispersed particles of liquid or solids. The oft-caricatured throat spray in fact generates a liquid-based aerosol that can soothe the throat. Drops in a throat spray are larger than a nebulizer-generated aerosol, and therefore they travel a shorter distance. Depending on how rapidly you inhale, you can get these droplets to land on the vocal folds. The water particles in spray bottles are rather large and will not normally travel below the larynx.

For tracheitis and bronchitis, you may need to use a nebulizer. This is a device that breaks up a solution into tiny particles. These particles have less weight than sprayed water droplets and are carried farther down into the lungs. Different methods are used to nebulize liquids (such as the ultrasonic nebulizer).

Nebulizers can be very helpful in true medical conditions, such as croup or asthma. But they also carry a potential danger: they allow you to inhale materials (not just water or volatile oil vapor) deep into the lungs, where they may actually cause harm. Dr. Wilbur Gould told me years ago that Renata Tebaldi's career ended because she was inhaling nebulized oil to lubricate her vocal folds and developed lipoid pneumonia, losing flexibility in the lungs. It is for this reason that I have no problem with patients steaming, but I get concerned when they buy nebulizers. Of course, if this is done to treat a pulmonary condition (under the supervision of a physician), it is acceptable. If you do choose to use a nebulizer, a small amount of normal (physiologic) saline should do no harm.

While on the subject of pulmonary disease: if you use inhalers to treat asthma, be sure you know what you are inhaling, both the medication *and* the vehicle. Advair, a currently popular asthma inhaler, has a high incidence of associated temporary hoarseness, probably due to the vehicle used to carry the steroid into the lungs.

In summary, all of these methods have benefits and are especially useful for acute inflammatory conditions; but be sure that what you take into your body will reach the area you are treating and will not cause harm.

The Common Cold

The common cold is a viral infection that normally begins in the nose. It may be associated with some systemic symptoms but usually confines itself to the upper respiratory tract. It is normally a benign and self-limiting condition that resolves within a week, although it occasionally progresses to a bacterial infection, as the bacteria take advantage of the weakened environment.

There are many suggested treatments for the common cold. Antibiotics, often given, really play no role unless a secondary bacterial infection has developed. Vitamin C has been advocated as preventive and therapeutic. If you take Vitamin C, take it in divided doses over the course of the day, around 4,000 mg per day. Liquid forms (powder or effervescent tablet dissolved in water) may be better absorbed, hence more effective. If you decide on taking larger amounts (more than 4,000 mg a day), be aware that any excess is excreted in the urine, pulling out water with it. The result may be a degree of drying of the singer's larynx. To counteract this diuretic effect, increase your water intake. Finally, if you have a history of kidney stones, check with your doctor before embarking on Vitamin C therapy.

Zinc has also been recommended as good treatment. Unlike Vitamin C, zinc is not preventive and should be taken only after the cold has started. It can be taken orally (zinc gluconate tablets) or used as nasal swabs. The majority of clinical studies (although not all) agree that zinc can reduce cold symptoms, shorten the illness, and decrease the likelihood of transmission to others.

Other home remedies include garlic, echinacea, and homeopathic remedies. Though we cannot discuss them all individually, one word of caution: more is not necessarily better. If you take home remedies for cold, take the recommended dosage, and be aware of any side effects or potential interaction with prescription medications.

Pharyngitis, tonsillitis

Infections of the pharynx and tonsils may be viral or bacterial. Be aware that streptococcus is not the only bacterial culprit here. In other words, if your strep test is negative, it doesn't necessarily mean the infection is *not* bacterial. Again, most of these cases are benign and self-limiting, and they do not invariably progress down into the hypopharynx and larynx.

Keeping the neck and chest warm is intuitive and helpful. In addition to gargling with warm salt water or baking soda, drinking hot ginger tea is an excellent remedy. You need to chop up and boil fresh ginger in water, and then decant it and mix it with honey before drinking. It's pretty spicy, but it usually reduces the throat pain quickly. The heat (both thermal and spicy) of the tea increases circulation to the affected area, while the honey has a soothing and osmotic effect, decreasing swelling.

A general suggestion: as with any infection, rest. Don't try to "exercise" your way through it. Your body is busy enough dealing with the bacteria or viruses without being further stressed on the treadmill!

Tracheitis, Bronchitis

The lower vocal tract is self-cleansing, but it depends on adequate moisture to be able to remove any infection. If you have a cough as part of your illness, it is important to make it productive, to help the airway clear out any infected mucus. The cornerstone of home treatment is increased hydration, up to ten glasses of water a day. Inhaling steam with a drop or two of eucalyptus oil is soothing. Commercially available menthol and eucalyptus vapors are also useful. The menthol symptomatically opens up the airway, although in excess it can be irritating. Excess menthol can also interfere with mucus clearance from the airways by impeding movement of the tiny cilia that sweep the surfaces. Heat applied to the chest, as either a hot pack or a poultice, increases the circulation and may speed recovery. Again, if you do use a nebulizer, use it only with physiologic saline solution (unless you have been prescribed medications by your doctor); nebulizing oils (including eucalyptus oil) can cause these particles to land and remain in the lungs, leading to long-term problems.

Acid Reflux

The best management for most cases of reflux is behavior modification. This includes changing your diet, eating smaller amounts of food more frequently, and not lying down for about two hours after your meals. Long-term medication with proton pump inhibitors (such as Nexium, Prevacid, Prilosec) should ideally be avoided, since these medications may cause osteoporosis over time, particularly in older patients. One good home remedy is licorice, which can be used alone, or in combination with antacids. The only side effect of licorice is that it can raise the blood pressure, although newer forms (DGL, or deglycyrrhizinated licorice) are now available that seem not to exacerbate hypertension.

Home Remedies vs. Medical Treatment

Although home remedies can help with benign and temporary problems, they are not the answer if your condition is persistent or worsening. They should be used to assist your body in getting better; if they don't work, you should see a doctor to make sure you are not in need of medical intervention. Remember also that there are potential side effects with even the most benign self-treatment. Monitoring your improvement (or your failure to improve) should sensibly direct you either back to the vitamin shop or to the doctor's office.

20

Medications and the Voice

YOUNGNAN JENNY CHO, MD, FACS

Medications, whether by prescription or over the counter, can have unintentional side effects. For singers, even the slightest of side effects can cause significant impact on the voice, altering speech production and voice quality by affecting any level of voice production, from the central level in the brain down to the peripheral level of the larynx. Although for most people these side effects may be just an annoyance, singers and professional voice users who are much more attuned to their vocal quality are more likely to be impaired by the unintentional side effects of medications. Physicians who treat singers should be aware of these pharmacologically induced problems, and singers who take these medications should be informed of possible untoward side effects.

Medications that cause dryness are a major concern for singers. Antihistamines, decongestants, antitussives, antiemetics, anticholinergics, and antidepressants can all cause dryness of the upper airway and larynx. The vocal fold consists of a "cover," a thin layer of mucous membrane overlying the "body," which in turn consists of the vocal ligament and vocalis muscle. The space between the vocal fold and the underlying ligaments, known as

Reinke's space, must be well lubricated to allow the surface membrane to slide freely during phonation. For proper function and smooth vibration of the vocal folds, the surface of the vocal folds must be moist and clear of any debris. However, the vocal folds themselves lack mucus glands. The mucus-producing glands are located in the surrounding area, the laryngeal ventricles, as well the rest of the respiratory tract. Mucus is squeezed onto the surface of the vocal folds as the larynx moves, and it must be thin and copious in amount. Any change in the amount or viscosity of mucus will affect the vibratory function of the vocal folds, hence vocal quality.

Mucus production varies, even in the absence of medications. Respiratory tract mucus production is controlled by the autonomic nervous system. The sympathetic system, also known as the "fight or flight" system, is stimulated during times of anxiety; it is controlled by adrenaline. Release of adrenaline causes vasoconstriction and decreases mucus production. This is why during times of stress, such as stage performance, the throat may feel dry. The opposing parasympathetic system is controlled by acetylcholine. High acetylcholine results in vasodilation and greater mucus production. If the larynx is too dry, it can cause a brittle sound, and difficulties when phonating softly at the top of the vocal range. Too much thick mucus overlying the vocal folds when phonating can cause glottal choking and incomplete vocal fold closure. The vocal fold mucosa must also oscillate smoothly over the vocal ligament.

Whereas hydration of the laryngeal structures controls voice quality, the laryngeal muscles control vocal pitch. The more contraction, the higher the pitch. For proper function, the larynx has to be well hydrated and laryngeal muscles well coordinated.

Antihistamines, both in pill form and as nasal spray, can be a significant cause of mucous membrane dehydration. They block H1 histamine receptors and inhibit acetylcholine effect. By lowering mucus secretion, they dry the upper respiratory tract mucosa. This causes more phonatory effort and produces harsher voice, with high jitter, shimmer, and hoarseness. Intranasal steroids can be used in lieu of, or in addition to, treatment of allergies in some cases and may reduce the need for antihistamines. Leukotriene inhibitors such as Singulair do not dry as much and can be used as an alternative to antihistamines.

Decongestants are sypathomimetics and cause vasoconstriction and less mucus production. Alpha-adrenergic agonists, such as pseudoephedrine and phenylephrine, cause reduction in blood flow and mucus secretion. The amount of mucus produced is less but is more viscous, causing phonatory impairment.

Although the mechanism is different, the result is similar to the antihistamine effect in causing harsh, dry voice. Additionally, oral decongestants can raise the heart rate and interfere with sleep, two effects that heighten the sensation of performance anxiety.

Antitussives such as codeine, hydrocodone, and dextromethorphan are either central or peripheral suppressants of cough. They are opioids or their derivatives, causing vocal fold dryness. Also, most cough suppressants are prepared with alcohol (which acts as a diuretic), producing further vocal fold dryness.

What about cortisone? Systemic corticosteroids such as prednisone are frequently used to decrease laryngeal swelling. However, this needs to be used with care. In long-term use, it can cause vocal fold edema, muscle weakness, and ultimately vocal fold bowing. This can result in a weak voice, lower vocal pitch, and vocal fold dryness. Inhaled steroids can be used to target the respiratory tract more specifically.

Steroids are also very useful in controlling asthma, chronic pulmonary disease, and reactive airway. Although in short-term use to treat temporary illnesses they may be used safely, with chronic use they too can cause untoward side effects, such as yeast infection of the throat and possible vocal fold atrophy. Gargling and rinsing the throat after using a topical steroid may minimize side effects. Intranasal steroids used to treat allergies, reactive runny and stuffy nose, and acute infections, by contrast, have been safely used in the long run with minimal side effects (nose bleed, sore throat, headaches). Although fungal infection such as thrush is possible, it is not commonly seen. Unlike with oral, injectable, or inhaled steroids, systemic absorption is minimal.

The beta-adrenergic agonists used as "rescue inhalers" for acute asthma attack such as albuterol and isoproterenol promote relaxation of the respiratory muscles. This decreases airway resistance, promotes lung compliance, and can improve vocal quality.

Both male and female hormone supplements can lead to dysphonia. Androgens (testosterone), the male hormones, can cause muscular hyperplasia and edema. This leads to limited upper range, vocal fatigue, and deep, dark voice. At an early phase this is potentially treatable, but once structural change has taken place the voice change is irreversible.

Women may be exposed to androgens either by prescription or inadvertently. Birth control pills containing synthetic progestins may be a problem, as this chemical breaks down to a hormone with androgenic (testosteronelike) activity. High and light soprano voices may darken with such birth control pills. Most of the newer birth control pills are free of androgen precursors, but female singers should avoid androgen use. A common dietary supplement, DHEA (dihydroepiandrosterone), is particularly problematic, since it is freely available without a prescription.

The effects of female hormones are bit more complicated. Estrogen causes water retention, edema, and lowering of vocal pitch. Progesterone is even worse in this regard, accounting for water retention and vocal problems experienced by women during the premenstrual period.

Medications taken for psychologic and psychiatric problems also can have a deleterious effect on the voice. In addition to the drying effect of antidepressants, which is due to their anticholinergic and adrenergic action, medications that sedate can also affect coordination and overall performance. Neuroleptics, such as haloperidol, used for its antipsychotic effect, work by blocking the central dopaminergic receptors. They can even cause a temporary Parkinson's-like syndrome with vocal tremor as well as harshness and limited phonatory modulation. Antianxiety medications such as diazepam and buspirone cause muscle relaxation and depression of senses. Neurostimulants can cause vocal tremor and abnormal speech pattern.

Diuretics, such as furosemide, frequently used for their antihypertensive effect, further water elimination. This causes overall dehydration. Angiotensin-converting enzyme (ACE) inhibitors, a common antihypertensive group of drugs, can cause persistent cough leading to hoarseness from vocal trauma. The mechanism is unclear, but the effect is reversible once the medication has been stopped.

Beta blockers such as Inderal slow heart rate and are used for heart disease and regulating blood pressure. They can also be used at times to control tremor and performance anxiety, but they should be used with caution since they can slow heart rate too much and cause lightheadedness and syncope. They are not generally advised for patients with asthma.

Many over-the-counter medicines and supplements are also known to affect the laryngeal tissue. Fat-soluble vitamins such as A, D, and E raise bleeding time and can accumulate in the body to a toxic level. Vitamin A derivatives such as Accutane, taken for severe acne, can be drying. Vitamin E can raise the potential for vocal fold hemorrhage in patients who may be at risk, such as those with dilated blood vessels on the vocal folds. Water-soluble vitamins (such as B complex and C) are not stored in the body and get excreted; therefore they need to be replenished daily. However, in large doses they too can cause side effects. Vitamin B6 is a known cause of vasodilation, of swelling and bleeding with vocal trauma. Megadoses of vitamin C act as a diuretic, causing drying effect. Therefore, when high doses of vitamin C are taken for immune boost (as during a cold), one needs to be vigilant about keeping the body well hydrated.

Aspirin is commonly taken for its analgesic effect as well as cardiac protection by thinning blood (reducing platelet stickiness). This very effect can however, also promote vocal hemorrhage with vocal trauma in predisposed singers. Factors predisposing to hemorrhage include the presence of dilated blood vessels on the vocal folds, menstruation, and the use of substances such as alcohol that further vascular dilation. Like aspirin, nonsteroidal anti-inflammatory agents (NSAIDS) such as ibuprofen and other blood thinners such as coumadin and Plavix also worsen bleeding time by reducing platelet clumping. This can cause greater risk for vocal fold hemorrhage, especially with extensive voice use and vocal trauma. Niacin, a B vitamin, dilates blood vessels can also aggravate bleeding. This vitamin is often taken by patients to reduce their cholesterol. If you have a history of vocal fold bleeding, these seemingly harmless and ubiquitous drugs should be taken judiciously.

Antibiotics are crucial in treating bacterial infections and are an essential aspect of medical management. However, with frequent application you may build resistance to future use. For this reason, it is important to complete the full course of the prescribed antibiotic regiment unless you discuss it with your physician. Antibiotics, like many other drugs, may interact with other ingested substances, causing an increase or decrease in their potency as well as untoward side effects. For example, tetracycline or doxycycline (often taken for acne) is bound by calcium, and therefore should not be taken at the same time as milk products or antacids such as TUMS. Most commonly, the unintended eradication of bacteria in the gut (both harmful and beneficial to our general system) may lead to diarrhea as a common side effect. Increasing dietary intake of live bacterial cultures such as yogurt or probiotics may be helpful in restoring normal intestinal flora.

When we consider the act of singing, we think of the larynx, or more specifically the vocal folds and their function. The voice box should be free of infection, swelling, and irritation and be well lubricated. However, the generation of voice requires much more. It involves the larynx but also trachea, chest, abdomen, pelvis, and central nervous system as well as fine neuromuscular functions of these organs. Hence, any medication that may affect these organs should be carefully considered before being taken.

Staying healthy by controlling one's life style and environment is important. Of course, when needed, medications are a necessary part of maintaining health. But with any medicine, one should be aware of possible side effects. Medications can affect vocal quality on many levels. Since minute changes in vocal function can alter vocal quality, a singer should be aware of the roles that various medications have in vocal pathology, and be especially cognizant of possible drug interactions. Hydration is an important factor in keeping the vocal folds healthy. Aside from treating underlying causes, adding a mucolytic such as guaifenesin may be helpful, as well as nasal irrigation with saline. For many singers who travel extensively and see a number of physicians in different cities, it is important to inform the treating physician not only of current medications being taken but also of recently discontinued medicines that may be still in the body. This of course implies that the singer should keep track of everything ingested, inhaled, or injected into the body. Preventing

TABLE 20.1

Medications		Effects
Antihistamine (e.g. benadryl/fexofenadin/ loratadine)		dehydration
Antidepressant		drying, sedation
Antitussive		dehydration
Antiemetic		dehydration
Antihypertension		cough
Decongestant		dryness, tremor
Corticosteroid		muscle weakness, yeast infection
Aspirin/Anti-inflammatory		vocal hemorrhage
Sedatives		dryness, sedation
Birth control		loss of high notes
Neurostimulant		
Neurolepic		vocal tremor
Anabolic steroid		loss of high notes
Vitamin	Vitamin B(niacin)	vasodilatation
	Vitamin C	diuretic in large doses
	Vitamin A	vocal dryness
	Vitamin E	vocal hemorrhage

duplication and possible overdosing can minimize potential side effects. On that note, keeping a medication diary may be useful in maintaining one's own health. Table 20.1 summarizes the pharmacologic effects of common classes of medications on the singer's voice.

21

Exercise Programs for Vocal Artists

An Effective Performance Enhancing Strategy

ANNETTE OSHER, MD

RICHARD A. STEIN, MD

Regular and moderately vigorous exercise is critical to one's overall health. Even though medical research speaks loudly and clearly to this issue, physicians may not emphasize adequately it to their patients.

Exercise is an essential part of a program to protect you from cardiovascular illness, heart attacks, and strokes. Although certain genetic factors in our makeup play a strong role in determining our individual risk of suffering and dying of heart disease, exercise and diet are of prime importance in modulating that risk. Recently the sciences of exercise and disease prevention have converged in recognizing the very strong positive role that exercise plays in improving both the duration and the quality of our lives.

For singers, exercise is particularly important. They focus on the voice, but their performances do not generally involve significant physical exertion (unless they are in the chorus line of a musical). Add to this a busy travel schedule and unpredictable day-to-day planning, and even with the best of intentions a regular, scheduled exercise program is difficult to fit in. And one important point we need to make is that, whatever your schedule, regular exercise needs to be a planned part, not left for "free time"!

This chapter addresses a clear and simple way to help you to design and start the right exercise program for you. We will discuss why exercise is important, how much, how often, and what types of exercise should be done. Additionally, once your program is in place, it is important to know how to increase your exercise at the appropriate time so that you can continue to improve your fitness and health.

There is a wealth of epidemiologic data to prove that exercise can make a real difference to both longevity and quality of life. One such study, done after World War II on English bus workers, compared the incidence of heart disease among bus drivers and bus conductors. On English double-decker buses, the driver sits all day, while the conductor moves through the bus, climbing stairs frequently to the second level to sell tickets to passengers seated there. Although this was not the only difference between the two groups, they were in many important ways (working hours, exposure to pollution, etc.) similar. Not surprisingly, Dr. J. N. Morris and colleagues[1] found that the nonactive bus drivers had a significantly greater incidence of heart attacks than did the active conductors.

A subsequent study done in the United States by Dr. R. S. Paffenbarger[2] on Harvard University alumni showed that those who exercised regularly had a much lower rate of heart attacks and strokes. Subsequent studies have shown that even if you already have had a heart attack, engaging in regular exercise under the supervision of your physician will lower your risk of having a second infarction.

How exercise makes you feel is also important. Studies that ask individuals about regular exercise and depression have shown that people who exercise regularly are more optimistic and less subject to depression. Individuals who exercise have more energy and are less anxious.

What kind of exercise, and how much, should you do? This question can be answered in terms of frequency (sessions per week) and duration (how many minutes per session). The intensity of the workout is also an important consideration.

The surgeon general of the United States has recommended that you exercise almost every day for at least thirty minutes at moderate intensity. Here are some guidelines to ensure that you are doing enough exercise to reap the benefits.

A brisk walk is acceptable, and recommended, moderate-intensity exercise. If walking is to be your main form of exercise, aim for 12–15 miles a week, at a moderately hard level (rated 7 on a 1–10 scale of perceived exertion, as described later). Some physicians consider this to be the best form of exercise, since it moves all parts of the body, is low-impact, and is enjoyable. The downside of walking for exercise is that it is somewhat time-consuming (an hour a day, four times a week), and once your heart is conditioned, it becomes more difficult to reach the target heart rate, even with brisk walking.

The second approach, recommended by the American College of Sports Medicine, is to exercise three times a week, for forty minutes at a moderately intense level. Examples of this aerobic exercise are treadmill exercise, step, elliptical trainer, climbing, rowing machines, dancing class, and vigorous walking. The intensity of the exercise should be monitored in terms of heart rate. Optimal benefits are obtained when you exert yourself at two-thirds of the maximum heart rate for your age. At this heart rate you will be able to exercise for thirty minutes, achieving the desired result, and becoming trained, fit, and able to do more exercise.

The formula used for this (and it is to be seen on the wall of many gyms), begins with an estimation of your peak heart rate, 220 minus your age. Applying this formula, a forty-year-old individual will have a peak heart rate of 180 (220 − 40) beats per minute. Optimal workout heart rate for this person is 70 percent of 180, or 126 beats per minute. Therefore, 126 beats per minute is the exercise intensity level that a forty-year-old should exercise at for the session. Of course, this is an average for all persons of that age, and it doesn't take into account preexisting level of fitness, or health risk factors.

Since the formula method is only an approximation, more commonly used is the cognitive method called the RPE (Rate Perceived Exertion). To use this method, ask yourself to subjectively rate the effort of exertion perceived while doing the exercise, on a scale of 1 to 10, with 1 being how you feel at rest and 10 equal to exhaustion. When you feel you are in the 6, 7, or 8 range, you are likely to be exercising at the correct intensity.

What kind of exercise is best for you? Picking your activity is important from the point of view of pleasure and satisfaction. Unless you feel good and find the exercise rewarding, you will stop exercising. Selecting the "best" exercise is not the point. More important is to choose from a list of activities the ones you enjoy; otherwise you may not stick with it, and despite your best intentions the benefits will be lost. So think about what activity you would like. For example, do want to have company, or do you prefer to exercise in solitude? Once such decisions are made, chose an exercise activity that is safe, easy, and acceptable.

Most of us think of exercise simply as aerobic activity, a way of maintaining our cardiovascular system. Recently, we have come to appreciate the value of combining strength training exercise with aerobic exercise. It is therefore also important to include strength training in the plan.

Strength training means using a form of resistance, like free weights, weight machines, resistance bands, or a person's own weight to build muscles and strength. A single muscle can be isolated, or a group of muscles can be strengthened. Strength training should be done twice a week, for a period of fifteen minutes;

it should involve ten to twelve exercises that work the major upper, lower, and core muscles.

The cumulative effect of strength training depends not only on the amount of weight but also on the number of repetitions and the frequency of exercise. Using lighter weights to exercise different groups of muscles simultaneously will provide gain without pain.

Like aerobic cardiac exercise, strength training is a gradual and cumulative process. Be aware that doing too much too fast may cause an injury. For the novice, it is wise to begin a program at a gym or the local "Y," under the supervision of a trainer to help with carefully setting up a program. For both aerobic and strength training, check with your physician before you begin an exercise program.

Okay, you have begun your exercise program, and more importantly, you are sticking with it. How do you increase your exercise level? As you improve your exercise capacity by exercise training, the exercise will feel easier. Using the RPE method is one approach. To work up to your 7 out of 10 level will involve more effort, and this will automatically continue to improve your fitness and your exercise program. This will keep you in an ideal training zone.

For the strength training program, you should begin by repeating each exercise ten times to fatigue. This initially means setting the weights or the tension of the machine to the level where ten repetitions cause muscle fatigue. Fewer repetitions to fatigue can be discouraging (or harmful), while more are unnecessarily time-consuming. Once you are able to increase this to fourteen repetitions, increase the hand weights by a small amount, and start again, going back to eight to ten repetitions. Work up to fourteen repetitions, again to fatigue, and repeat.

Your exercise schedule is now in place, and you have begun to feel the benefits. Now, beware of the "program busters"!

Trainers, coaches, and physicians have learned some of the reasons for which people stop their exercise programs. On the top of the list is the pain and soreness from initially overdoing the exercise. We all tend to be impatient for results, thinking that doing more, but less often, will achieve the same results. The "weekend warrior" is a classic stereotype, the sedentary person who gets injured by trying to become a Sunday triathlete. If you push ahead too fast and too hard, you can develop pain in your joints and muscles, and it will be natural to want to stop the activity. The problem is that, once they are hurt or in pain, most people will not restart the exercise program despite their original best intentions.

The number one rule to avoid this program buster is to start at a low and comfortable level and work up slowly. Coaches use the 10 percent rule, increasing each activity by less than 10 percent at a time and staying at this level for several weeks.

Another program buster is wedging your exercise between two important obligations. The exercise will be skipped if you are running late, and you will give up on it. Be sure to pick a good time and place, and avoid conflict in scheduling. Your exercise time is also an important obligation, since staying in shape powers you to attend to all those other obligations!

Yet another way to sabotage your exercise program is to pick an activity that will become uncomfortable or unsafe. Running in the park at the time of year when darkness is coming earlier, you may find yourself avoiding running until there is more light—but then not restarting exercise at all.

Convenience is still another factor: if you use a gym or club, pick one that is close by and has generous hours. Nothing sinks an exercise program more quickly than the thought of having to travel a long distance to get there, or the need to rearrange your schedule to accommodate that of your exercise facility.

If possible, leave the cell phone at home. Taking a phone when you exercise is a great way to introduce stress and distraction and increase your risk of injury. Since for many of us the time we spend exercising is the only time we have for ourselves, maximize the benefits of "me" time by parking the Blackberry in the locker or car.

These are just some potential saboteurs. Take a few minutes and think of the numerous ways you could bust your exercise program, and then plan around those activities.

The rewards of your exercise program are many, in terms of longevity, quality of daily life, and psychological outlook. As you do more walking, running, rowing, climbing, cycling, or dancing, the physical work of everyday life and the work of performing will be easier and less fatiguing. You will have more stamina and endurance. You will feel better and stronger.

If you choose an activity and a setting that you enjoy, you will feel that you are doing something for yourself. What a wonderful choice, and you deserve it! If you then combine the exercise program with a healthy diet, you will see the result in terms of attaining your desired weight.

Exercise and diet can also lower elevated blood pressure. If you take medication to lower your blood pressure, you may find that the treatment is now working better than it did prior to exercising and diet changes. Other risk factors for heart disease such as elevated LDL and high triglycerides may decrease, while HDL, a factor thought to be cardioprotective, may go up with exercise and an improved diet. These changes move you into a lower risk zone for heart disease and stroke.

Your health, energy, and spirit will be elevated to meet the demands ahead. After all, the purpose of good health is to allow yourself to fully actualize your potential as a human being. Keeping your body healthy is a "sine qua non" of a long and successful life.

Recommended Websites

www.oshermd.com
www.americanheart.org
www.goredforwomen.org
www.acsm.org
www.choosefitness.com
www.health.msn.com

Notes

1. Morris, J. N., Heady, J. A., Raffle, P. A. B., Roberts, C. G., and Parks, J. N. "Coronary Heart Disease and Physical Activity of Work." *Lancet* ii (1953), 1053–1057, 1111–1120.

2. Paffenbarger, R. S., Jr., Wing, A. L., Hyde, R. T., and Jung, D. L. "Physical Activity and Incidence of Hypertension in College Alumni." *Am. J. Epidemiology* (1983) 117(3):245–257.

22

Mental Health for Singers

DAVID M. SHERMAN, MD

Would that the lives of singers played out harmoniously! If you have already embarked on a singing career, you are probably painfully aware that, to the contrary, yours is a challenging journey that can be as stressful and bruising as it can be attractive and exciting. On the one hand, singers are humans like everyone else, susceptible to the range of mental health concerns to which all people are vulnerable. On the other hand, as a singer you face a unique set of stresses that are particular to your trade. A singer once told me, "The things that are most wonderful about this career are also the most difficult." The challenges of being a singer really do cut both ways. In this chapter we look at the common emotional challenges that singers face, with an eye to maintaining emotional health.

Note: I thank my mental-health colleagues, especially my fellow therapists at the Juilliard School Counseling Service, as well as Anthony Tommasini, chief classical music critic at the *New York Times,* for invaluable input in preparing this chapter. Above all, I thank my patients, without whom I would not have a clue.

Owning Your Career Choice

Singers launch their musical careers at different ages. For some of you, the "choice" occurred at such a young age that it might feel more like an assignment in life than an autonomous choice. This is true for some pop singers (think Michael Jackson or Judy Garland). It is also true for opera singers, who may enter the classical world as prodigy string players or pianists. For children, singing (and music in general) is something that is simple and joyous, even instinctual. But then, perhaps a parent urges you further, or a teacher suggests that you have talent. As time passes, singing might become more complicated; not only is it something that is fun, but it is also something that others are encouraging you to do. Either an abundance of attention or a deficit of it is often seen in the early childhood experiences of performers. These opposite experiences can both spur a child to strive to be noticed, to win people over. And budding performers of all stripes thrive on praise for their talent. But a few years later, the questions may arise, "Whose idea was this anyway? Is this what I want to be doing with my life?"

Psychologists have studied the effect of praise on child behavior. Children who are overly praised for accomplishments, whether it be "successfully" building a tower of blocks or singing a song, tend to be more anxious and less likely to take chances with further pursuits out of the fear that they won't be able to match their previous effort. Excess praise over time can sap true playfulness and creativity.

When musical careers are launched early amidst praise, urging, and even coercion, it is common to wrestle later with a musical career choice, and to feel confused. This confusion may surface in late adolescence, but it can happen after that as well, and even be a recurring question: "Is singing *right* for me?" Perhaps framing the choice as one of right and wrong, in such fundamental terms, only serves to make the question that much more pressured. In reality, you may have been thrust into singing under one set of circumstances (e.g., family expectation) but later discover as an adult your own intrinsic attraction to singing. Or alternatively, you may have loved to sing in your youth (without any clear outside coercion), but at a later age you may develop a new set of priorities and interests that propel you into another career. Regardless, it is important that you take *ownership* of your career choice, be it singing or another life path.

The Challenges of Late Career Development

Although the choice to become a singer happens all too fast for some, it may unfold all too slowly for others. This is especially true for opera singers. First, opera talent is often discovered late, perhaps plucked from a church chorus or college musical. Second, opera singers may spend decades discovering and honing their voice, not fully coming into their own until age forty. What this means is that while your musical peers may be reaching the heights of their career, you, as an aspiring opera singer, are in much a earlier stage of development, contending with years of uncertainty, your ultimate destination unknown.

If and when your success is fully realized, there is then the common experience of having a limited shelf life. (Athletes and dancers face a similar situation, but in their twenties). The singer Renee Fleming noted at age forty that she probably had fifteen years of singing at her best before her brilliance would begin to fade.

Practicing

Then comes the practicing. Musicians, especially those who are classically trained, develop a complicated relationship with practicing that often has early roots. Practicing can be laden with emotion, whether pleasure, wonder, and a sense of mastery, or anxiety, boredom, self-loathing, and resentment. Some of these more painful emotions may be remnants of power struggles with parents.

Practicing can also feel isolating and like a painful sacrifice. As a child you may have spent long hours in practice, on top of your regular school studies. In some cases this can lead to a sense of delayed development in other aspects of life such as relationships and love. And even though those in other fields might leave school or work at the end of the day with a sense of closure, it can be much more difficult for you as a musician to know when you have "finished" your work. Setting limits to practice time and maintaining balance is extremely important for emotional health in a musical career.

And the self-directed nature of practicing often lends itself to procrastination. This is especially true if you tend toward perfectionism. A common barrier to getting started in practice may be harsh self-expectation of, for instance, mastering a difficult piece in one sitting. For this type of block, it is often helpful, if paradoxical, to set expectations low—to contract with yourself to practice for only one hour a day, and stop after the hour no matter how little you feel you have accomplished. Two helpful books on procrastination are *The Now Habit* by Neil Fiore and *Procrastination: Why You Do It, What to Do About It* by Jane Burka and Lenore Yuen.

Performing: Harnessing Stage Fright

You might expect that all singers are born performers who should feel at home on the stage. Surprisingly, this is sometimes far from the truth. That to which we are most drawn—for instance, performing—is also that which elicits the most fear. After all, you as a performing artist often have the most *self-worth* invested in your performance, and thus the greatest reason for performance anxiety.

It is well known that a certain level of adrenaline is good for performance, rousing a high level of motivation and focus. This is why your performance on opening night often surpasses your performance for a dress rehearsal; this is why recordings are often made before a live audience. But there is a level of excitement felt to be optimal for performing at our best. Too much adrenaline begins to lower performance; those who study performance anxiety have proposed an inverted-U relationship between performance and anxiety.

What do people mean when they talk about stage fright? They actually experience stage fright in a variety of dramatic ways. Some experience stage fright as merely a state of restlessness and jitters. Jitters may be uncomfortable and somewhat compromising of performance, but they can be worked through in a number of ways and ultimately harnessed to good effect.

Others, however, may experience stage fright as a more catastrophic reaction, a state of all-out *panic* (more of a steep inverted V than an inverted U). Panic is a condition where the sympathetic nervous system, the source of the fight-or-flight response, is fully activated. (Imagine anxiety controlled by a switch rather than a gradual dial.) Symptoms of panic include racing heart, constricted throat, shortness of breath, blurry vision, tingling, feelings of altered reality, and a subjective sense of terror or impending doom. Needless to say, performance during such a state can be *severely* compromised.

Whether you experience jitters or panic, there are a number of ways to overcome stage fright. Choice of one approach over another depends to some extent on the scope and intensity of the anxiety. But it also depends on your personal inclination.

First, there are numerous readings on how to harness anxiety in a pressured situation, with the goal of performing at one's best; see, for example, the books by performance coach Don Greene. You may also consult with a performance coach in person. Second, an effective method of overcoming performance anxiety and other phobias, whether it is fear of flying or fear of snakes, is through *exposure therapy*. This involves a well-planned program of exposing oneself to performance situations in order to gradually be desensitized to performing. This is sometimes accompanied by learning relaxation techniques such as progressive muscle relaxation. Exposure therapy is best done with the guidance of an experienced behavioral therapist. In New York, clinics with qualified therapists include the Center for Cognitive Behavioral Psychotherapy and the American Institute for Cognitive Therapy. Third, it may also be helpful to take a broader approach to an anxiety through psychodynamic psychotherapy. See the section "Seeking Help" below for a description of some types of psychotherapy. Fourth, other practices that can be helpful for stage fright and other forms of anxiety as well include guided imagery, exercise (such as aerobic exercise and yoga), focus on healthful diet, and adequate sleep.

Finally, medication is also an option, particularly if you have been struggling with stage fright for a long time without relief. Many performing artists are familiar with the use of beta-blockers (e.g., Inderal, whose generic name is propranolol) for performance anxiety. Most commonly, beta blockers are taken on an as-needed basis prior to big performances. They work by temporarily blocking the effects of norepinephrine and epinephrine, which are the fight-or-flight chemicals that surge through the body when one is experiencing significant anxiety or panic. Beta blockers thus damp down on the racing heart, the tremors, etc., and in this way also help one feel calm. They are taken thirty to sixty minutes before a performance and, in the case of propranolol, last about four hours.

Beta blockers and other prescribed medications are by far a better option than self-medicating with sedatives or alcohol, all of which have been shown to worsen performance because of their sedation and clouding of cognitive processes. In fact, research has well documented the negative effects of alcohol and sedatives on objective measures of performance, even as the performer subjectively rates his or her performance as improved. Obviously, another reason to avoid alcohol or other sedatives in managing anxiety is that these are substances to which people form addiction.

Though beta blockers are often traded casually among performers, it is better to consult with a doctor about taking these medications. Beta blockers are relatively safe, but there are a variety of instances necessitating caution (e.g., where asthma, diabetes, or low blood pressure is a factor). Also, there are numerous beta blockers to choose from, so one size doesn't fit all. Once prescribed, it is often helpful to try a test dose of a beta blocker either on a day off or at a less important performance to evaluate its effect.

There are situations where beta blockers may not be the right medication option. Performance anxiety is sometimes a part of a broader difficulty, formally labeled by psychiatrists as social anxiety disorder—generalized type. This involves a pervasive, persistent discomfort with a variety of social situations and is due to fear of being scrutinized, embarrassed, or humiliated. It usually results in avoidance of many such situations, to the detriment of relationships and career. Here, beta blockers have *not* been shown to be effective. Instead, psychotherapy or a class of antidepressants called serotonin reuptake inhibitors (such brand names as Prozac, Paxil, Celexa, Zoloft, Lexapro, Effexor, Cymbalta) are often helpful.

Relationships with Teachers

A good teacher is someone who facilitates learning, growth, and mentorship in an atmosphere of safety, calm, nurturance, mutual respect, and freedom from shame and judgment. A good teacher also responds helpfully to feedback from the student.

Having the right teacher is probably more important for a singer than for any other musician. Whether you are speaking or singing, it is literally impossible to hear the way your voice sounds to others. Thus, singers are extremely reliant on the trained ear of their teacher for feedback. With this reliance comes intimacy. And with this level of intimacy comes a high potential for disappointment, or even for feeling that the relationship is not working. Considering leaving a teacher can be fraught with fear and anxiety ("if I decide to leave will my teacher hate me," or even "if I leave, will he retaliate and somehow bar my career path?"). Though this may have some reality to it (a teacher might be particularly powerful and narcissistic), students more often overplay these concerns.

Ultimately, you owe it to yourself to find a good-enough working relationship with your teacher. At the same time, it is important to consider that the relationship is, by definition, a two-way street. In other words all relationships require work from both sides!

Because of a teacher's authority, it is normal (and only sometimes problematic) to *transfer* onto our teachers feelings and patterns of relating from other figures in our past. For instance, the desire to please a teacher may in part be a re-creation of our desire to please a parent. But all sorts of transferred feelings and patterns are possible, from love and idealization to competition, fear, hate, and anger. Again, these feelings are inevitable and normal. Indeed, they are often beyond our awareness. They can feel manageable and even constructive in the relationship (the stirrings of fear motivating one to be a little more prepared for a lesson). But they can also be powerful and destructive (overwhelming anxiety causing one to shy away from the constructive give-and-take of a lesson). Particularly intense feelings may be a clue that an experience from childhood is being triggered.

If a relationship with a teacher is not going well, it is helpful to consult with trusted colleagues or mentors for their input. To work through the deeper psychological aspects of relationships, it may be helpful to consult a psychotherapist.

Is This Art or Work?

Then there is the question that musicians sometimes have: Is this an artistic pursuit, or is this a way to make a living, or both? People consciously or unconsciously define their singing in different ways. One performing artist that I worked with felt like a fraud whenever she was not inspired to practice. If she was not inspired, she though this must mean she was not a true artist and that surely she should be doing something else. But everything else seemed like a meaningless pursuit, because to her singing was uniquely perched on a pedestal. Thus it may be an important task to be mindful and accepting of one's relationship to singing. Perhaps this involves allowing that singing may be art, but it may also be work, and work, any work, has its drawbacks and drudgery.

The Stress of Taking Care of One's Voice

An opera singer told me, "When it comes to one's voice, every singer is a hypochondriac." Like no other musical instrument, your voice is invaluable and irreplaceable. You may spend a lot of time worrying whether your voice will be in tip-top shape for performance time. At the same time, the voice is a delicate creature over which we have limited control. It is susceptible to illnesses, hormonal change, medication, and aging. It is a challenge to accept this uncertainty and lack of control.

Dealing with Failures

Many singers hold themselves to reaching or maintaining impossibly high, self-set standards. It is these singers who may be prone to feeling that theirs is an unforgiving profession, but it is often their own internalized critic that is the least forgiving.

There is also something especially personal about being evaluated on your voice. Your voice may feel more an expression of your intimate self than, say, your piano playing. (When you play the piano, it is you and the piano; when you sing, it is just you!) Having a voice and being heard are important psychological themes for some people, perhaps especially for singers. Thus criticism, failing auditions, and periods without work can be especially hard for many singers.

The fear of failure can be an obstacle to practicing and reaching for different opportunities. But the reality is that for almost everybody, successes come in dribs and drabs; in between are failures, from which we may learn and build. It is important for some singers to work on framing failures in a healthy way. If an audition does not go well, say to yourself, "That audition didn't go well, maybe I can do better next time," as opposed to "Wow— I'm really bad! I may as well stop trying!"

Success at All Costs?

At various points in your singing career, you may face decisions about what you are willing to sacrifice in order to succeed. There may often be a tension between pursuit of success and compromising other personal goals, comforts, health, or even integrity. Common examples:

- I have an offer to tour in Europe this summer, but it would be disruptive being away from my partner and children for an extended period.
- I've been asked to sing a piece that is taxing on my voice, but I really need the money right now.
- The opera company is always pointing out that I will need to lose weight in order to get better parts, but I've been struggling with my weight my whole life and I don't think this kind of pressure is healthy for me.
- My teacher is coming on to me, and I'm disgusted, but I'm worried about what rejecting him will mean for my career.

Conflicts like these arise in any profession, but they are probably more common in a singing career because of the sense that in order to survive one must make extraordinary compromises. There is no clear road map that reveals what is worth the compromise and what is not. But for your inner sense of wellness, it is important to consider your priorities and consciously answer questions about what you are willing to do for your singing career. Talking it through with family, a trusted friend, a mentor, or a psychotherapist can be helpful. The goal is to be at peace with your decisions, with yourself, and with what's around you.

Avoiding Burnout

Singing is a profession where a high level of skill, discipline, and training is often "rewarded" by low pay, poor treatment, and a sense of expendability. Moreover, professional singers typically need to promote themselves to get gigs and deal with long periods of unemployment, lack of health insurance, low job security, and a periodic need to move to a new city or country for a stint. At least some of these qualities may be exciting (travel, and the "thrill of the chase"), but they can also feel demoralizing and lead to burnout. If you are feeling burnt out, it is time to consider ways of coping with the stress and restoring balance. Exercise, mediation, breathing techniques, yoga, taking time for leisure, and socializing may all be helpful in managing stress. Psychotherapy may also be extremely valuable for centering yourself and examining your life goals.

Issues of Body Image and Aging

On leaving her performing career, a middle-aged cabaret singer once told me, "What a relief it is to not have to worry about my appearance, and now I feel I can age like everyone else!" Whether you are singing opera or rap, whether you are young or old, whether you are man or woman, it may feel—and may, to a varying extent, be the reality—that success rides not only on your voice and talent but also on your looks and youth. For many, it is stressful to be judged on appearance. Singers often spend considerable time wondering if their successes and failures have to do with their physical presentation, and so they may feel burdened by concerns about attractiveness, imperfections, youthfulness, weight, and clothes. It can feel maddening, cheapening, and anxiety-provoking. In their more benign forms, these concerns can consume time energy and money; but in the extreme, they may contribute to life-threatening conditions such as eating disorders or body dysmorphic disorder (a disabling preoccupation with a slight or imagined defect in one's appearance).

Even Stardom Has Its Perils

You may assume that once success comes, it is all smooth sailing. There is no doubt that success can alleviate many stresses, especially in the areas of finance, job security, and autonomy. But making it big does have its own challenges. And these challenges mount as one enters the realm of stardom. With great success, some people find themselves subject to great fluctuations in sense of self, and they may have crises in their marriages, friendships, and identity. Others may treat you differently because they objectify you, are intimidated, or assume you need your privacy. Paradoxically, stardom may lead to loneliness and isolation. Also lost may be your sense of privacy, freedom of mobility, and perceived safety. And it is often the situation that singers and other artists are in the public eye one day and then abandoned the next, again leading to a rollercoaster ride for the psyche. David Giles wrote about these issues in *Illusions of Immortality: A Psychology of Fame and Celebrity*.

The Decision to Exit the Stage

Some singers sing for a lifetime, but many others decide to stop, whether at age twenty or sixty, to pursue other endeavors. In any profession, people change careers, but it is probably a more common experience for singers and other musicians thanks to the many unique challenges posed by a musical career. Singers may shift to music-related endeavors (say, conducting or teaching), or they may leave music altogether. Regardless, leaving singing may involve feelings of sadness and disappointment at putting aside a passion, or at least putting away something in which one has invested sweat and tears. Common expressions of anxiety about making a change include "I don't have any other marketable skills," "There's nothing else I feel as passionate about," and "How am I going to go back to school at my age?" There may also be the possibility that the decision to exit brings a sense of tremendous relief and rebirth. When making such a change, it is natural to feel a combination of sadness and relief. But if you are overly wrought with feelings of self-blame, failure, and depression, it would be helpful to seek psychotherapy to ease a difficult life transition and explore its unique significance for you.

When to Seek Help

Psychotherapy can be an extremely helpful approach to resolving any of the questions and stresses discussed here. You need not feel that life has become completely unmanageable, in order to benefit from psychotherapy. In fact, psychotherapy can be an enriching experience that may well help free up your full voice as a singer. After all, singing is a challenging combination of control and letting go.

There are also certain situations when it is absolutely essential that a person seek professional help. Here is a list that, even if not exhaustive, highlights a few of the more common treatment-necessitating conditions that a singer may face:

- Concerns about eating and body dysmorphic disorder
- Alcohol and drug problems
- Depression and bipolar disorder
- Severe anxiety
- Difficulties with emotional regulation (sometimes related to abuse or trauma)

Discussion of these conditions is beyond the scope of this chapter. A useful U.S. website for reliable and unbiased information on illnesses and medications (including herbal medicines) is Medlineplus (www.nlm.nih.gov). Run by the National Library of Medicine and National Institutes of Health, it is an enormous site, which includes a medical dictionary and encyclopedia as well as directories of doctors and clinics. It also has links to other medical sites. More information on substance abuse can be accessed at www.drugabuse.gov (the National Institute on Drug Abuse).

How to Seek Help

First there is the question of choosing the "right" psychotherapy. Over the decades there has been a proliferation of types, such that today therapists themselves are hard-pressed to describe how their colleagues work. In reality, many practice an eclectic type of therapy (and even use the term "eclectic" when asked to describe their approach), and the practices found among therapists have more commonalities than differences. The two biggest traditions in psychotherapy are *psychodynamic* psychotherapy and *cognitive behavioral* psychotherapy (CBT). Psychodynamic psychotherapy has roots in the field of psychoanalysis, originated by Sigmund Freud and further elaborated by thinkers over the last 120 years. Psychodynamic psychotherapy explores feelings about oneself and others within relationships past and present (including within the psychotherapy relationship, a concept termed *transference*), with the goal of identifying unconscious conflicts, motivations, defenses, and wishes. By bringing the unconscious into awareness, one can become more flexible and fulfilled in love and work.

CBT is a more recent form of psychotherapy. It is an approach that focuses on identifying and challenging negative assumptions about oneself in the world, with the goal of improving mood and functioning.

Studies have attempted to determine the relative effectiveness of a number of types of psychotherapies, but the "active ingredient" in good psychotherapy remains elusive. It is very likely that a variety of psychotherapies are effective and that the most important goal is finding a therapist with whom you are able to build a constructive therapeutic relationship. And as long as the therapist is professionally trained, you need not be overly concerned by credentials: in the United States psychiatrists (MDs), psychologists (usually PhDs or PsyDs), nurse practitioners (NPs), and social workers (usually MSWs) practice psychotherapy. Only psychiatrists and nurse practitioners have the training and license to prescribe medication. Before you choose a therapist, it is wise to meet with a therapist or two, and then don't be afraid to trust your gut in making your choice.

The second challenge is accessing *affordable* mental health care. If you are fortunate enough to have insurance or adequate funds, then seeing a recommended private practitioner is usually the best option. (Note that in some locations there are clinicians who do not participate in insurance panels.)

Alternatively, if you have limited or no health insurance, there are some tricks to getting low-cost psychotherapy or psychiatric services. Larger cities have university-based psychology departments as well as independent psychoanalytic institutes where you can get psychotherapy for a low fee. There are also psychiatry departments within major medical centers where low-fee psychotherapy *and* psychiatric services (such as medication) are available. Most of these clinics have information online for scheduling an intake.

A third, last-resort option for medication and sometimes psychotherapy is to consider participating in a clinical research trial. In the United States all clinical trials are registered at www.clinicaltrials.gov, where you may search by medication, disorder, and geographic area for trials that are recruiting volunteers. You need not feel too much like a guinea pig, as clinical studies must pass stringent ethical guidelines and help subjects find effective treatment if a subject is not benefiting from a particular research protocol. Finally, if you have difficulty affording medications it is often possible to solicit medication directly from a pharmaceutical company on the basis of need. The relevant applications can be accessed through the website www.needymeds.org.

Distinct from treatment, but also potentially extremely helpful, are support groups. It may be possible to find support groups for singers and other musicians in some localities. Then there are illness-based support groups: for depression and bipolar disorder, check out www.dbsalliance.org; for other severe mental illnesses, see www.nami.org; and for twelve-step-based addiction support groups, see sites such as www.aa.org, www.na.org, and www.ca.org.

A Final Thought

For any pursuit, the truest satisfaction can be discovered in the *process* rather than in the ever-elusive final *result*. In singing, this may entail learning to find pleasure or meaning in every sung verse. If you are able to strive toward this sort of engagement, fulfillment will be yours no matter where the music leads.

23

The Alexander Technique for Singers

PEDRO DE ALCANTARA

Frederick Matthias Alexander was born in Tasmania, an island off the coast of Australia, in 1869. In 1904 he emigrated permanently to London, where he died in 1955. In his late teens, Alexander decided to become a professional actor. Despite his many talents, he tended to become hoarse and lose his voice on stage. He consulted medical experts and singing teachers, whose first advice was simple: "Rest your voice." As long as he spoke little or not at all, his voice was indeed fine. But if he recited for any length of time, he became hoarse again. The second advice he received from his doctors was as simple as the first: "You might try an operation." Alexander was far from persuaded. "Would the operation solve my vocal problems once and for all?" "We don't know," his doctors said. Alexander then did something revolutionary for a young man in Tasmania at the end of the nineteenth century. He decided to ignore the authorities' advice and find out for himself what was causing his problems.

Alexander's Discoveries

He watched himself in front of several mirrors, speaking, reciting, and moving, until he began to discern certain patterns. He gasped for air whenever he took a breath, pulling his head back and down and depressing his larynx. But when he directed his head forward and up, his vocal problems disappeared, and the coordination of his whole body improved as well. He had stumbled upon a great discovery: The relationship among the head, the neck, and the top of the back works as a kind of "primary control" in coordination, movement, posture, and behavior. Observe a baby taking her first steps: it's only when she finds the poise of her head and neck that she manages to keep her balance and walk.

Sing a short melody using your habitual posture. Now pull your head back in space, scrunching the neck. Sing the same few notes as before, and the quality of your voice will be significantly altered. This demonstrates that an "abnormal" position of the head and neck affects the voice negatively. Just as you can go from this abnormal position back to normal, however, you can progress beyond the normal position to an ideal poise of the head and neck, thanks to which you'll find the ideal state for your whole body and for your voice as well.

Body and Mind

While working through his vocal problems, Alexander remained well coordinated at rest, but the moment he decided to speak or recite, his old habits asserted themselves. In time, he understood that the problem was not so much in what he did but in what he *intended* to do. As long as he held on to a fixed goal or end, he would misuse himself and damage his voice. He called this "endgaining," and he realized he needed to give up on his intended goals and let a new identity emerge, one based on different decisions, choices, and gestures.

The interaction of body and mind is intimate and constant. You can't access those energies of yours that you normally call "physical" without engaging those that you normally call "mental." The most banal physical gestures from daily life—brushing your teeth, for instance—contain depths of psychological and emotional content. Suppose you direct your head and neck in a new way, and your voice vibrates more freely as a result. How do you react to your new voice? This isn't the habitual voice you've used for speaking and singing over years and decades. Most likely you'll perceive the new voice as a threat to your sense of self.

Changes in coordination and posture are synonymous with changes in personality and character; changes in vocal technique are synonymous with changes in aesthetics. Alexander considered that our daily task was not to use our bodies well, but to react intelligently and constructively to a given situation. To our overall manner of reacting, he gave the name "the use of the self."

Nondoing

A singing teacher gives you a suggestion or a bit of feedback. If you act immediately and habitually, you risk engaging in patterns of eagerness, hesitation, anger, doubt, and so on. By endgaining, you might not even hear the suggestion altogether! At all times, we need to be able to "do nothing," that is, not act in the old, habitual manner. To do nothing means to become able to choose among many possibilities: many reactions, many sounds, many interpretations, many phrasings, many ways of interpreting whole roles. . . . From that space where you do nothing, an adaptive response arises: you try your teacher's suggestion, or you consider the feedback without dismissing it at once or embracing it slavishly.

Ask your accompanist to play the piano part to something you are working on. Listen to the whole piece from beginning to end, without singing, humming, or mouthing the words, without trying to figure anything out, without responding to spots that you consider difficult or challenging, without getting excited or depressed. If you suspend all these reactions, you'll sense the sounds, rhythms, and bass lines much more clearly than you would otherwise. Then this listening function, receptive and nonjudgmental, can inform your actions when you rehearse and perform. In short, you "act" better if you know how "not to act." This applies to all experiences: taking singing lessons, practicing, rehearsing, performing, and everything else in your daily life. It's not a matter of becoming passive, but becoming ready: ready not to act, and ready to act in a thousand ways at a moment's notice.

Alexander named the capacity not to act "inhibition" (meaning the contrary of "excitation," rather than the common meaning of "suppressed emotion"). Since the orientation of the head, neck, and upper back affects the coordination of the whole body, a good way of inhibiting your habitual misuses is by becoming attuned to your primary control. Every decision from your will passes through the conduit of the primary control and determines how you act and react. To inhibit means to keep the conduit free, so that your decisions can flow unimpeded from will to action—or nonaction, as the case may be.

Energy and Direction

With the help of a partner, do this exercise. Stand and lift an arm, as if to hail a taxi. Have your partner gently hold your arm with both hands. Without changing the arm's position, imagine that the arm becomes heavy, then light; long, then short; stiff, then supple. Most likely your partner will report significant changes in how your arm behaves. These qualities of heaviness, lightness, contraction, and expansion, which are wholly independent of positions in space, represent types of energy at your disposal. Pouring from your imagination and irrigating the body, so to speak, these energies inform every one of your actions. You can energize every single body part, and you can energize different body parts in parallel, opposing, or complementary ways.

Alexander teachers often use verbal formulations to help these "nondoing energies" irrigate the body. One such formulation is, "Let the neck be free, to let the head go forward and up, to let the back lengthen and wide, all together, one after the other." Repeating formulations mechanically won't energize the body—and might even hinder it. But infusing the formulations (be they spoken or silent) with rhythm, meaning, and kinesthetic feeling will turn them into triggers for energy flow or "direction," as Alexander teachers call it. Some teachers believe that specific verbal formulations are fundamental in getting the energies flowing, while others use visual, tactile, or similar means.

The voice itself is a form of energy, emanating from your body and propagating all around you in the form of oscillating waves. Just as you can make your arm heavy or light, long or short, you can make your voice heavy, light, expansive, contracted, diffuse, condensed, warm, cold, and so on. Learn to "direct" your voice by generating, holding, gathering, projecting, or otherwise employing your innate energies. The better you become at directing your whole self, the better you'll direct your voice.

Imagine a magnet pulling your head heavenward, and another magnet pulling your coccyx earthward. Your body might respond to these imaginary magnets by lengthening in opposite directions. Attune yourself to the principle of "oppositional forces," and you'll stabilize and strengthen your body with no muscular effort. Gravity provides a permanent downward pull, and your directions and energies counter it with a permanent upward thrust. Create oppositions within yourself—for instance, by pointing the head in one direction and the back in another, or by pointing your elbows away from your shoulders or your wrists away from your elbows. Establish oppositional pulls within the face by directing your cheeks up and out and your jaw forward and down. When balanced, these oppositions energize the face and facilitate the work of lips, tongue, and jaw. Look at a young child smiling in happiness: her face is lit with muscular oppositions, and yet she isn't tense in any way.

The voice itself is made of oppositions. If the vocal folds don't oppose the breath to some degree, there can be no sound. The very muscles involved in phonation create antagonistic actions, one muscle opposing another within the larynx and throughout the vocal mechanism. Your task as a singer, then, is not to become totally relaxed but to balance out all the tensions and energies that your voice requires to be strong and free.

Faulty Sensory Awareness

Your pianist rushes, but she's sure she doesn't. Your tenor sings flat but swears he is perfectly in tune. Your conductor gives a wildly confusing upbeat, but claims to be as clear as day. Very often there's a gap between what we're doing and what we *feel* we're doing—a universal phenomenon Alexander called "faulty sensory awareness." You can observe the phenomenon in others, but because of its very nature you might not notice it in yourself until you hear a recording of your voice or watch yourself on video.

If you misuse yourself—that is, if your body is out of whack, or if body and mind don't quite work together, or if you're not fully present in the moment—you're likely to misread information, receive it in an incomplete and distorted manner, and interpret it through a filter of assumptions, fears, and desires.

Proprioceptors are nerve endings in muscles, tendons, and joints that allow the body to sense itself, as it were. They help you monitor your position in space, movement, balance, tension, effort, and so on. The neck is particularly rich in proprioceptors. If you stiffen your neck and misdirect your primary control, it's only logical for you not to perceive yourself accurately. By the same token, freeing your neck will help you develop your sensory awareness and narrow the gap between what you do and what you feel that you're doing.

To be sure of yourself when the facts stand in contradiction to your certainty is destructive. But being insecure in your thoughts and gestures is just as counterproductive. A good solution to the conundrum of faulty sensory awareness is to embrace uncertainty at the outset, and then act with confidence. ("I've been wrong in the past and I'll be wrong again in the future, but this is how I see it right now.") Having acknowledged the possibility of being wrong, you act with clarity and conviction. If it turns out that you're wrong in some way, change your mind and start the cycle of "acknowledged uncertainty, forthright action" all over again.

Breathing

Early on in his teaching career, Alexander was known as "the breathing man," as his students routinely overcame plenty of breathing difficulties. Yet not only did he pay little attention to breathing itself, he discouraged his students from doing so too.

Cross your arms tightly in front of the chest, raise your shoulders, and collapse your head and neck downward. If you stay too long in this position, you risk suffocating. Now straighten up and assume your everyday posture. What happens to your breathing?

Breathing is a function of coordination: you breathe as you coordinate yourself. The posture I invited you to assume is "abnormal" and leads to an abnormal and unhealthy breathing pattern. Your postures in daily life are "normal" and lead to normal breathing patterns. Logically enough, ideal postures lead to ideal breathing patterns. Since your postures are inseparable from your attitudes, breathing is in effect a function of how you use yourself, or how you react to every situation in your life. Don't lose your head, and you won't lose your breath. In other words, react constructively and you'll breathe freely.

Do another experiment with a partner. Smile gently, open your mouth, and whisper the vowel "ah" quietly. Then close your mouth and let air come in through your nostrils. What happens to your body in the process? Your partner might tell you that you collapse your spine when you whisper the vowel and pull your head back and down when you inhale. Now point your head gently heavenward and your coccyx earthward, keep your spine elongated and still, and perform the exercise again. What happens to the whispered "ah" and to the inspiration that follows it? They both become stronger and easier.

Air rushes into every open space as the result of atmospheric pressure. If you expand your thorax by letting your ribs move, you create a space inside your body that is automatically filled with air. You need never "take a breath," since the breath takes itself! The difficulty lies in *letting* the ribs move, instead of *making* them move. Direct your primary control and establish an opposition of forces throughout your body, and consider most of your work done.

In Conclusion

The art of living lies in knowing how to react in every situation, or how to "use yourself." The source of your difficulties lies not in what you do but in your end-gaining, when you hew rigidly to disorderly intentions and goals. Make room for the new by non-doing the old, or inhibiting it. Good coordination requires not relaxation but a balance of opposing tensions, energies, and directions. Navigate faulty sensory awareness by acknowledging your uncertainties even as you work confidently. Don't lose your head, and you won't lose your breath or your voice.

Readings

Frederick Matthias Alexander, *The Use of the Self* (London: Orion, 2001; first published in 1932).
Pedro de Alcantara, *Indirect Procedures: A Musician's Guide to the Alexander Technique* (Oxford: Clarendon Press, 1997).
Jane Ruby Heirich, *Voice and the Alexander Technique* (Berkeley: Mornum Time Press, 2005).

Resources

American Society for the Alexander Technique (AmSAT), www.amsat.ws.
Canadian Society for Teachers of the F. M. Alexander Technique (CanSTAT), www.canstat.ca.
Society of Teachers of the Alexander Technique (STAT, United Kingdom), www.stat.org.uk.

There are national organizations for the Alexander Technique in many other countries. You can access them through links in these same sites.

24

Eastern Philosophy

Practical Implications for the Singer

STEVEN K. H. AUNG, MD, OMD, PHD, FAAFP, CM

To better understand the practical implications of Eastern philosophy for professional singers, it is crucial that we carefully define which areas would be most helpful. By briefly examining practical implications in terms of self-knowledge; focus; equanimity; maximal performance; being in the present; and healing, loving kindness, humility, and gentleness, we will hopefully provide professional singers with relevant insights.

Self-Mastery and Self-Knowledge

A professional singer can learn from Eastern philosophy that if she could *actually* bring all of her talents to a challenge, very little would stand in the way. As the magnificent Sun Tzu said, "Can you imagine what I would do if I could do all I can?"[1] How does one truly bring all of one's natural talent and skill to bear on a problem?

The singer can learn from Eastern philosophy that even though he may *like* praise and *fear* criticism, he creates the most autonomy by living for neither, because to be dependent on either can be dangerous. Eastern philosophy can remind us to *listen* very carefully to our intuition or inner voice. Our inner wisdom can be infinitely more on target than we often give it credit for. This inner voice can often capture things far sooner and more accurately than intellect does alone. Eastern philosophy can help us appreciate that if we can imaginatively grasp what things are about in their earliest stages, then it might be possible to begin creating things of great merit. Lao Tzu stated, "To see things in the seed is genius."[2] This is, of course, far easier said than done.

Focus

By limiting our attention to one small piece or by compartmentalizing, we can make the seemingly overwhelming manageable and nonthreatening. Nothing is unmanageable or beyond understanding when broken down into appropriate parts. Eastern philosophy is helpful in reminding us of this.

Respond rather than react. Eastern philosophy reminds us that it is hard to be focused on a challenge when we are in a highly reactive state. If we can tone down how we experience something, by responding instead of reacting, we greatly increase the odds of dealing with something quite handily.

Practice, practice, practice as if you were a monk in a temple learning a national martial art. Or perhaps the Western equivalent is as mentioned by Abraham Lincoln and others: prepare, prepare, prepare. Appropriate practice or preparation can do wonders for making it easier for the singer to focus on the performance *and* enjoy the moment in all its beauty. Although Eastern philosophies certainly do not hold a monopoly on the idea of practice or preparation, there is definitely *deep* appreciation for them. There is an element of acceptance; it is necessary, and without this discipline the whole undertaking is at best diminished.

Eastern philosophy reminds us that we need to be focused throughout the entire endeavor. It only takes a moment of inattention to destroy an entire song, performance, or work. There is an unfortunate human tendency, on seeing the finish line, to just let up, and then instead of succeeding one fails, sometimes even quite miserably. In Eastern philosophy there is an appreciation that humans can invest remarkable effort, energy, and time in pursuing goals, but they can still fail, despite being tantalizingly close to succeeding. It is really quite sad, and certainly a tremendous waste. If singers were more aware of this tendency, they might more likely avoid it.

In Eastern philosophy everything may be considered a little dot . . . and a little dot can be everything. It is useful to focus and to make this so intense that it becomes crystal-like. This is called by a Hindi name, *Samathi*. Deep Samathi represents a whole person *and* the entire universe. The concept of Samathi is reflected in modern computer design, with chips that have become ever smaller and yet ever more potent. To elevate focus to the next level of intensity, the professional singer may also use Samathi.

Equanimity

Lao Tzu said, "Nothing is softer or more flexible than water, yet nothing can resist it."[3] Like water, you as a performer can learn to be supremely adaptable, while having remarkable mental toughness that can carry you through any situation. Learning how to be flexible will help you be resilient in the face of what to others would seem like crushing circumstances. In Chinese thinking, bamboo has come to symbolize this characteristic: it bends easily, but it cannot be broken. Contrary to many commonly held Western stereotypes, having the ability to adapt or change shapes makes one stronger, not more vulnerable.

To truly be able to weather the public attention, scrutiny, and (for some) almost perversely intense public fascination, a professional singer needs to learn how to deal with enormous stress.

This pressure is bound to be multiplied tenfold during performance, especially a live show. Eastern philosophy can help the professional singer develop balance and equilibrium so that it is easier to face a performance with less stress and far more ease.

Eastern philosophy would tend to view the professional singer holistically and as a complete person. If the singer can *truly* love another person and be loved by someone, she will tap into a potentially inexhaustible source of power, strength, and courage. This force of life (love) will serve her extraordinarily well when she performs. Eastern philosophy recognizes that a professional singer who feels unloved, disconnected, and in love with no one is much more likely to be a person who is vulnerable to the ravages of loneliness, or its sinister cousins depression and addiction.

To have grace under pressure, the professional singer can learn from the Eastern philosophical emphasis on function and control being inextricably wrapped up with physiological harmony. If the throat, tongue, vocal folds, and other primary structures producing a singing voice are *not* working in perfect harmony, or if even one of the key structures is impaired, then the singer's performance will suffer.

Maximal Performance

Lao Tzu stated, "The snow goose need not bathe to make itself white. Neither need you do anything but be yourself."[4] Use this idea as a guiding principle: that you will be the greatest and most arresting professional singer possible by being you. Only by being you can you be at your best.

Eastern philosophy teaches us that life may present many challenges and surprises. The trick is not to impose one's desires on reality, but rather to accept it in a way that makes sense. By going with the flow of these challenges, one can maximize performance given the circumstances. By fighting realities, we exhaust ourselves and inevitably undermine performance, without touching the other realities that are disturbing us.[5]

Learning to maximize performance is certainly an area that Eastern philosophies can be helpful with. There is the notion in Eastern philosophy that one can get better results by being more relaxed, at ease, or in a flow . . . rather than just trying, harder and harder, more and more. This is quite similar to some of the highly successful techniques used in sports psychology to help athletes be focused—trying, of course, but above all being in tune with flow and absolutely at ease.

Eastern philosophy can help the professional singer value being *patient*, and this can pay huge dividends. By acknowledging that many human endeavors start with small steps and only later grow to become huge undertakings, singers will benefit from this in their own performances. This may be used to balance the omnipresent perfectionistic, workaholic, obsessive-compulsive, or driven behaviors that characterize some professional singers.

For optimal performance, the singer has to have body, mind, and spirit in good alignment. Having a beautiful voice physically is of course important, but also mentally the singer has to be able to connect with the audience. On a spiritual level, the singer ideally needs to make the audience feel joy and be healed and free of emotional burdens.

Being in the Present

Like Guan Yin Tzu, the professional singer cannot waste precious attention by thinking about possible successes or failures, but instead must be completely in the present activity . . . the present moment of performance.[6] With freethinking and having a mind at ease, it will be much simpler for the professional singer to *do what he is doing.*

A professional singer always needs to be aware of being in the moment. Eastern philosophy may be used to enhance lung capacity so that a performance is more natural and efficient. This sense of physical ease tends to translate into the singer being totally immersed in the present, in the performance. By being in the moment, he or she can interact better with the audience. This creates more happiness, relaxation, excitement, and peace. In many performances, the singer and the audience are continuously exchanging healing energy and improving the whole positive energy in the auditorium.

Healing, Loving Kindness, Humility, and Gentleness

An individual singer may have a voice that is gentle yet powerful enough to have a healing effect on the heart and soul of audience members. The singer can also help the listeners release stress and tension. The job of a singer is not only to entertain but also to play a major role in healing people. Singing with loving kindness is quite different from singing solely to entertain. A singer who has genuine loving kindness can ease the impact of disease, illness, suffering, or loss. *Ideally*, all singers ought to have a healing voice.

Eastern philosophy can help singers understand it is a *strength* to admit they do not know or understand something. Unfortunately, some people may be totally unwilling to admit they really do not grasp something, or even know that it exists. This humility before truth(s) ultimately serves the singer and others well. Eastern philosophy may help professional singers cultivate an awareness that is kinder and gentler.

Conclusion

In Eastern philosophy, the Yin and the Yang have to be balanced. This concept of balance has profound implications for professional singers. A singer has to find balance between his or her life as an entertainer and personal life. Part of this balance may be found in learning to appreciate nature.

In addition to Yin and Yang, balance, and nature, professional singers may find it helpful to consider the five elements of personality in Eastern philosophy. Although the framework for five elements is certainly different from Western thought, singers unfamiliar with it may find it helpful to think about concepts from popular psychology, such as introversion and extroversion, astrological types, or sibling birth order types.[7] We are not saying they are the same thing, but the five-elements approach will likely seem more accessible if a singer realizes it is not so far removed from things that most of us already have some familiarity with.

Every singer has a personality type that can be defined in terms of five elements: wood, fire, water, earth, and metal. Some singers may be metal-type personalities and would like to have everything very precise and accurate. Some singers may be water-type personalities and would tend to be very flexible and easygoing. Some singers may be wood-type personalities, tending to appreciate or focus on nature.

Generally singers who share a five-element personality type tend to associate with one another and be comfortable working together. Some singers may have difficulty and feel very uncomfortable working together if their types are not a good match. Generally, *all* of a singer's emotions are associated with what type of five-0element personality he or she has.

In Eastern philosophy, the *heart* is viewed as the ultimate source of *spirit*. Within Eastern philosophy, singing is considered to be from the heart. Indeed, singing is of a very spiritual nature.

It is well known that anatomical and physiological explanations are notoriously inadequate in revealing why one singing voice sounds like Aretha Franklin's and another person's singing voice is quite shabby.

Suggested Reading

Aung, Steven K. H. "The 'Pearls' of Medical Acupuncture: Six Vital Energetic (Qi) Alignment Procedures." *La revue française de médecine traditionelle chinoise,* 168 (1995): 203–207.

Aung, Steven K. H. "Loving Kindness—The Essential Buddhist Contribution to Primary Care." *Humane Health Care International,* 12 (1996): 81–84.

Aung, Steven K. H. "Traditional Chinese Medicine: Physical, Mental and Spiritual Approaches." *South African Journal of Natural Medicine,* 4 (2001): 26, 27, 59.

Aung, Steven K. H. www.aung.com.

Cohen, Kenneth S. *The Way of Qigong: The Art and Science of Chinese Energy Healing.* Foreword by Larry Dossey. New York: Ballantine, 1997.

Davies, D. Garfield, and Jahn, Anthony F. *Care of the Professional Voice: A Guide to Voice Management for Singers, Actors and Professional Voice Users.* 2nd ed. New York: Routledge (Theater Arts Book), 2005.

Gardner-Gordon, Joy. *The Healing Voice: Traditional and Contemporary Toning, Chanting, and Singing.* Freedom, CA: Crossing Press, 1993.

Gaynor, Mitchell L. *The Healing Power of Sound: Recovery from Life-Threatening Illness Using Sound, Voice, and Music.* Boston: Shambhala, 2002.

Gimbel, Theo. *Form, Sound, Colour, and Healing.* Essex, UK: C. W. Daniel, 1987.

Kaptchuk, T. J. *The Web That Has No Weaver: Understanding Chinese Medicine.* Chicago: Congdon and Weed, 1983.

Liang, Shou-Yu, and Wu, Wen-Ching. *Qigong Empowerment: A Guide to Medical Taoist Buddhist Wushu Energy Cultivation.* Providence, RI: Way of the Dragon, 1997.

Maciocia, G. *The Foundations of Chinese Medicine.* Edinburgh, UK: Churchill Livingstone, 1991.

Motoyama, Hiroshi. *Theories of the Chakras: Bridge to Higher Consciousness.* Wheaton, IL: Theosophical Publishing House, 1988.

National Cancer Institute, National Institutes of Health, Department of Health and Human Services. http://www.cancer.gov.

National Center for Complementary and Alternative Medicine, National Institutes of Health, Department of Health and Human Services. http://nccam.nih.gov/.

Ni, Maoshing. *Secrets of Healing: Harness Nature's Power to Heal Common Ailments, Boost Your Vitality, and Achieve Optimum Wellness*. New York: Avery (Penguin), 2008.

Pike, Geoff, and Pike, Phyllis. *Chi: The Power Within: Chi Kung Breathing Exercises for Health, Relaxation, and Energy*. Pymble, Australia: Bay Books, 1993.

Porkert, M. *The Theoretical Foundations of Chinese Medicine: Systems of Correspondence*. Cambridge, MA: MIT Press, 1974.

Reid, Daniel. *Harnessing the Power of the Universe: A Complete Guide to the Principles and Practice of Chi-Gung*. Illustrations by Dexter Chou. Boston: Shambhala, 1998.

Sohn, Robert C. *Tao and T'ai Chi Kung*. Rochester, VT: Destiny Books, 1989.

Wu, Shen. *Musical Qigong: Ancient Chinese Healing Art from a Modern Master*. Dumont, NJ: Homa & Sekey Books, 2001.

Notes

1. http://www.brainyquote.com/quotes/quotes/s/suntzu382397.html. Quote by Sun Tzu. Viewed December 22, 2008.

2. www.answers.com. Quotes by Lao-Tzu. Viewed November 30, 2008.

3. www.thinkexist.com. Quotes by Lao-Tzu. Viewed December 22, 2008.

4. www.answers.com. Quotes by Lao-Tzu. Viewed November 30, 2008.

5. It is important that this concept be applied only to appropriate matters or issues in life. This thinking must *not* be taken out of context and applied in a manner that signifies the acceptance of evil, amoral or immoral acts, or injustice.

6. http://quotations.about.com/cs/inspirationquotes/a/Focus9.htm. Quote by Guan Yin Tzu, inspirational quotes and the subtopic "focus." Viewed December 22, 2008.

7. For a truly insightful discussion of sibling birth order, we recommend reading *Born to Rebel: Birth Order, Family Dynamics, and Creative Lives* by Frank J. Sulloway.

25

Meditation and Relaxation Techniques

STEVEN K. H. AUNG, MD, OMD, PHD, FAAFP, CM

Singers are engaged in an extraordinary calling. These gifted performers do not only entertain but create a flow of sounds designed and intended to touch the hearts and spirit of an audience. Sound and silence are like yin and yang to the singers' healing arts. If singing is healing, then listening is transformation.

In the course of their professional and personal lives, singers experience many forms of acute and chronic physical and psychological stress. It is also important to emphasize how essential singers' health is for their voices. The effects of nutrition, sleep, weight, and exercise will show in singers' voices over time. The more physically, mentally, and spiritually healthy the singer, the more focused he or she can be on the passion and beauty of the song, rather than the mechanics of vocal production. This chapter is concerned with alleviation of vocal stress, due to the subtle strain of constant use, or of the acute vocal damage of intensive performing. The meditation and relaxation techniques presented in this chapter will help singers thrive.

The Chinese word *Qi* is probably best understood as vital energy. Qi needs to be balanced and in harmony if the body, mind, and spirit are to be in optimal alignment. Techniques such as meditation, qi gong, tai chi chu'an, and yoga may prove useful in improving alignment. Singers may choose to work on these meditation and relaxation techniques individually, or in groups. Individual exercises are best for self-cultivation, while group exercises are well suited to motivation; yet either approach will balance or harmonize vital energy, or Qi.

Meditation

Meditation is a noninvasive, compassionate, and healing-oriented approach to health and wellness. Many people find meditation essential to feeling rejuvenated, reconnected, aligned, revitalized, and deeply relaxed. Meditation is a traditional natural approach to regaining energy, balance, harmony, and equilibrium.

There are many types of meditation, each based on certain techniques. Some use breathing exercises as their primary guide. Others use concentration exercises as the basis of a mental exercise. Meditation can be done while sitting, standing, walking, or running. It typically involves breathing, concentration, or stretching. Meditation is a physical, mental, and spiritual approach to well-being. The mental side of meditation may be used to eliminate emotional contamination. Meditation may also help create a state of therapeutic emptiness, which reduces stress, increases relaxation, and makes it easier to be creative.

Breathing exercises are generally considered the foundation of all meditation. They control the airways and bring about deep tranquility through using the diaphragm. They also help singers focus, develop awareness, and heighten concentration. Breathing exercises increase lung capacity, enhance energy, and enrich vocal quality. Many kinds of breathing exercises variously use chest, abdominal, and nasal types of breathing.

In traditional Chinese medicine (TCM), breathing exercises are the most powerful way to start and regulate the flow of energy through the entire body. Every time humans breathe, energy flows within them. Every time humans cease breathing, energy stops at this specific area. Every time humans breathe out, the energy intensifies at that location. Therefore, breathing exercises are essential in daily living. Singers need to follow proper breathing exercises to enhance energy and strengthen the voice.

Concentration exercises give direction to energy movement in specific areas. This not only enhances the flow of Qi in the body but also provides harmony and balance. There are many types of concentration exercises. Some use the meridians, which connect with the organ systems. Concentration exercises may also help the sound become clearer, more focused, and more distinct. These exercises keep the mind very sharp and clear. Concentration exercises direct Qi to the area that needs to be trained and stimulated. The key component of concentration exercise is to control the mind, so that one can control the body. For the singer it is essential to have good concentration so that energy is directed to the tongue, throat, and lungs. In this way the singer can control the voice according to his or her needs.

Spiritual exercises involve the entire autonomic nervous system, as well as the organs of special sense (vision, hearing, taste, smell, and touch). They may also use Mother Nature or natural settings to enhance the circulation of vital energy (energy that exists on three levels: body, mind, and spirit).

Medical Qi Gong

Qi means energy. *Gong* means ability. Together they mean the ability to build up one's own energy. Qi gong has existed for more than three thousand years, in TCM. Qi gong includes precise breathing, posture, movement, stretching, and concentration exercises. Above all, the objective is to attain balance and alignment in physical, mental, and spiritual energy. With commitment, discipline, and practice, many singers find that integrated practice of qi gong leaves them feeling rejuvenated, relaxed, revitalized, regenerated, and realigned. All singers will benefit from having good Qi or energy.

For our purposes, there are five schools of medical qi gong that we should mention. The Taoist schools are useful for strengthening both mind and body in life and nature. Buddhist schools tend to emphasize cultivation of mental discipline. Confucian schools attempt to calm the mind, so that it is more tranquil and peaceful. Medical schools focus on preventive self-care, wellness, and prolonging life. Finally, boxing schools promote preparedness in the practitioner's self-defense and combat skills.

Medical qi gong is safe, natural, and holistic. Qi gong exercises focus on prevention, self-care, and discipline. To a large extent medical qi gong is based on understanding the flow of energy in the organ and meridian systems of the body. Medical qi gong emphasizes awareness and appreciation of nature. To be effective, medical qi gong needs to be done daily. Responsibility, compassion, and taking care of oneself as well as others are all emphasized. In medical qi gong, healing begins as more harmony is established among body, mind, and spirit.

Qi gong may be divided into several primary constellations of exercises. Breathing exercises are used to initiate Qi or energy through the body. Concentration exercises are used to direct energy to various specific locations in meridians and organs, or the body in general. Movement and posture exercises enhance Qi flow at specific energy centers (chakras), meridians, and organ systems. Phonation exercises are also used to increase Qi at precise energy centers, organ systems, acupoints, and meridians. Color visualization exercises are done to enhance various organ and meridian systems. Mantras are used to enhance deeper concentration and create additional healing energy. Mudras are hand positions, used for better alignment, energy, and concentration.

Qi gong is much more than a seemingly simple set of exercises. Like certain martial arts, yoga, and other health disciplines, qi gong is a way of life that contributes to better health and wellness. It is best done every day.

The four basic breathing exercises (Figure 25.1) help singers develop concentration and improved lung capacity.

These breathing exercises help the singer perform better. At the same time, the exercises give deep relaxation. Breathing exercise number one in the figure is especially useful for lung capacity. Breathing exercise number three is excellent for building up Qi and enhancing immune system functioning.

Concentration exercises direct qi to the appropriate areas and organ systems. There are four basic concentration exercises (Figure 25.2).

For the professional singer, it would be wise to perform the small circle concentration exercises. This exercise serves to enhance concentration, increase energy in the throat and vocal folds, and at the same time improve the capacity of the lungs. The figure eight concentration exercise is helpful for singers' energy, and to enhance immune functions.

Color visualization exercises (Figure 25.3) also help the singer. By stimulating chakras (energy centers), singers can be enhance their abilities.

More specifically, singers should focus on working with the crown chakra (on the top of the head), the throat chakra (in the middle of the throat), and the chest chakra (in the middle of the chest). By stimulating these three energy centers, singers can improve their singing quality. Every organ system has its own characteristic and direct association with a specific color. White is associated with the lungs, yellow is associated with the spleen,

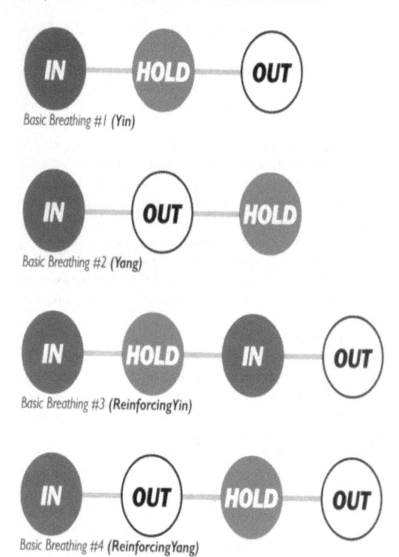

FIGURE 25.1 The Four Basic Breathing Exercises.

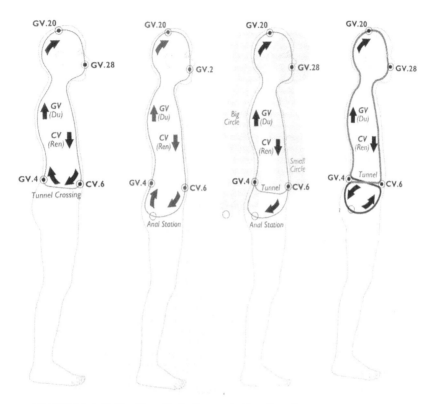

FIGURE 25.2 The Four Basic Concentration Exercises.

green is associated with the liver, and purple is associated with the pericardium. In traditional Chinese medicine, the lung meridian includes the whole vocal tract. Thus, if singers visualize white while meditating, they can improve the capacity of their lungs and throat. It might also be wise for the singer to visualize blue, which is used to enhance the healing of the body.

Phonation exercises (Figure 25.4) enhance specific organ systems and energy centers (chakras).

All of the chakras in the body have corresponding phonation sounds, which enhance their energy. For singers to harmonize

chakra

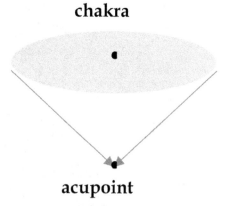

acupoint

FIGURE 25.3 Acupoint and Chakra Comparison: a Chakra is More Powerful than an Acupoint.

their whole body system, it would be wise to produce the "alll" sound. In order to make the vocals strong and clear, the "hammm" sound in the throat energy center is very beneficial. The "yammm" sound in the chest energy center promotes the capacity of the lungs. In addition to phonation for the chakras, all of the organ systems in TCM have corresponding sounds. The "sheee" sound is useful to build capacity for the lung system. The "wooo" sound helps to enhance kidney energy, which is responsible for healing and immune response. Although every singer has a distinct vocal quality, the phonation exercises discussed here will improve the quality of singing, in addition to contributing to overall health and wellness.

Tai Chi Chu'an

Tai chi chu'an (or Tai chi) is a slow-motion, meditationlike exercise. It involves stretching, physical movement, mental aware-

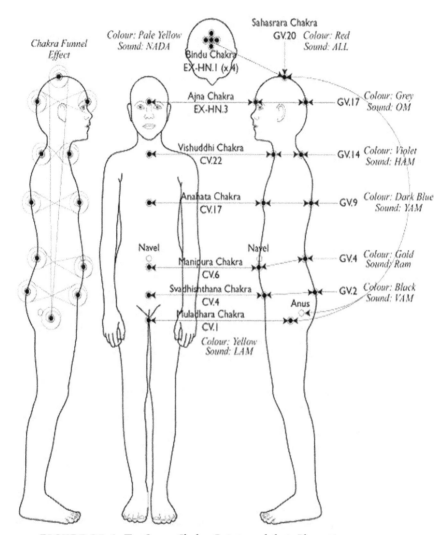

FIGURE 25.4 The Seven Chakra Points and their Phonations.

ness, and spiritual stability. Because of its slow, repetitive nature, it keeps the body balanced and in harmony. Stretching joints helps unblock and maintain energy. Tai chi chu'an has many forms, according to the ancient masters. There are yang, wu, tsun, and Taoist schools, and each has its own style of stretching. Of course, individual styles have their own characteristic movements. Some are softer, whereas others are considered harder or more militant, like a martial art. Tai chi chu'an is very popular outside of China, because it is easy to learn, low in impact, and gentle.

Tai chi chu'an can help build balance in the organ systems very quickly, thanks to the emphasis on stretching and soft, controlled movements. In this way, the body becomes more balanced, because the organ and meridian systems, as energy pathways, have better harmony and better health overall. Lung capacity is also improved by tai chi chu'an exercises, so singers can concentrate on delivering more enriched vocal performance. The quality of slow movement in tai chi chu'an is perfect for bringing about deep relaxation.

With regular practice, tai chi chu'an will balance singers' energy flow to maintain their health and well-being. It only takes twenty to thirty minutes of practice per day for these effects. Given the discipline that singers broadly are capable of following, twenty to thirty minutes is a modest amount of time to invest in the many health and vocal benefits of practicing tai chi chu'an.

The practice of tai chi chu'an will improve singers' physical, mental, and spiritual balance. TCM holds that it is always better to follow a preventive regimen than to have to follow a curative one. Tai chi chu'an can play a very important role in keeping the professional singer healthy, joyful, and functional. As Lao Tzu has it, we should anticipate difficulty by managing the easy.

Conclusion

Meditation, medical qi gong, and tai chi chu'an are all excellent for singers' self-care, responsibility, and motivation. It is important that singers consider these techniques part of their daily regimen of strengthening and relaxation. Every singer should develop a regimen of these activities, as best suited to his or her nature, culture, and temperament.

Suggested Reading

Aung, Steven K. H. "The Vital Importance of the Qigong Tree Hugging Experience and Installation." *Qi: The Journal of Traditional Eastern Health and Fitness*, 15(1) (2005): 36–43.

Aung, Steven K. H., and Lee, M. H. M. "Music, Sounds, Medicine, and Meditation: An Integrative Approach to the Healing Arts." *Alternative and Complementary Therapies*, 10(5) (2004): 266–270.

Aung, Steven K. H. "Qigong Sounds: Medical Therapy Through Phonation." *Journal of Traditional Eastern Health & Fitness*, 11 (2002): 39–46.

Aung, Steven K. H. (1996). The concept of Qi in traditional Chinese medicine: An overview and elucidation. *Journal of the Australian Medical Acupuncture Society*, 14 (1996), 6–13.

Aung, Steven K. H. "A Brief Introduction to the Theory and Practice of Qigong." *American Journal of Acupuncture*, 22 (1994), 335–348.

26

Yoga for Singers

JUDITH E. CARMAN, DMA, RYT

The connections between yoga and singing are many and intimate. Both rest on a foundation of awareness, control, and use
of the breath. Both require control of a strong and flexible body
developed for freedom and endurance. Both demand mental concentration and the ability to coordinate mind and body. Both
lead to knowledge and expression of the soul. Both open the
heart. They are natural partners. This is the foundation of using
the practices of yoga as tools to develop, maintain, and greatly
enhance the art of singing in all its facets: physical technique,
breath control, mental focus, musical flow, expressive communication, and radiant performance.

The philosophy and structure of yoga match the art of singing at almost every point: "Yoga is the control of thought-waves
in the mind" (Yoga Sutra I.2., tr. Prabhavananda and Isherwood).
When the mind can be made still and calm as a clear lake whose
surface is undisturbed by any motion, "then the inner self rests
in its true nature" (Yoga Sutra I.3, paraphrase). This clarity of
mind, which provides accurate perception of things as they are
and leads to union with the higher self, is the goal of all yoga
practices.

To this end, yoga works from the outside in, beginning first with acceptance of five rules of respectful behavior in all relationships (abstaining from violence, falsehood, theft, extreme behavior, and greed) and five principles of relationship to oneself (purity, contentment, self-discipline, study of scriptures, and worship of the Divine). Building on this foundation of ethical behavior and personal growth, a yoga practice includes physical postures (*āsanas*), breathing practices (*prāṇāyāma*), concentration practices, meditation, contemplation, and deep relaxation.

The practices of yoga can be designed specifically for many purposes and activities. The therapeutic benefits of yoga are becoming well known in relation to injury and illness; numerous sports now use yoga as a complementary practice to their particular physical activities. But for no other population is there such a complete match between yoga and specific needs as for singers. Yoga in its purest form is like singing, and singing in its purest form is like yoga.

For the student singer, yoga practices are developmental in nature as well as productive in the areas of self-confidence and performance anxiety. For the working singer, yoga practices can support and continue to refine all the elements of the art of singing, culminating in confident and radiant public performance.

Two important areas of concern for working singers are prevention of accumulated tension, which interferes with ease in singing, and relief from the accumulated stresses encountered in rehearsal, performance, and the vicissitudes of daily life. A basic daily āsana practice consisting of gentle stretching in all positions and directions keeps the body both toned and relaxed. In areas where tension tends to accumulate, such as the jaw, neck, shoulders, or lower back, specific āsana sequences can be designed to prevent the buildup or relieve the effects of these tensions. Developing a keen awareness of specific areas of the body helps the singer relax problem areas at will. This awareness is developed both in mentally focused physical practice and in deep relaxation practices that move combined breath and awareness from point to point throughout the body.

Equally as important, and sometimes more important, is a daily breathing practice (prānāyāma), the techniques of which will vary according to the needs of the moment. There are breathing practices for energy, calmness, balance, and even heating and cooling. Almost all kinds of stress can be relieved to some degree by slow, deep breathing through the nostrils. The exhalation phase of the breath, when slowed as much as possible, is the primary reliever of stress as it calms the nervous system. Daily practice of conscious control of the breath creates the ability to use the breath in whatever way is needed, including singing long legato phrases.

A primary mode of breath practice involves the use of ratio, in which the breath is treated in four separate parts: inhalation, suspension with the lungs full, exhalation, and suspension with the lungs empty. Inhalation and suspension with lungs full are energizing; exhalation and suspension with the lungs empty are calming. Each part of the ratio can be lengthened for development of that part of the breath. Lengthening exhalation (and suspension with lungs empty) develops both the muscular and mental ability to sing long phrases and the ability to calm the nervous system at will.

Working body and breath daily is only one side of the equation. The other side uses what has been developed physically as preparation for working with mind and emotions. Āsana practice conditions the body to sit comfortably. Prānāyāma practices lead to calmness and prepare the mind for concentration. Concentration practices develop the mind's ability to focus on a single point without distraction, by learning to let go of thoughts and emotions that naturally arise, in an unending stream, every waking moment. Singers require this ability to focus solely on *what* they are doing without being distracted by thoughts and feelings that raise questions about *how* they are doing, which often undermine confident performance. This ability can be consciously developed in the yoga practices of concentration.

Beyond the ability to concentrate lies the ability to enter into the inner stillness at the core of every person. "All true artists, whether they know it or not, create from a place of no-mind, from inner stillness," writes Eckhart Tolle. The way into this inner stillness is the practice of meditation, the state of mind that appears following prolonged concentration. The practice of letting go of thoughts and feelings that arise uninvited, of watching them disappear of their own accord, eventually brings the mind to brief moments of stillness and silence. Here is the entrance to our intuition, our inner knowing of the way to live a fearless and balanced life. It is the accumulated effect over time of these brief moments that begins to change resistance into acceptance, reaction into response, fear into confidence. Every singer needs self-acceptance and responsiveness to all situations in order to experience the joy of singing untainted by previous conditioning or present distractions. The practice of meditation has the power to free the mind and emotions from tension and stress and open the singer to the wealth of creative possibilities.

Tension and stress frequently contribute to, and sometimes cause, physical strain and even injury to various parts of the body affected by the complexities of performance. Working on the modern operatic stage is a good example of a sometimes hazardous environment for the singer. In addition to staging that often requires considerable athletic ability (especially for male singers), opera sets can include steep stairs, varying floor levels, and uncomfortably raked stages. The ability to negotiate these areas physically demands a body developed for strength, flexibility, and balance. Yoga postures that strengthen feet and legs, lower back and torso, and shoulders and arms as well as those that keep hips flexible and the neck free to rotate will help prevent injuries that might occur in the course of a particular role.

Equally important is the ability to sing in any position (kneeling, prone, or supine, as well as standing in awkward postures) and to move into and out of that position in character. The practice of yoga postures provides the strength, flexibility, and balance required for these movements.

Another hazard for the working singer is travel, especially by air. After a long flight, it is important to restore circulation in the legs. An excellent yoga posture for this purpose is to lie on the floor with the legs resting straight up against a wall ("Legs up the Wall" Posture) for several minutes.

As bodies age, muscles and joints become less flexible, and connective tissue thins and becomes more vulnerable to injury. At this stage of a career, it is more important than ever to keep all systems in the best possible shape and both sides of the body equally strong. An ongoing complete yoga practice, adjusted to the needs of the particular singer, is possibly the best way to stay in excellent physical and mental health and remain at peak performance ability as long as possible. If illness or injury does occur, an enduring yoga practice will have developed the qualities of body, mind, and spirit that assist greatly in recovery.

Although the examples given here refer to the operatic singer, all performing singers encounter various difficulties and hazards in the course of a career, and all can benefit from the practices of yoga.

In addition to their relevance to the act of singing, yoga practices promote good health on every level: physical, mental, and emotional. The physical postures (āsana) promote stability; smooth function of muscles, tendons, ligaments, and joints; strength; flexibility; balance; and refinement of structural alignment. As all postures are coordinated with the rhythm of the breath, the entire breathing mechanism is expanded and strengthened. Moreover, the many breathing practices (prāṇāyāma) contribute to overall good health, as deeper, fuller, and slower breaths provide full oxygenation of (and reduce stress levels in) the whole system. Taken together, the physical postures and breathing practices promote excellent circulation in all the body systems and strengthen the immune system with regular exercise.

Mentally and emotionally, the concentration and meditation practices are avenues for changing negative thought patterns and, therefore, attitudes and behaviors that obstruct productive and joyful living. Deep relaxation techniques yield the profound rest and clear awareness that are crucial for the health of the entire mind-body system.

A style of yoga that is perfect for singers is *Viniyoga,* in which postures are taught and practiced with a combination of "repetition" and "stay": repeated movement into and out of each posture for warming muscles and promoting flexibility, and "stay" in the posture for building strength and refining alignment. The central focus is always the breath, which is used in specific patterns that are metrical in structure and that correspond closely to the metrical structure of music. In this respect, yoga practice reinforces many of the musical elements of singing. Viniyoga is a complete system of classical yoga practices and contains all of the elements described as being useful to the singer at different stages of a career.

Although this is only an introduction to the value of a regular yoga practice for singers, a few practical tips may be helpful. First, a daily yoga practice should include several physical postures that work the body in all positions (standing, kneeling, prone, supine, and seated; inversions should be practiced only after working directly with a competent teacher) and in all directions (upward extension, forward bending, backward bending, lateral bending, and twisting). It is important to use forward bending postures as the transition between postures that move in differing directions, for example a backward bend and a twist. Three examples of standing postures that are excellent for singers:

1. *Tadāsana* (Straight Tree or Mountain Posture) with arm and heel raises—for spinal extension; opening the chest; loosening the shoulders; deepening inhalation; strengthening the feet, ankles, and calves; and balance (Figure 26.1).

2. *Virabhadrāsana* (Warrior Posture) facing forward with arm variations—for strengthening the postural muscles of the upper back, opening the chest, deepening inhalation, and strengthening and stretching the legs (Figure 26.2).

3. *Parśvottanāsana* (Intense Side Stretch Posture)—a forward bend over one leg at a time, for stretching the hamstrings and greatly strengthening the lower back (Figure 26.3).

There are many postures that can be used to good effect. The important thing is to construct a workable sequence with the help of a book on yoga or a teacher who is also a singer, and then practice and adjust the sequence to fit your particular needs.

Two other postures necessary for the singer are an easy seated posture (*Sukhāsana*, Figure 26.4, or any other comfortable seated posture) for breathing practices, concentration, and meditation; and *Śavāsana* (Corpse Posture), the supine posture for deep relaxation, in which the feet are comfortably apart, arms slightly away from the torso, palms up, spine straight, and eyes closed.

Two books that give extremely clear information, both written and in photographs, on all the practices helpful to singers are *Yoga for Wellness* and *Yoga for Transformation* by Gary Kraftsow (see "Further Reading"). Two other excellent books are *The Heart of Yoga* by T. K. V. Desicachar and *Yoga: Mastering the Basics* by Sandra Anderson and Rolf Sovik (see "Further Reading").

Specific breathing practices that are very helpful to singers are (1) *Anuloma Ujjāyī* for calming the nervous system, (2) *Viloma*

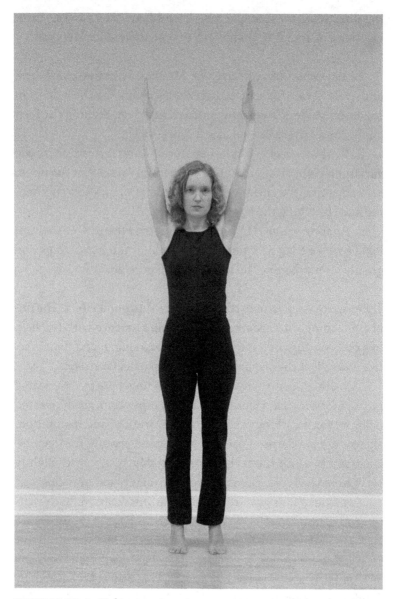

FIGURE 26.1 *Tadāsana*

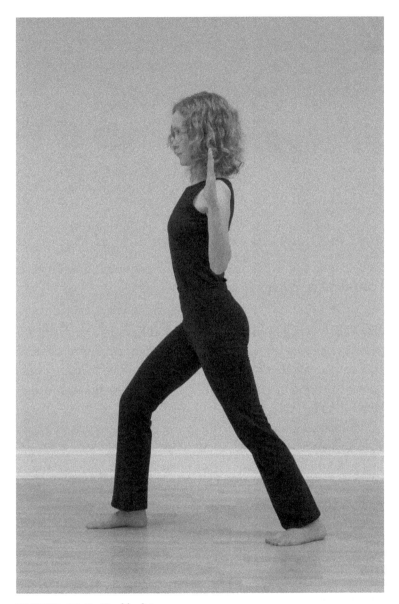

FIGURE 26.2 *Virabhadrāsana*

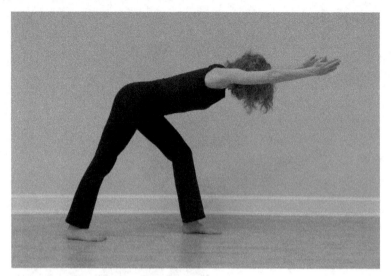

FIGURE 26.3 *Parśvottanāsana*

Ujjāyī for increasing energy, and (3) *Nadi Śodhana Prānāyāma* for restoring a sense of balance to the body and mind. Any concentration practice that uses the breath as a mental focus not only quiets the mind but continually reinforces the singer's relationship to the breath.

Maintaining a yoga practice on tour is not easy, but it pays rich dividends in stress reduction and a sense of overall well-being. Beginning the day with a complete yoga practice goes a long way toward having a productive and satisfying day. Three DVDs under the collective title *YogaAway* ("the workout: feeling great again" for strength, "finding focus: feeling clarity of mind" for concentration, and "stress reduction: feeling at home" for relaxation), originally designed for traveling business people who stay frequently in hotels, are an excellent source of help for singers on tour.

For special needs of the lower back and sacrum and the upper back, neck, and shoulders, Gary Kraftsow's DVDs of practices for

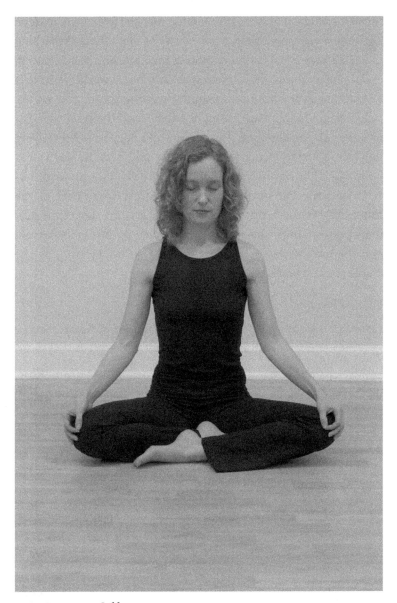

FIGURE 26.4 *Sukhāsana*

these areas are highly recommended. For performance anxiety, nothing brings greater relief and clarity of mind than a breathing practice followed by concentration or meditation, and relaxation.

In our increasingly technological and noisy world—where it seems that everything is constantly gaining speed, and we are called on to do more and more in what is still the same amount of time—the ancient practices of yoga fill a deep need for slowing down and experiencing inner stillness and silence. The mind-body system is naturally resilient if given a chance to restore itself regularly. The practices of yoga address every part of the mind-body complex that the singer uses all at the same time during a performance. The act of singing engages the whole person, and the practices of yoga complement that act by training the whole person: body, breath, mind, and spirit.

Further Reading

Anderson, Sandra, and Rolf Sovik. *Yoga: Mastering the Basics.* Honesdale, PA: Himalayan Institute, 2000. Very clear exposition of the full range of yoga practice; excellent photographs of poses.

Carman, Judith E. "Yoga and Singing: Natural Partners." NATS *Journal of Singing* 60, no. 5 (2004): 433–441. An article detailing the advantages of the practice of yoga for voice students.

Desicachar, T. K. V. *The Heart of Yoga: Developing a Personal Practice.* Rochester, VT: Inner Traditions International, 1995, 1999. A wonderful book by the son of Krishnamacharya, the Indian yoga teacher who fathered most of the schools of yoga taught in the West today, presenting a complete approach to practicing yoga.

Kraftsow, Gary. *Yoga for Wellness.* New York: Penguin Compass, 1999. The basic textbook of the American Viniyoga Institute, an excellent resource with more than one thousand photographs.

———. *Yoga for Transformation.* New York: Penguin Compass, 2002. A superior text that illuminates yoga beyond āsana—those aspects of yoga that promote transformation of the whole person on all levels.

———. *Viniyoga Therapy for the Low Back, Sacrum and Hips.* DVD. Pranamaya (www.pranamaya.com), 2007.

————. *Viniyoga Therapy for the Upper Back, Neck and Shoulders.* DVD. Pranamaya (www.pranamaya.com), 2007.

Prabhavananda, Swami, and Christopher Isherwood (trans. and commentary). *How to Know God: The Yoga Aphorisms of Patanjali.* Hollywood, CA: Vedanta Press, 1953, 1981.

Tolle, Eckhart. *The Power of Now.* Novato, CA: New World Library, 1999.

YogaAway. the Workout: Feeling Great Again. Strength. YogaAway (www.yogaaway.com) 2006.

YogaAway. Finding Focus: Feeling Clarity of Mind. Concentration. Yoga-Away, 2006.

YogaAway. Stress Reduction: Feeling at Home. Relaxation. YogaAway, 2006.

Yoga Journal. Issues contain many articles with excellent information on various topics.

Yoga + Joyful Living. Published bimonthly by the Himalayan International Institute. An excellent source of information with in-depth articles.

27

Acupuncture for the Vocal Performer

ANTHONY F. JAHN, MD

GERTRUDE KUBIENA, MD

Acupuncture is an ancient form of medical treatment. It consists of modulating the flow of life energy through the body using small needles inserted at specific points.

The practice of acupuncture originated in China thousands of years ago. The exact date is not known, but the oldest acupuncture needles found (thus far) date back to the New Stone Age. Over the ensuing millennia, acupuncture therapy has become increasingly sophisticated, and it has spread from China through the rest of Asia and, over the last century, to the West.

Although acupuncture is the best-known aspect of traditional Chinese medicine (TCM), it is only one of many important branches (see Table 27.1). Two of the most important, meditation/exercise and Chinese herbs, are covered elsewhere in this book. Though seemingly different, all of these treatment methods are connected by a common set of beliefs about health, illness, and life. These beliefs are in turn grounded in the Taoist philosophy, the oldest religious system in China and still active.

TABLE 27.1 Branches of Chinese medicine (TCM)

Acupuncture
Acupressure
Chinese Herbs
Diet and Nutrition
Tuina (Medical Massage)
Meditation (Qi Gong)
Tai Chi

Taoism, Health, and Disease

Taoism believes that the essence of life is change, a constant flow of energy from one manifestation to another. The opposite extremes of these manifestations, called Yin and Yang, are in fact opposite only in appearance: they are aspects of the same process, which is the ever-flowing energy that is life. Nothing remains the same, and everything is in the constant process of changing into something else. The only thing constant, in fact, is the process of change.

Everything in the universe is interrelated through this series of energy transformations, and we humans are an inextricable part of this process. We are affected by the weather, the seasons, the time of day, and any number of other influences both outside and inside our bodies. Taoist philosophy holds that we exist normally in harmony with the rest of the world, and our bodies and minds (two aspects of the same energy) maintain our health through constant, free, and unimpeded circulation of life force (called Qi). If this flow is obstructed, if the balance of energy is disturbed, illness results. Acupuncture restores the healthy flow of energy through the body by unblocking any obstruction and by relieving excess and restoring deficiency, both states of energy imbalance.

How does acupuncture work? Clinical observation over thousands of years has identified specific pathways of energy flow, called meridians, that form a network interconnecting all parts of the body. The meridians cover the body's surface, but they also form a three-dimensional network linking the surface to the internal organs. Needles are inserted into points along these meridians to modulate the flow of energy, and they can have a powerful effect on distant areas of the body that seem to be unrelated to the point of insertion.

How can a needle inserted into the lower leg relax the shoulder? In modern times, a great deal of scientific research has been done on acupuncture. Many mechanisms have been demonstrated, including a change in electrical potential energy at the insertion level; activation of nerves, the spinal cord, and the brain; and release of endorphins and hormones. Furthermore, the medical effects of acupuncture take place independently of the patient's awareness or will: studies on animals and unconscious patients have proven that the effects of acupuncture are real, not merely placebo. Today, in an era of integrative medicine, acupuncture is an important treatment modality that can make any other therapy, Western or otherwise, more effective.

Acupuncture and the Singer

Acupuncture is especially useful for the vocal performer, for several reasons. It often works immediately. Properly done, it has a very low rate of ensuing complications. It can be repeated as necessary and over time has a cumulative benefit beyond the immediate effect. Acupuncture can avoid the need for (often costly) prescription medications, many of which have unintended side effects. For example, acupuncture treatment of pain can be dramatic and immediate, without the side effects of stomach irritation and potential vocal fold hemorrhage that may result from excessive use of aspirin or other analgesics. Nasal and sinus congestion can be effectively managed without using vocally drying antihistamines or decongestants. Lower back pain and menstrual cramps can significantly impair singing, and these conditions can often be relieved with a twenty-minute acupuncture session. Anxiety and tension can also be greatly reduced, without the sedating side effects of conventional medications.

Another benefit of acupuncture (and TCM in general) is that it focuses on function, rather than just structure. This is a different paradigm from conventional medical treatment. Western medicine tends to emphasize the physical properties of things, such as appearance, size, and shape. But singing is not a body part; it is a process. Its components, such as breathing and muscle contraction, are also physiologic processes. Structure is by and large determined by function. In fact, how things look is often just a reflection of how they function. An example is the vocal nodules, which develop as a consequence of chronic voice abuse. The true "disease" is the process: excessive muscle tension and abnormal laryngeal posturing. The visual correlate (nodules) is in reality an indicator of this process, not the so-called disease itself. Removal of the nodules doesn't address the true problem of abusive voice use, which, if untreated, continues, with likely recurrence of the nodules.[1] By dealing with the flow of energy, Acupuncture addresses abnormal function directly and immediately.

Most important, acupuncture treats both the body and the mind. Every physical illness has an emotional component. The physical and emotional components can reinforce each other, resulting in a greater degree of disability. By treating only the physical problem, the physician leaves the emotional state still impaired, and complete recovery may be delayed. For example, laryngitis—a physical condition—leading to a canceled performance or audition can create anxiety, which can lead to increased muscle tension in the larynx, neck, and shoulders; insomnia; and even some depression. Even after the physical problem resolves, lingering muscle tension can continue to cause discomfort or hoarseness. Taoism considers the mind and the body dual manifestations (Yin and Yang) of the same entity, and acupuncture can treat both simultaneously, enhancing more rapid and complete restitution of health.

How Is Acupuncture Done?

The acupuncturist first takes a detailed history, much as a Western physician does. Chinese diagnosis additionally involves checking the radial (wrist) pulse and looking at the tongue. In TCM, both the pulse and the tongue reveal a great deal about the kind of dysfunction (excess, deficiency, stagnation) from which the patient may be suffering. The Chinese word for "listen" is *ting* (Figure 27.1), a composite character that incorporates the symbols for not only "ear" and "eye" but also "heart"—meaning, the good Chinese practitioner examines his patient not only by looking and listening but also with an open mind and a compassionate heart.

Once the diagnosis is made, a plan of treatment is developed. Acupuncture treatment can be used to improve states of energy deficiency, reduce excess energy, and relieve sites of energy blockage along the meridians. Needles are used close to the area being treated, but distant sites are also stimulated. In fact, distant points may have a more powerful effect. The stimulation can be administered by manipulating the needles, by gently heating

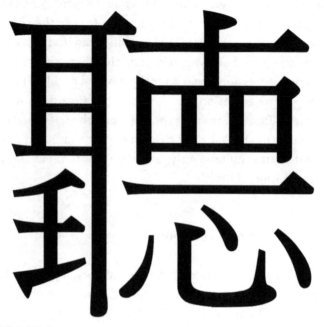

FIGURE 27.1

them (with a heat lamp or moxibustion), or by stimulating them with electrical impulses. Some therapists use soft laser beams to activate acupoints. Since laser acupuncture is painless, it is a good alternative for children, and for particularly sensitive parts of the body. Sometimes cupping is used: attaching small glass or plastic suction cups to areas of the body where excess heat is believed to cause dysfunction.

A typical acupuncture session lasts twenty to thirty minutes. The results are often immediate, but also cumulative, increasing with repeated sessions. A typical course of treatment may involve two sessions per week for four weeks. In addition to treating specific problems, acupuncture has also been used preventively, to improve immune function, increase energy, and balance and harmonize normal bodily processes.

TABLE 27.2 Some Common Medical Conditions among Singers which Respond to Acupuncture

Allergies	Depression	Menstrual Cramps
Anxiety	Dysphonia	Neck strain
Asthma	Fatigue	Rhinitis
Bronchitis	Headaches	Shoulder tension
Colds	Insomnia	Sinusitis
Cough	Lower Back Pain	TMJ

Conditions That Respond Well to Acupuncture Treatment

Table 27.2 lists some conditions commonly affecting vocal performers that often respond dramatically to acupuncture therapy. It is important to consider, however, that acupuncture should be used in conjunction with, and not instead of, conventional medicine. The main reason for this is that some symptoms are due to potentially serious illnesses, which are best diagnosed and treated using modern Western medicine. If a condition fails to completely resolve with acupuncture, or if a symptom recurs, worsens, or extends to greater impairment, the patient needs to be evaluated by a physician.

Ideally, acupuncture should be used in an integrative fashion, to manage problems that impair normal function, but in the context of a full medical evaluation and plan of treatment.

Notes

1. This is yet another illustration of the Zen admonition, "Do not confuse the finger pointing at the moon with the moon."

28

Chinese Herbal Remedies for Singers

GERTRUDE KUBIENA, MD

Because the voice is a singer's greatest stock in trade, this chapter discusses some applications of traditional Chinese medicine (TCM) for vocal problems. TCM is a very complex system, based on its own contemporary theory of science and emphasizing the individual's condition. Nevertheless TCM offers some very simple possibilities to facilitate a singer´s life. Although there are a number of measures you yourself can take in this regard, let me start with a note of caution: if you have a complex problem, let a real specialist for Chinese medicine make the optimum prescription for you. Furthermore, make sure that he or she is collaborating with a safe pharmacy, where the Chinese herbs, coming in from the wholesale trader, are proven as to their identity and potency, and free of insecticides and toxic substances.

A Survey of Methods of Traditional Chinese Medicine for Singers

In any discussion of TCM, most people first think of acupuncture. Acupuncture is certainly a very efficient method, but TCM offers far more possibilities. There are various branches of TCM:

- Chinese medicated diet therapy
- Chinese herbal therapy
- Acupuncture
- Acupressure
- Meditative exercises

Acupressure can help to relax and strengthen vocal folds. Meditative moving exercises, such as Qi gong and Taiji quan (Tai chi), are very effective because of their harmonizing effect. The Chinese idea is to smooth the flow of qi—vital energy—a precondition for health in general and especially for singers, who are constantly under pressure.

Chinese Medicated Diet and Herbal Therapy

There are very simple possibilities in medicated diet and very effective prescriptions in Chinese herbal therapy. Chinese dietary and herbal formulas can be used to facilitate the effect of conventional treatment, and hasten resolution of conditions such as the common cold, sore throat, laryngitis, tonsillitis, and pharyngitis. These measures can also help with managing reflux esophagitis, edema and nodules of the vocal cords, dry throat, and a condition called "plum stone qi." This is the description of a subjective feeling of a lump in the throat, as if a piece of meat or the pit of a plum is stuck in your throat. With this condition, called "globus syndrome" in Western medicine, there are often no objective findings. In the absence of apparent physical causes (such as reflux), this condition is considered by many to be caused by the autonomic nervous system.

Chinese Medicated Diet

Chinese traditional medicine addresses every aspect of life, since a life lived in harmony with the rest of nature is a life lived to the fullest. Whereas in the West we do not think much about what we eat (except in terms of calories), in TCM various foods are considered to have therapeutic properties and are classified according to these properties, such as heating or cooling. Practitioners of TCM therefore "prescribe" certain foods to assist in the treatment of specific conditions, much as they would prescribe medicinal herbs or acupuncture. Since the treatment involves foods generally available without a prescription, singers can use this modality on their own, to facilitate the effectiveness of whatever other Eastern or Western therapeutic measures are taken.

Chinese Dietary Treatment of Hoarseness

TCM recognizes different sorts of hoarseness and classifies them according to symptoms and patterns. Hoarseness may present as part of an infection, an acute condition with low and harsh voice and abundant, thick, yellowish phlegm. The Chinese pattern referring to this condition is called phlegm heat, that is, a common cold with yellow sputum.[1]

There are various recommended dietary treatments for this type of hoarseness. One is a tangerine peel drink: cook 9 grams of tangerine peel (*chen pi*) in water and drink the decoction in small doses at short intervals. Or—and this is my secret formula—soak tangerine peel in champagne and just enjoy the delicious drink. An important qualifier: the tangerine peel should be fermented, and therefore you would need to buy it at a dealer of Chinese remedies, rather than use tangerines from a grocery store. If the Chinese remedy is not available, use sliced kumquat fruit.

Another dietary prescription: slice white radish, run it through the blender, and strain it through a cotton cloth to preserve the juice. Drink the juice either with sea salt and fresh ginger or with honey. (I personally prefer the first version.) You may also cook the sliced radish, drink the soup, and eat the radish.

Another clinical presentation is gradual loss of voice, associated with dry mouth and pharynx, itching pain, and sore throat. In the West, this may be considered an allergic type of condition. For this form of hoarseness, you can take tea leaves and cook them together with honey until the honey has dissolved; then take small amounts to lubricate and soothe the throat.

For the prevention of hoarseness, and protection of the voice of singers, speakers, and announcers, TCM recommends a rice porridge made with pear juice. Take three to five pears, 50 grams of polished rice, and crystal sugar (as much as you like). Cut the pear into slices, put it into the blender, and obtain the juice by straining it through a cotton cloth. Combine the strained juice with the rice and the sugar in an earthenware pot, and add about half a liter of water to make a thin porridge.

Treatment of Globus Syndrome (Lump in the Throat)

For "plum stone qi" (globus syndrome), seaweed is a very effective medicine. Seaweed, or nori in Japanese, can be purchased at Asian grocery stores. Alternatively, go to the sushi restaurant and have your sushi wrapped in sea weed. Mussels and other seafoods are also beneficial.

Chinese Herbal Therapy

Hoarseness and Sore Throat: Prevention and First Aid

There is a very safe and simple remedy every singer should know and always at hand: Sterculia seeds, in Chinese *pang da hai* (literal translation: fat big sea). These can be purchased in Chinese grocery stores, usually in the tea section. The application is very simple: if you suffer from sudden hoarseness or just feel it coming on, take two Sterculia seeds, soak them in a cup of hot water, wait until it is cooled down to drinking temperature, sift the fluid, and drink it. The seed at this time should have unfolded into a jellylike flower. You may use the same seeds to prepare another tea by soaking them once more with hot water. Some singers sip their Sterculia tea over the course of the day. By the way, since Sterculia tea does not have any specific scent or flavor, it is neutral and so you may even use the "sterculia water" to prepare your favorite tea, such as Earl Grey.

Because prevention is an important aspect of traditional Chinese medicine, you may use one seed a day during the common cold season and as well before you are going to sing—no matter if as a soloist at the opera or with your local chorus. Why? Because this herb is considered to be very efficient at eliminating phlegm, and at the same time moistening your vocal cords. So it should enable you to sing with a wonderful, clear voice even in aggressive air conditions. Furthermore, it "moistens the intestines," meaning it prevents constipation, which frequently occurs during traveling; nevertheless it does not cause diarrhea. This herb is especially effective if combined with Oroxylum seed (in Chinese *mu hu die*, literally translated "wood butterfly" because of its butterfly shape).

Apart from these harmless first aid and prevention measures, you should never apply Chinese remedies without consulting an expert! One reason for this is that TCM prescriptions are based on a different diagnostic system from that of Western medicine. For example, a cough in Chinese medicine can be caused by both excess and deficiency. Without identifying the correct syndrome, the right "cough medicine" cannot be properly prescribed. Chinese herbal therapy is highly effective and so along with healing it can harm if not applied correctly.

So, without advocating that you self-prescribe these herbal medications, and just to give you an idea what Chinese herbal therapy can do for you, I shall give you some examples.

Hoarseness and Sore Throat Due to Reflux of Stomach Acid

This is a relatively frequent disorder, especially in obese persons. If there is pressure in the belly, the stomach may be pushed upward through the diaphragm when the patient lies down. Consequently the stomach acid flows upward into the gullet, and in reaching the throat it can damage the vocal cords as well as the pharynx. Subhuti Dharmananda points to a very simple formula, called "minor Pinellia decoction plus Poria" (*xiao ban xia jia fu ling tang*):

• Pinellia (*ban xia*) is a phlegm-transforming herb with the positive side effect of harmonizing the digestive system. As well, it impedes uprising tendencies of substances from the stomach, i.e., it has an antiemetic effect.

• Poria (*fu ling*) is a parasitic mushroom, growing around the roots of conifers, very effective in eliminating dampness and at the same time calming the mind and strengthening the metabolic system. Poria increases diuresis, but in contrast to modern diuretics it never will dry you out. So we call it a "thinking diuretic."

• Fresh ginger (*sheng jiang*), last but not least, assists Pinellia in harmonizing the stomach.

This formula is a precursor to the most-used phlegm formula, a decoction of two old drugs, *er chen tang*. Added are citrus peel (*chen pi*), licorice, and occasionally mume fruit (*wu mei*).

Hoarseness and "Plum Pit" Due to Nervousness

This is a commonly seen pattern, originally associated with problems of women. Nevertheless this pattern may be found in both women and men. Conventionally it is treated by psychopharmacology, which may cause addiction. Fortunately it responds outstandingly to a prescription called "Pinellia and magnolia combination," in Chinese *ban xia hou po tang*. It consists of the same ingredients as the aforementioned formula with the addition of magnolia bark (*hou po*) and Perillia leaf (*zi su ye*). Both herbs are good for "moving the vital energy qi." In Chinese medicine, life is equal to movement; in this formula movement is especially important because one wants to get rid of stagnant fluids. This formula was proven not only to be effective in treating nervous or neurotic vocal disorders but as well to have an antidepressant effect.

Hoarseness Due to Either Common Cold or Overuse of the Vocal Cords

"Gasping formula" is literally "the pill for people whose voice sounds like a broken whistle" (*xiang sheng po di wan*). This is a patent remedy, and it treats sudden hoarseness stemming from common cold with fever, causing laryngitis. Although the target of the formula is to fight the effect of an infection of the respiratory system, it is nevertheless frequently applied successfully for hoarseness due to overuse of the vocal cords, occurring in singers and speakers. It includes these ingredients:

- Forsythia fruit (*lian qiao*), a heat-clearing herb with antitoxic effect.
- Licorice (*gan cao*), the most used ingredient in Chinese prescriptions. On the one hand it is a qi tonic; it gives strength. On the other hand, it harmonizes the drugs within a formula and causes a sort of "time release" effect; the blood level of the herbs in the formula stays constant over a longer period. Furthermore it has an antitoxic effect, as long as it is used unprepared. Fried with honey, it loses this effect in favor of reinforcing its ability to guide the other herbs to the digestive system.

- A sort of cardamon (*sha ren*), very aromatic and thus trans-formative of interior dampness. It helps with digestion of the other herbs in the formula.
- Terminalia fruit, as well called chebulla. In spite of stabiliz-ing properties, it helps to transform phlegm and stops cough.
- Chinese mint (*bo he*), of a cold nature and thus able to "re-lease the surface." The Chinese idea is to get rid of exterior patho-gens by opening the pores and letting them evaporate.
- Platycodon root (*jie geng*), the root of a beautiful flower, serv-ing as a mucolytic (phlegm dissolver) and benefiting the throat. One of the most valuable herbs for singers.
- Rhubarb root (*da huang*), at the same time a laxative rem-edy and stimulant of blood circulation. To say it in the Chinese way, it "moves the blood." The former property is destroyed by cooking the herb for a long time, though, while its blood-moving property is preserved.
- Chinese lovage root. Cnidium or Chuanchiong rhizome is another blood-moving herb.
- Catechu (*er cha*), made from either Acacia catechu or Un-caria gambier. Nowadays it is applied externally.

This formula does not at all influence the autonomous nervous system but only addresses physical symptoms.

Hoarseness and Sore Throat Associated with Vocal Cord Nodules

This condition may be treated by an herbal combination, again according to Dhamanander[2]:

- Terminalia fruit (*he zi*), stabilizing, transforming phlegm, and stopping cough.
- Platycodon root (*jie geng*), phlegm dissolving and benefit-ing the throat.

- Adenophora root (*nan sha shen*), a so-called yin tonic. In the preceding chapter you heard about the two universal components Yin and Yang. In symbolic terms, Yin is a synonym for substance, moistness, coolness; in contrast Yang stands for action, dryness, warmth, and so on. Note that Yin and Yang are inseparable, the Yin-Yang principle emphasizing the fact that all matter in the universe may be considered from material (Yin) and functional (Yang) aspects. In this formula, the Yin tonic adenophora serves to protect the vocal cords from damage by the other remedies.

- Borax (*peng sha*), not really toxic but nevertheless to be applied only with caution and normally only externally.

These four ingredients are mixed with honey to make small pills, which can be dissolved and swallowed very slowly to work as a local application for the vocal cords.

Hoarseness Due to Vocal Cord Polyps

Vocal cord polyps and nodules are considered in TCM to be an accumulation of dampness and phlegm. So the treatment principle is to remove dampness in the first place.

I can't say that the following prescriptions are 100 percent effective. But if you have the opportunity, try them! They will certainly not harm patients; on the contrary, they will likely benefit general health.

In the treatment of vocal cord polyps, the principle of removing dampness is emphasized. As an example, here are formulas for devising a mixture for inhalation:

Vocal Cord Nodules, Decoction for Inhalation

- Licorice (*gan cao*): Harmonizes, consoles, guides the digestive system.

- Chinese mint (*bo he*): Disperses wind heat, which is to say, relieves febrile diseases with headache, cough, red eyes; soothes the throat, relieves constraint.
- Safflower (Carthamus, *hong hua*): Moves blood, breaks up blood stasis.
- Citrus fiber (*zhi luo*): Promotes the flow of qi, unblocks plugs and therefore is used for phlegm, cough, trauma, thoracic pain.
- Mume (*wu mei*): Preserves the lungs, binds up the intestines, stops bleeding and diarrhea, generates fluids. Quiets internal parasites. As well, a very good remedy for any sort of nausea or vomiting (morning or travel sickness, chemotherapy), if stuck into the umbilicus.
- Green tea (*cha ye*): Clears head and eyes, calms nervous irritation, dissolves food stagnation (e.g., overeating, eating unaccustomed food during travel) and phlegm, antitoxic, diuretic, reduces blood fat, lowers cholesterol level.

Vocal Cord Nodules, Decoction for Internal Application

Take the preceding formula and add:

- Rose flower (*mei gui hua*): Regulates qi mildly as well as blood; harmonizes liver, digestive system, and menstruation.
- Oroxylum (*mu hu die*): Benefits the voice by relaxing the throat.

And finally, an herb for women who sing:

- Radix angelicae sinensis, a root known in Chinese as *dang gui*, may be useful for female singers on many levels. It tonifies and moves the blood and regulates menstruation. It helps with the abdominal pain that may occur with a period. It reduces inflammation and facilitates wound healing. And finally, in cases of dry cough it supports the effect of other medications.

If you are interested in pursuing Chinese dietary and herbal therapy, I recommend that you consult with a qualified TCM practitioner, who can evaluate you, arrive at a TCM diagnosis, and prescribe the appropriate treatment. As mentioned earlier, some of the measures discussed here are harmless and often helpful, while others can have a strong effect, whether therapeutic or potentially harmful. One of the hazards of uninformed self-treatment is the use of herbs or proprietary mixtures that contain ingredients of variable purity and potency.

For further reading, see http://www.itmonline.org/arts/throat.htm. There you will find extremely valuable advice for herbal therapy, as well as for acupressure and massage, the latter pair illustrated with pictures.

References

Bensky D., and Randall Barolett. (1990). *Formulas and Strategies*. Eastland Press, Seattle, WA.

Bensky D., S. Clavey, and E. Stöger. (2004, 1st ed. 1986). *Chinese Herbal Medicine: Materia Medica*, 3rd ed. 2004. Eastland Press, Seattle, WA.

Hsu Hong-yen, Chen Yuh-pan, Shen Shuen-jyi, Hsu Chau-shin, Chen Chien-chih, and Chang Hsien-chang. (1986). *Oriental Materia Medica*. Keats, New Canaan, CT.

Hsu Hong-yen, and Hsu Chau-shin. (1997). *Commonly Used Chinese Formulas: Companion Handbook*. 2nd rev. ed. Oriental Healing Arts Institute, Long Beach, CA.

Dharmananda, Subhuti. http://www.itmonline.org/arts/throat.htm. This is a very useful link to treatment and literature for singer's problems.

Zhang Enqin (ed.). (1992). "Chinese Medicated Diet." In *A Practical English-Chinese Library of Traditional Chinese Medicine*. Publishing

House of Shanghai College of Traditional Chinese Medicine, Shanghai, 1992 (1st ed., 1990).

Notes

1. Zhang Enqin (ed.), "Chinese Medicated Diet (1992), pp. 562ff.
2. http://www.itmonline.org/arts/throat.htm.

29

Self-Screening for Vocal Injuries

ANAT KEIDAR, MA, PHD

NANCY KLEEMANN MENGES, MA

The voices of the most famous singers in the world are instantly recognizable to their fans by their style and tone. In the pursuit of their desired sound, singers range from prudent self-preservation to extreme self-mutilation. The knowledge and use of healthy vocal habits and the motivation to seek recommendations for vocal health maintenance vary greatly among singers. Yet the effects of even subtle vocal impairment can be devastating, particularly to classically trained singers, who strive for a smooth, mellifluous, and maximally effective sound. Singers in the genres of pop, rock, and punk cultivate a sound that is often marked by raspiness, growls, grunts, and screams (think Janis Joplin). The trademark sounds of popular music can ultimately induce laryngeal damage, mostly to the mucous membrane covering the vocal folds. Although in the short run such trauma can actually enhance the breathy, husky, and diplophonic sound the singer is trying to achieve, in the long run the combination of injurious stylistic demands and the resulting laryngeal damage can severely compromise the singer's vocal longevity.

Factors Affecting Vocal Longevity

Vocal pathology is often the culmination of an escalating spiral of faulty technique, mechanical injury to the vocal folds, and attempted (pathologic) compensation. These factors are affected by voice use, environmental influence, and the individual's health. The amount and manner of phonatory output, both singing and speaking, as well as general health, technical training, and availability and quality of medical care determine vocal pathology. Environmental factors include inadequate dietary and hydration habits, substance abuse, abnormal sleep patterns, and exposure to environmental pollutants. Health-related factors include genetic predisposition, coexisting conditions or diseases, hormonal changes, and age.

Even though the presence of these elements all can contribute to vocal damage, clinical experience indicates that vocal behavior is the dominant factor in most cases. Most voice problems in singers and actors result from vibratory trauma, and they reflect a cumulative process of chronic misuse or overuse (Keidar, 1997; Bastian, 1990, 1993, 2002).

We estimate that, at some time in their career, 10–20 percent of singers develop some form of chronic voice disorder, the most common category of which is benign mucosal disorders (BMD). Singers generally try to deny, trivialize, or ignore warning signs of vocal injury (Bastian, Keidar, and Verdolini-Marston, 1990). They attribute their vocal deterioration to allergies, reflux, postnasal drip, phlegm, or stress. Some voice teachers abet their students, ascribing the symptoms that arise from physical impairment to "poor vocal technique," "undeveloped instrument," "inferior vocal apparatus," "improper classification," or even "emotional impediment" (Bastian, 1990; and Vaughn, 2001). It is true that any or all of these conditions can cause, aggravate, or prolong vocal dysfunction. Nonetheless, the presence, nature, and severity of any disturbance must be addressed as soon as it is detected.

Recognizing Symptoms Associated with Vocal Fold Swelling

Though there is an extensive list of symptoms related to the various types of vocal pathology, this section concentrates on describing some of the warning signs of BMDs: vocal fold polyps, hemorrhage and vascular lesions, and polyps and cysts. As with so many disorders, early detection and diagnosis is the key to effective treatment.

More Effort and Diminished Endurance in Singing

Singers who report that their singing voice (and in extreme cases their speaking voice) has lost flexibility and agility and feels "heavy" and unresponsive may be suffering from mucosal damage. Other symptoms include loss of vocal stamina and a sense that once-easy vocal tasks now require a great deal more effort. The ability to sing high notes or perform tasks that call for rapid changes in vocal fold length and stiffness (such as coloratura, fioratura, and trills) is severely compromised. The singer compensates by "pushing" the voice to sing louder and harder. This often results in a change in fach (voice classification) to a heavier, lower classification as the singer adapts his or her repertoire to accommodate the ability of the compromised voice.

Compromised Performance of Rising Fundamental Frequency (F_0)

The singer may find it difficult or impossible to perform tasks that combine singing at a low-amplitude oscillation ($\leq$ *pianissimo* dynamic level) and a high frequency oscillation of the vocal folds (high pitches). Adult males will typically experience difficulty in the *passaggio* region (the natural transition between chest and falsetto registers), even if the falsetto remains largely intact. If impaired phonation is present in both the *passaggio* and falsetto, swelling is clearly present. The *voix mixte*, also referred to as the "head voice" or "light chest mechanism," is particularly susceptible. In women, the falsetto register is most affected, and so as they sing higher and softer the problem becomes more evident.

Escaping Air, Breathiness, and Respiratory Overdrive

Any of these qualities throughout the F_0 range may reveal muscular tension dysphonia. MTD is a laryngeal posturing abnormality that is characterized by a vertically elevated laryngeal position and tight coupling between the thyroid and hyoid. There is excessive tension in the supra-hyoid musculature and incomplete closure of the vocal folds during the adduction phase of the vibratory cycle, culminating in a posterior glottal chink. These qualities can be indicators of poor vocal technique, but when breathiness and air leakage vary directly with F_0 (i.e., the higher one sings, the breathier one becomes), swelling may be a cause. Since chronic MTD often leads to vocal fold swellings, the two conditions often occur together.

Normal phonation involves approximating the vocal folds with a certain amount of tension. This is called prephonatory posturing. When the folds are swollen, the normally anticipated level of approximation and tension may not be adequate to produce a voice, and only escaping air is heard. The larynx is then rapidly adjusted (using greater force and tighter approximation) to produce an actual sound. This phenomenon, delayed phonatory onset, is another common feature of vocal fold swelling.

Unpredictability and Waning Dependability of the Voice

All singers suffer from some day-to-day fluctuations in vocal capability, but the singer with mucosal swellings will experience growing inability to depend on the voice to perform previously simple tasks. Deterioration proceeds exponentially; singers with more serious mucosal disturbances will sustain more immediate, graver, and long-lasting consequences.

Squeaky Vocalizations

Often erroneously referred to as the "whistle register," high-pitched "squeaks," particularly in the extreme upper F_0 range, are an aberrant phonation caused by dampened oscillation at the site of stiffness (swelling) that denotes segmental vibration. Only a part of the vocal fold's length oscillates, depending on the location of the lesion. In other cases multiple simultaneous oscillations occur, usually at different frequencies, anterior and posterior to the restricted section or sections, resulting in perceived diplophonia (simultaneous multiple pitches). The phenomenon is analogous to a string on the cello, if the segments both above and below the point of contact where made to vibrate simultaneously at different frequencies. This segmental oscillation, especially when appearing simultaneously with a diminished ability to sing in the upper register, is a clear indicator that stiffness, and most likely swelling, is present.

Hoarse, Raspy, Gravelly Quality

When the singing voice displays any or all of these characteristics, and the notes lack brilliance, clarity, and resonance, vocal swelling may be the culprit. When the speaking voice is also affected, it can be surmised that the swelling has progressed beyond the subtle or mild stage (Bastian 1990).

Volatile Vibrato

When excessive or improper use of the musculature is present the vibrato will be compromised, with potentially devastating consequences. Warning signs of this situation are a slowing of the vibrato rate, widening of vibrato extent (wobble), and unsteady vibrato. Without proper attention the muscles can be overloaded, even resulting in premature senescence.

Addition of Compensatory Behaviors to Sound Production

While trying to regain the former sound of the voice, the singer may introduce tension-producing actions into the sound production. He or she may begin to add pharyngeal constriction, supralaryngeal valving or tightening, "clamping" with the false vocal folds, squeezing in the back of the throat, retracting the tongue, and tucking or overextending the jaw to the production of sound. Attempting to initiate phonation (attack) by scooping, glottalizing (also called a glottal attack or *coupe glottique*), pinching, and aspirating (especially on high notes) are common compensatory behaviors, especially if these behaviors were not present prior to the onset of symptoms. It can be difficult for the singer to abandon these behaviors, once established, and this will only further the deterioration of the voice if not properly corrected.

Vocal Tasks That Reveal Vocal Fold Swelling

Bastian, Keidar, and Verdolini-Marston (1990) have devised and tested simple vocal tasks that both trained and untrained singers may perform to reliably ascertain whether vocal fold swelling is present. The singer can use these vocal tasks, two of which are reproduced in Figure 29.1, to convert the information given here

(A) STACCATO

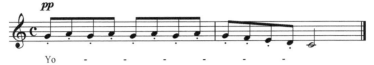

Yo - - - - - -

(B) TWINKLE TWINKLE LITTLE STAR

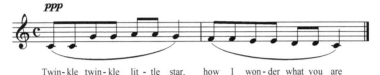

Twin-kle twin-kle lit-tle star, how I won-der what you are

FIGURE 29.1 Vocal tasks.

into practical application. In addition to revealing the existence and severity of swelling, they can show whether the source of the impairment is physical or technical.

Correct Performance of the Tasks

It is understood that a vocal exercise is only effective if it is performed correctly. Close attention to vocal execution is imperative, lest the results lack validity. Each task given here represents a type of musical phrase, the staccato and the legato. Because problems can be concealed with louder singing, the singer is advised to complete the tasks as softly as possible, in the higher pitch range (a high-frequency oscillation, low-amplitude oscillation combination). Other exercises may be substituted for these, as long as they fit the same criteria. Poor results are not a diagnosis in and of themselves, but merely an indicator that there is a problem that needs proper attention. If the singer demonstrates inability to adequately perform these tasks, it is highly recommended that he or she schedule a formal consultation with a qualified and experienced laryngologist, speech and language therapist, or vocologist.

Focus on the Upper Register

The musical examples have been printed in an arbitrary key. The singer is advised to transpose the starting note to a key that fits in his or her midrange, and then repeat, ascending in half- or whole-tone intervals. Men should highlight the *passaggio* (depending on classification), the *voix mixte*, and the lower part of the falsetto. Women should focus on the C5–C6 octave, although high sopranos should continue testing their capabilities past high C.

Emphasize Accuracy of Articulation and Phrasing

To accurately perform the staccato task, the singer must maintain a *pianissimo* dynamic level on the vowel /o/, while preserving precise rhythm, tempo, and intonation. Each note must be detached, brief, and equal in duration to the others. The singer is cautioned against slowing down, delaying challenging notes, or employing glottal attacks or excessive airflow to initiate sound.

To accurately perform the legato task, the vibrato should be checked; singers, especially females, should strive for the clear, straight tone production of the boy soprano. The phrase should be sung *pianissimo*, on one breath, and the notes joined smoothly from start to finish.

Interpreting the Results

Mucosal swellings should be suspected if:

- The task can be completed only if sung loudly. If the singer perceives that "nothing comes out when I sing softly," there is cause for concern.

• As frequency increases so does breathiness. Aspiration (/h/ sound) and audible air emission, faint noise in the sound, and a "busy buzzing bees" sound are all forms of breathiness. The breathiness can be constant or transitory. If it can be heard clearly on initiation of sound, on prolongation or termination of sound, or in ascending progressions, swelling may be present.

• Delayed phonatory onsets (DPA) and intermittent aphonia (IA) are observed. In DPO the actual voicing of an utterance may lag almost imperceptibly behind its intended starting time and be preceded by a slight "hiss" of air. In IA, the sound actually ceases sporadically for a fraction of a second or longer, creating spontaneous interruptions or cessation of sustained utterances. These gaps may be silent or include spots of air leakage and aperiodicity *(irregular vocal fold vibration)*.

The singer is advised to use these "swelling traps" to establish a baseline. Having done so, the singer can continue testing himself or herself daily. According to Bastian et al. (1989), "a sudden noticeable change in baseline performance of the tasks would indicate the need for relative or complete voice rest, whereas persistent sub-standard performance would indicate the need for consultation with a laryngologist".

The singer may also use these tasks to verify or question the results obtained from a visual examination of the vocal folds. According to Bastian, Verdolini, and Keidar (1989), "occasionally a singer's poor performance on the staccato and 'Twinkle, twinkle little star' tasks, in spite of a clean bill of health from the otolaryngologist, may inspire another look." Although inability to perform these tasks well does not always mean there is swelling (breathy singing can also be a symptom of incorrect laryngeal posturing), it does suggest that the singer is unable to easily approximate the vocal folds, whether the cause is structural or functional. If a diagnosis of swelling is made, these tasks can also be used to monitor progress during behavioral rehabilitation, assess phonosurgical results, and supervise the voice as it transitions back into performance.

Assemble a Medical Scrapbook

When it comes to voice disorders, all the answers to the questions of the present can be found through careful examination of the past. Therefore, it is imperative that the singer assemble a medical scrapbook, ordering all pertinent medical documents chronologically. These may include contact information for health care providers, color prints of vocal folds, videotapes from laryngeal imaging, evaluation summaries, surgical reports, clinical progress notes, and medical prescriptions. The documents can be scanned into a computer data file or simply kept in a paper file, to be brought to future medical consultations. As a companion to medical records, the singer should also make a recording containing short selections that exemplify the phases of his or her vocal development. These documents will give the health care provider a complete history from which to create a treatment plan.

Keep a Vocal Health Journal

In addition to constructing an up-to-date document file detailing the singer's medical history, it is recommended that the performer maintain a vocal health journal. Keeping precise daily records will assist the singer in recognizing how his or her vocal behavior affects vocal pathology.

Since it is the entire body that is the instrument, the journal must contain records of anything that affects its daily productivity. These entries need not be lengthy; a rubric system of 1–5 is efficient in establishing a basis from which patterns can be revealed. The singer should structure the entries in whatever manner is most comfortable, because if the structure is well tailored to the singer's comfort level, he or she will be most likely to maintain the document.

The journal should include information about the amount and frequency of prescription and nonprescription drugs being taken. General information about physical health—symptoms of allergies, cold, and reflux—should be noted. Sleep patterns, diet, and hydration should also be part of the journal; many times examination of these often-overlooked factors can explain a decreased sense of well-being. Pre-menopausal women should keep track of their menstrual cycle or pregnancy.

Specific to singing, the journalist should carefully document the amount of time the voice is used and the manner in which it is used. The amount of talking should be recorded as well as singing time. The latter can be subdivided into categories of voice lessons, auditions, and practice time, with attention to repertoire.

The journal should also detail the singer's mental and emotional health. For many performers, the outer voice is a reflection of the inner voice. If there is conflict or turmoil in the singer's life, the strain can be transmitted to voice production. Examining and expressing one's emotional and mental status in a journal entry may redirect tension from a physical manifestation to the written page.

Whether from defense mechanisms or simple forgetfulness, the mind is a self-filtering organ, consciously or subconsciously editing past experiences. Ordering the past in document form and detailing the present in a journal can ultimately provide history and answers to questions that may arise in the future.

Bibliography

Bastian, R. (1990). "Prevention of voice disorders." In K. E. Miller (ed.), *The Principles of Singing* (2nd ed). Prentice Hall, Englewood Cliffs, NJ (chap. 11, pp. 48–56).

Bastian, R. (1993). "Benign mucosal and saccular disorders; Benign laryngeal tumors." In Cummings et al. (eds.), *Otolaryngology—Head and Neck Surgery*, 3, 1897–1924.

Bastian, R. (2002). "The vocal overdoer syndrome: A useful concept from the voice clinic." *Journal of Singing*, 58 (5), 411–413.

Bastian, R., Verdolini, K., and Keidar, A. (1989). "The team approach to management of patients with voice disorders." *NATS Journal*, 45 (5), 16–19.

Bastian R., Keidar, A., and Verdolini-Marston, K. (1990). "Simple vocal tasks for detecting vocal fold swelling." *Journal of Voice*, 4 (2), 172–183.

Keidar, A. (1997). "Occupationally related injuries in singers." In Michael McCann (ed.), chapter on Entertainment and the Arts (Performing and Media Arts), *Encyclopedia of Occupational Health and Safety*, 96.25.

Vaughn, S. (2001). "A singer's guide to vocal care." *Journal of Singing*, 57 (3), 53–60.

30

Crossing over Safely

JACKIE PRESTI, MA, CCC-SLP

As a young singer, I was often advised, "Study and train classically, and you will be able to sing any type of music." This advice may have been true during the early years of American popular music and it may still hold for the vocal demands of many "legit" Broadway shows, but classical singers wishing to work outside the classical world now need to learn to adapt their vocal skills in order to understand the distinction between classical singing and contemporary commercial music (CCM). The linguistic and musical traditions, stylistic considerations, and tonal differences of the various aspects of the CCM genre are as important as the vocal and stylistic differences that exist between Purcell and Puccini.

Historically, CCM (it was once called "popular music") was sung by singers with little vocal training if any. However, for today's CCM professional the vocal requirements and competitive nature of the field have changed. The demands upon the vocal apparatus are formidable, requiring singers to have a clear and extensive understanding of how to perform CCM with the power, range, and vocal agility demanded by the rigors of difficult music, all the while maintaining a sound that is "natural" and "untrained" in the classic sense. Adding to this challenge, subsets of CCM carry with them their own distinct physiological, tonal, musical, and vocal demands: jazz, rock, blues, gospel, folk, musical theatre, pop, reggae, heavy metal, country, rap, and alternative all require a pedagogic approach to teaching voice that has only begun to be explored through the use of modern technology and the experience-derived teaching techniques of those of us who have "been there and done that!"

My work as a studio session singer and stage performer required that I become a vocal chameleon in order to be true to the many styles of music I was asked to sing. Later, as a speech-language pathologist, voice therapist, and voice teacher, I had to adopt a teaching approach to communicate these vocal and musical styles in order to both train and heal the voices of performers who currently perform in these genres. Though I am a staunch advocate of laryngeal synergy (having all registers and muscular activity equally balanced) no matter what type of singing one does, in recent years I have worked with more and more classical singers who wish to broaden their work opportunities by learning to sing contemporary commercial music in an authentic and healthy way. In an attempt to make this chapter as practical and useful as possible (and unfortunately, being unable to model these sounds for you), I have compiled a guide for Classical Singer Crossover Styles 101.

Because CCM singers manage their vocal registers somewhat differently from classical singers, I have dealt with the topic geared a bit more to the female voice, as women have to negotiate these registers more dramatically than men. However, I hope that the male singers out there will be able to learn more about CCM in regard to the very important aspects of tonal considerations, styles, and musicality. I have intentionally left out the topic of "belting," with the understanding that this is being covered in another chapter. Much of what I have written about here, however, will remain the same in regard to belting.

There are many obvious differences between classical and CCM singing. Remember that, although amplification in opera is uncommon or not accepted, CCM singers always (yes, even on Broadway) use microphones as part of their resonance arsenal. This confers some advantages, but it also brings its own problems. If singing in front of an orchestra is considered challenging, try singing in front of amplifiers, huge horn sections and back-up singers without a microphone. Impossible!

Let's begin with the language and terminology of CCM, and hopefully you will be able to find a voice instructor who will guide you in learning how to produce these sounds safely and effectively.

Chest Voice

It has been my experience that many classical singers have difficulty finding their true chest voice. Many have been trained to carry down the head or upper register (soft palate elevated, larynx dropped) in a smooth, unbroken, and strong manner with consistent tonal quality. They will often insist that they are singing in their chest voice when in fact they are not. This is simply low head voice, dominated by the cricothyroid muscles, a different mechanism and tonal quality from true chest voice.

Why is chest voice the common currency of CCM singing? Chest voice (thyroartenoid dominant, vocal folds shortened and thickened) is used extensively in CCM in order to produce tones that are more natural to everyday spoken speech. Chest voice also easily lends itself to the bright, twangy sounds of American speech. All of the other CCM styles also fit into this category (speechlike), with more or less weight and tonal sweetness or roughness.

Again, the idea is to find your true chest voice. This initially needs to be accomplished (especially for sopranos) by making sounds that are not all that appealing! They will often be heavy and rough, but with enough practice and guidance you will be able to find height to the resonance (hard palate) that minimizes the "clunkiness" and static feeling of those initial sounds. Practice speaking one syllable, nonsustained open vowels or words, in the lowest part of your range. Gradually move on to extend these notes to F4/G4, while still maintaining the height of the hard palate resonance. The goal is to be able to achieve these sounds so that they blend easily into the middle voice, or mix (more about this later) with little or no tonal difference, and with the ability to take the weight off them and easily maneuver through the passaggio with no perception of a register break. Many CCM singers can actually soften and take the chest voice up through the middle voice without sounding like they are belting. The tonal quality may be "colored" by added breathiness, twang, rasp, straight tone, vibrato, etc., depending on the type of CCM being sung and the particular style of that music. These "colors" are often added to specific words and notes to better communicate the emotional intent of the phrase. This is especially effective on a microphone with a bit of delay (echo). The trick is to be able to do this without adding excessive laryngeal pressure and without muscling the sound. Add more body, twang, and range to this register and you're on your way to belting!

Mix Voice and Middle Voice

Since very little CCM is actually sung in the upper register (head voice) outside of some musical theatre pieces, the maneuvering from the chest voice into the middle register (mix) is the key to singing CCM. The trick is to be able to sing in the middle register with the same tonal quality, control, and blend as the chest voice. Although the "covered" voice (*voix couverte*) is part of the classical singer's bag of tricks, the "mix" voice in CCM should not sound "dark," "covered," "hooty," or "swallowed." At the beginning of learning to produce these easy, bright sounds, many classical singers will exclaim: "But I'm not really singing." Exactly! After a time, you begin to see the challenge of keeping the breath under the middle sounds with ease, connecting into the chest voice with no register breaks, and gaining power in the middle voice for loud passages while still maintaining the natural tone quality they have acquired. Does it have some "nasal" ring to it? Absolutely. The hard palate is the party wall between the mouth and the nose, and it actually forms the floor of the nasal cavity anatomically, so some sounds will ring and feel slightly nosey—but should not sound nasal. Should air be escaping from your nose? Absolutely not. Should your tongue be tight and pushing the sound forward? Jaw weighed down and locked? Absolutely not. All of the basics of good technical singing remain the same. Once you have gotten really good at this, it will be hard to tell what's being sung lightly in your chest voice and what is being sung in your newfound mix voice.

Remember, there is no fixed point for transition from chest into mix and head. With practice, you will be able to pull the chest voice up and the mix voice down depending on the phrase, vowels, and emotional feeling you wish to impart. These sounds will eventually become equally strong and interchangeable. This is an exciting technical vocal journey and can be used in singing all styles of CCM.

CCM Vowels

Unlike in opera, where the entire story is being told through singing, in modern musical theatre recitative (verse) usually follows a dialogue between characters or a spoken monologue. Singing the verse is meant to be an extension of this communication, not a separate "now I'm singing" approach to the scene.

Many of these verses and music were purposely written in the lower part of the singer's range and designed to be executed in a natural, speechlike manner using American English vowels. Italian-shaped vowels sung in American English usually have nothing to do with the character and always sound out of place and affected. This also applies even more importantly to other styles of CCM. I cannot express this strongly enough. Just as a classical singer works to perfect her accent in the many foreign languages she sings in, nonclassical music written in American English requires its own language. The vowels are not elongated, but brighter and more horizontal, while the consonants are softer and sometimes even slurred. All too often, classical singers singing CCM overenunciate their consonants (especially fricatives and plosives, which sound obtrusive and disruptive in a microphone) in a dramatic manner that no one would use outside of reciting Shakespeare! Remember that the microphone is helping to carry your voice and lyrics. Musical theatre, jazz, rock, pop, heavy metal, R&B, country, and gospel were born in the U.S.A. (with apologies to the Brits) and need to be sung that way!

Vibrato

In order to authentically and effectively sing CCM, one of the most important vocal abilities that the classically trained singer must master is singing without vibrato. It is my understanding and experience that except for very early music (Renaissance, Gregorian chant) and some very modern music (atonal, sound design) 99 percent of classical singing involves the use of vibrato throughout every note and phrase. In CCM, however, vibrato is generally used sparingly, as a coloring device to add emphasis (warmth, excitement, energy) to a particular note, phrase, or word and spins exactly on the given pitch at the place of resonance in an easy and nonconstricted manner. It is, in a perfect world, not wobbly. You will often hear singers of CCM use vibrato that has a distinct rhythmic feel to it. Gospel singers will pulse their vibrato as a triplet; folk singers will often use a slower, lilting version of it; and jazz singers may rarely use it or reserve it to color the end of a note or phrase. Musical theatre singers traditionally use it more consistently throughout an entire song; however, it is not considered a "must have" for singers of CCM, while the ability to sing without vibrato is!

Musicality, Phrasing, and Rhythmic Considerations

As I mentioned earlier, each style of CCM carries its own historical, musical, and vocal stylistic and technical considerations. The degree of artistic freedom granted to the performer from show to show varies greatly. Of all the CCM categories, musical theatre probably maintains the strictest traditions of CCM; once the show is "set" and the musical direction has been given, it usually stays that way for the entire run. The composer, musical director, and performer have made specific decisions about how each song is to be sung technically (is this mixed? belted? head voice?) as well as musically phrased. Other CCM styles however, have a much more "improvised" approach and may never be sung exactly the same way twice. Jazz more than all of the other styles carries with it the most improvisational approach and applies a more instrumental mind-set to singing and phrasing the musical line. Jazz singers, at least the good ones, not only communicate the lyric with the natural rhythmic inflection of the syllables of everyday speech but incorporate the rhythmic element of swing, which sets the "groove" and overall feeling of musicality to the music. Beats 2 and 4 of the bar are accented and considered the key to the "feel" of the music. Eighth notes may become triplets and are "laid back" within the musical phrase. Pitches may be bent and phrases may be delayed, rushed, or stretched over bar lines at the emotional and musical discretion of the singer, with little regard to how the music was originally written.

This same improvisational musical approach to the melody and phrase apply strongly to gospel and blues, but it is usually applied to a lesser degree in other styles of CCM. It is important to note that the gamut of human emotions enters into the musicality and attitude of each style. Singers may convey aggression, sexiness, sadness, etc., from song to song without having to follow any rules with regard to characterization, tradition, or tonal consistency. There is a freedom of individual expression that is critical to each performance. This enables the performer to keep performances fresh not only for the listener but for himself as well.

Listen, Listen, Listen

There is no substitute for sitting in a quiet room and listening to music. Make sure you can snap your fingers in a relaxed manner on beats 2 and 4 of each bar. Try to figure out what each singer brings to the performance technically, musically, and emotionally. Listen for changes in tone that match attitude and emotion, improvisational changes in melody that "move the performance" in energy and feeling, and technical vocal abilities that leave you asking, "How do they *do* that?"

Practice Advice

All singers know that practicing is often a humbling, nerve-wracking experience. The new sounds you will be making may not reflect the seasoned singer you are, but try to start with simple songs (ballads, folk, easy standards, pop) and pick keys appropriate to that style. No key should move you above C5/D5, which should still be mixed and not moved into your head voice. There is no easier way to betray your classical background than to sing a popular song in head voice. Remember that when you began singing classically, you didn't start with difficult arias! Get together with your CCM singer friends, and experiment with the concepts mentioned in this chapter. Try to match their tone and approach to a song. Join a nonclassical singing group and learn to match and blend your voice with the other singers. Learn some simple songs on piano or guitar that you can sing and play. Experiment with your new sounds on a microphone, getting used to the volume and effects that work best with your individual sound. And most of all, have fun!!

31

That "Somebody Done Somebody Wrong" Sound

Production, Diagnosis, Treatment

TOM CLEVELAND, MA, PHD

Voice disorders have many causes, both functional and organic. Abuse, misuse, and overuse—accidental and purposeful—are catalysts for voice problems. Although abuse, misuse, and overuse can be associated with all voice genres, some genres are apparently more prone to create voice disorders than others. Contemporary commercial singing and country and western singing are some examples. Gospel singers who tell the clinician that an audience does not appreciate their singing performance unless the singer is hoarse two-thirds of the way through the concert are obviously prime candidates for voice problems. Certain techniques of singing within different vocal genres can predispose a singer to problems as well. One such harmful technique that will eventually send the singer to the clinic for professional help is what we call *hyperfunction underclosure* (HU).

HU results in a strained and breathy voice. It is a debilitating vocal technique that gets its name from both the appearance and the resulting sound of the vibrating vocal folds. HU is a popular, usually unwittingly employed sound used by singers in many styles that come under the umbrella of contemporary commercial singing (the newest term encompassing all nonclassical vocal genres). Very likely facilitated by electronic media, that is, studio recording and audio reinforcement in live venues, hyperfunction underclosure is a laryngeal posture that allows the singer to create breathy sounds featuring a quality of excessive closure that, according to the users, creates emotion, sensitivity, and intimacy. But this popular vocal sound can, over time, rob the user of projection, clarity, endurance, and range.

The purpose of this chapter is to present a physiological description of this debilitating vocal style, give examples of sound production, present diagnostic methods, and suggest corrective approaches, by addressing a number of questions.

What Is the Physiology of the HU Sound?

The vocal folds, the doorway into and out of the lungs, provide openings and closures in varying degrees for bodily processes, including respiration, phonation, and other physiological functions. For respiration, the vocal folds open to allow air into and out of the lungs, while in phonation the folds assume degrees of approximation necessary for voicing. Voicing is dependent on the transfer of a sufficient amount of energy, in the form of air pressure beneath the folds, to set the vocal folds into vibration. Tightly closed folds require more pressure to overcome the resistance of this compression. Folds that lack closure, on the other hand, require greater effort to create pressure because a leak always exists. Valving, the process of varying the degree of vocal fold opening and closing, can be represented on a continuum ranging from a wide-open glottis to one of tight closure (see Figure 31.1).

However, the multidirectional mobility of the cricoarytenoid joint, as well as the different vectors of muscle pull that posture the arytenoid cartilage, allow a complex variety of vocal fold positions. Therefore a one-dimensional representation of the glot-

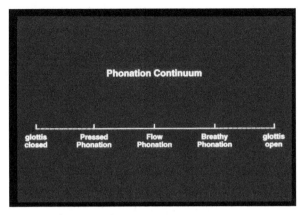

FIGURE 31.1 Phonation Continuum.

tis, suggesting that uniform movement exists between the ends of the continuum, does not include other possible combinations of vocal fold configuration. Such is the case with the configuration required for hyperfunction underclosure.

HU stems from a vocal fold approximation that has properties that appear to belong to both breathy and pressed phonation. The vocal folds are held with significant muscle effort, but not fully approximated. An urgent, husky intimacy is conveyed when the voice is used in this way.

Why Do Signers Sing This Way?

There are at least three reasons. First, it is a way to sing softly. Because the glottis leaks, it is difficult to sing very loudly. Second, singers report that they like the emotion in the sound. Third, most have never been trained to correctly produce sound and this production amounts to a default, in part perhaps because it is being modeled by so many other singers. It is part of the culture. Most singers feel that this is just "their singing voice." Beyond that, they never think much about it. And more importantly, they usually never think that the way they are singing is causing the problem they are experiencing.

Singers with HU are usually surprised when they develop a problem: the voice has not caused them difficulty before. Since it did not cause problems a year ago, the assumption is that they must be a victim of something. The concept of "Something happened to me" is more comfortable than "I have been doing something to cause this." It must be an accident, they usually say; there must be a medicine for this, or there must be a surgery for this. They also say, "This never happened to me before."

However, once their proprioceptive awareness is heightened, they realize that they have a lot of work going on in the throat. Singers are not aware of the price they pay to produce the sound; they simply think this is the way to produce their sound. If the price is high, they pay. Alternatively, once singers understand that the sound can be produced without much effort, they begin to realize how hard they have been working to produce the sound. They begin to distinguish the sensation of work in the throat, and they learn techniques necessary to not feel effort in the throat.

What Are the Singer's Major Complaints?

The singers reiterate three major complaints: my voice fatigues when I sing, I lose my upper range, and I eventually get hoarse. Singers will often say that they do not enjoy singing anymore because the voice is unreliable and more difficult to produce. Sometimes it will be there, and sometimes it won't. In the midst of a song, they do not know "if a high note will be there or not"; consequently, they will do whatever it takes to produce the desired sound, imposing a posturing strategy on the larynx that relies on greater effort, which can only add to the problem. Loss of vocal clarity is an early casualty here, but since voice purity is not necessarily the goal of many of these singers, they are typically in dire straits by the time they seek professional assistance.

Most singers perceive the onset as gradual, and they delay seeking help. Why? Because of more pressing commitments, they don't have time to check out the problem. The problem is inconsistent; sometimes the voice works and sometimes it doesn't, and even though tonal clarity is an early casualty, clarity is not their main concern. If the voice is rough, then the roughness is incorporated, intentionally or unintentionally, as part of the style. They usually report the problem only when they can no longer accomplish their singing goals.

How is HU diagnosed? Stroboscopy with a rigid transoral endoscope does not help in the diagnosis of HU. This is because most of these singers have a vastly different speaking voice compared to their singing voice, and they use their speaking voice during the stroboscopic exam. In other words, when they sing an "eee" for the doctor, it is in the speaking position of the larynx, not in "performing" position. Though it is easier for them to produce HU with the less intrusive flexible scope in place, and though it could be elicited, the chief means of diagnosis is via *auditory* evaluation, *simply listening*. The singer should be asked to produce her singing the way she usually does ("Sing a song in the way that is representative of how you normally sing"). Be aware that the loudness may not be the same, but this should not obscure the diagnosis: although softer in volume, the quality of voice production is unmistakable. The lack of clarity and degree of "press" will be obvious.

What Types of Lesions Are Developed from the HU?

Unlike in cases of muscle tension dysphonia, HU only rarely gives rise to vocal fold nodules. Rather than nodules, the results of excessive HU voice production are growing hoarseness, loss of range, vocal fatigue, and eventually a singing larynx that is in a pathologic state of almost tonic muscle contraction. This may be due to the fact that, although excessive muscle force is used with both forms of voice production, in HU the vocal folds are held in a less adducted and pressed position. But the final word is not yet in; our center has been evaluating this type of production for the past ten years, and more research is necessary.

How to Correct HU?

Our basic approach to treatment involves several techniques. First, the singer should be made aware of the difference between sound in their speaking and their singing vocal sound.

We have them speak a line in monotone. Then we have them speak the line with different inflection pattern, speaking and singing voice, from both a sensation and a sound. Next, we ask them to speak the line making the melody the inflection pattern. They must maintain the speech approach and not change anything but the inflection pattern, making it the melody of the song, somewhat like *Sprechstimme*. When they sing, they must continue to think they are speaking so that they will not revert to their "usual" way of singing. They must practice speaking as they use the melody as the inflection pattern.

As you can see, the actual corrective therapy is rather simple. More difficult is teaching the singer to make conscious choices regarding the employment of HU, rather than having this type of voice production be his default setting. Just as a covered voice is a conscious interpretive decision for operatic singing, HU needs to be employed consciously, and to attain a specific effect. In other words, a performer needs to sing mindfully, using certain technical maneuvers consciously and sparingly when appropriate.

In conclusion, Hyperfunction Underclosure is a popular, usually unwittingly produced sound, that is characteristic of many singers who perform contemporary commercial music. HU is diagnosed by auditory evaluation and treated with simple, understandable techniques. Because it is such a popular singing device with potentially debilitating effects, singers need to be mindful of how to use (and how not to use) this type of singing voice.

32

Musical Theater I:
The View from London

Pearls and Pitfalls for the Performer

LEONTINE HASS, BA, DIP RAM

As a vocal coach, I have worked for many years with West End musical theatre performers, recording artists, pop and rock singers, and the odd opera singer who turned to me when in trouble. During this time I have increasingly specialized in solving vocal problems, teaching a sound, healthy, reliable technique and training singers in the various aspects of the singer's craft.

I firmly believe that, regardless of which type of music a singer specializes in, good technique is the foundation of a beautiful and professionally sustainable tone, and that an informed understanding of the main principles of vocal physiology should underpin a singer's career. If it does not, the life of a singer becomes stressed and riddled with anxiety, professional goals seem forever out of reach, and singers become unhappy, confused, and unfulfilled.

Singing is a beautiful and rewarding activity to engage in. It stimulates the production of endorphins ("feel-good hormones") in the body, it makes other people happy if we do it well, and as an art form and vehicle for self-expression it is equally full of strength and vulnerability, summing up the human condition in all its myriad complexities. Although "singing naturally" is the goal, the actual mechanics of a good singing technique are frequently shrouded in mystery. Coaches often rely solely on artistry and metaphor in order to communicate their message to the singer. This is unquestionably an important aspect of training, but I am convinced that the starting point in a working relationship between vocal coach and singer should be for the vocal coach to provide technical solutions based on a sound understanding of the physiology of the larynx and body. It is vital that this be tailored to the physical characteristics of each individual artist.

As a broad generalization, I have found that there is a "right way" and a "wrong way" of singing. However, although there are facts there are various methods of imparting them. Singers learn in different ways. The vocal coach's teachings have to be conveyed in such a way that they can be absorbed, and most importantly put into practice, by each individual singer. Throughout this process, it is always good for both parties to hang a question mark on their beliefs from time to time and keep an inquiring mind, for voices, like human beings, are at once rationally explainable as well as forever mysterious. All too often, singers do not find a teacher who can show them how to use their voices with a technique that produces an easy facility. As a result, their technical limitations do not allow them to enjoy their craft and be freed up sufficiently to focus on their artistry and their musicality as expressive performers. Rather, they remain shackled by the inhibiting and restricting consequences of poor technique.

Writing generally on the topic of vocal technique is in itself a rather dry task, as is reading it. Rather, I shall proceed by focusing on specific problems I have encountered most frequently, and suggest their solutions. Of course, no essay can replace a session with an excellent, experienced vocal coach, but I hope the information that follows might at least begin to address some of the challenges singers encounter. Whether you are an aspiring or a professional singer, you have already won my utmost respect, as you are putting yourself out there, baring your soul to the world.

To be a singer, to have the gift of a voice and the ability to express yourself emotionally and physically while connecting to an audience with all the vulnerability and openness a human being is capable of must surely be one of the greatest of privileges. And yet, there is truth in the old adage that when God gives you a talent in one hand, he gives you a whip in the other. This is why I believe a practical, informed approach must lie at the heart of teaching.

Bertrand Russell said, "Never believe anything because you wish it to be true." You may have a wonderful relationship with your teacher, but if the technique you are learning is not working, then something is wrong. You may wish with all your heart to be a professional singer, whether in the world of musical theatre, pop/rock, or opera, and if you are producing a clean sound, have full command of your range, understand how to use your voice in various ways appropriate to specific repertoire, and have a flexible, healthy instrument, then you are probably on the right track. But if this is not the case, you need to start by finding someone who can pinpoint your vocal problems and, quite simply, "fix" them. With the right coach, this process is remarkably speedy and relatively painless, as long as you put in the concentrated practice. Persistent and correct practice in combination with regular lessons from a good coach will reset your muscle memory over a period of weeks rather than months. The more you put in, the more treasures you can take back for yourself. Singers should behave like vocal athletes. A better singer becomes a happy singer. Success breeds success. It is a self-perpetuating process. You just need to get off to a good start.

The Basis of It All: Support

Support, or anchoring the muscles of the abdomen, pelvic area, and back, allows us to hold back excessive air pressure from our vocal folds; it is a *sine qua non* of an easier vocal facility without excess vibrato or a breathy tone. Support essentially means to release air from the lungs in a controlled, slow, and sustained way for the purposes of singing. It is the management of breath for easy vocalization. Good support encourages efficient vocal fold closure, which means production of a stronger, more focused, sustainable, and clean sound.

Where does our voice come from? It comes from our vocal folds, which are located in our larynx and are attached to the thyroid cartilage, or Adam's apple, at the front of the throat, and to the arytenoid cartilages at the back. It does not come from our stomach, our uterus, or anywhere else (laugh not, I hear it often). When air passes through a narrow passage, the flow of air exerts negative pressure on the walls of the passage (the "Bernoulli effect"). Thus the vocal folds are pulled together when we sing and then vibrate at a terribly fast rate. At an A above middle C, there are around 440 closures of the vocal folds per second. A high C will require around 1,024 closures per second. In order to vibrate freely at such a fast rate, the airflow passing through the folds must be slow and sustained. If a singer sucks vast amounts of air into the top part of her lungs, there will be so much subglottic pressure, or air sitting right under the tiny folds, that singing becomes more difficult and there can result excessive vibrato and a whole host of other negative side effects.

So how do you support effectively? Support should be a flexible system. Support is not about rigidity. Although enough air has to pass through the vocal folds, too much air, or a rush of air passing through the folds, makes for a breathy tone; the voice can crack as the folds are literally blown apart by air, making singing difficult and long phrasing impossible. In order to support production of a long, sustained airflow at the same time as holding back a rush of air, it is important to use the muscles in the pelvic floor, abdomen, and back. How it *feels* to use these muscles is especially important for singers. If you imagine lengthening and widening, you are engaging your trapezius and are half way there.

The way singers support also depends on their individual physique. Try singing through your range on a "V" fricative sound, going from the lowest pitch all the way to the top. You will find that the higher you go in pitch, the stronger and higher your support has to be. Singers who are not very fit will feel as if someone is grabbing their stomach and slowly pulling it upward, all the way from the groin. The pelvic floor should be engaged as it would be in Pilates, rather than heavy weight lifting. To balance this action at the front of your body, you must also engage your lats (latissimus dorsi). Imagine you are holding ski poles and now push your elbows down. You will now feel these muscles engage. After you have found your lats, try finding your quadratus lumborum. These muscles sit slightly deeper than where your "love handles" might be. If you lean forward and imitate a gorilla (undignified but it works!), you should find them sitting deeply in the sides of your back. Remember: support is a slow "bracing" rather than a grip. I have found that many dancers grip inward, and this forces air out rather than releasing it slowly.

It is important for all singers (and especially for dancers) to release their lower abdominal muscles completely before and during the in-breath. Sometimes singers start to engage their support muscles before finishing the inspiratory cycle. This brings about constriction in the larynx. Do not take in more air than you need—no "hoovering." Otherwise you will have excess air pressure. Overstretching your abdominal muscles reduces their contractile efficiency and your control during release. Your intake of air is your chance to set yourself up correctly with openness and retracted vocal folds. Your in-breath should be silent, through the mouth, wide and low. If your in-breath sets you up with tension, you know you need to change this. You should feel open, as if you are inhaling a delicious scent.

Also, note that the way your support should vary for different voice qualities and pitches. Oversupporting while singing a low tone tends to cause too much vibrato in the tone. Sing through your range, focus on your body, and see how various pitches are best supported for an optimum sound. If you are singing in head voice, good low breathing and support are essential. However, supporting "belt" is quite different. In belt the vocal folds are short, vibrating on a thick edge, and closed for about 60–70 percent of the cycle. If the vocal folds are almost shut, the air has nowhere to go. Too much air pressure would blow the folds apart (the voice cracks). Therefore, belt requires only a very small amount of air. It almost feels as if you are coming off your airflow, as you would be when holding a heavy object. So in belt, support is felt much higher, the muscles come out right under your armpits, and your intake of breath is quick and high. You will also find that opera requires a much stronger support than does singing light musical theatre repertoire. Finally, although the diaphragm is integrally involved in your breathing, it is not helpful for singers to focus on it as such. Like your heart, the diaphragm is an involuntary muscle, and it can not be controlled in isolation.

One good exercise for a singer is to pair up with someone and allow him or her to pick you up. Don't resist the first time; your partner should find it relatively easy. Now imagine that you do not want to be picked up; root yourself into the ground, and anchor all your muscles. Although you weigh exactly the same, your partner will find it very difficult to shift you. This is quite similar to how it feels when you are supporting for singing. Rooting yourself into the ground does actually work, as this exercise shows. Now sing your songs through on the consonant *V* (do not repeat lots of *V*s but sustain the one sound throughout). This will encourage you to support efficiently. Then, sing your songs through on a voiced lip trill (like making a horse sound).

Make sure your knees are soft and not locked. From the groin up, imagine you are putting up a fence, pulling up from the groin to the belly button. Once this imaginary and flexible fence is up, imagine you are leaning against it. This tends to avoid any tendency to "grip," which pushes air out rather than holding it back. Now engage the muscles in your back. While keeping your neck long, imagine you are pulling ski sticks out of cement. If you cannot feel your back engaging, push your elbows down into the ground.

The image that you are on the end of a rowing machine is also a useful one.

The Greatest of Evils: Tongue Root Tension

If you stick your tongue out, you will see only one-third of it. The tongue is a very strong, large muscle, and it gets in the way constantly. It really is quite amazing how many singers I come across who have serious vocal problems, all to do with the tongue gripping downward. If you feel the area under your chin and above the Adam's apple with your thumb, you will be feeling your tongue root. Now try gripping or tensing it, so that it goes hard against your thumb. It is very difficult to sing like this and almost impossible to have an easy top to the voice. If the tongue is gripping down, the larynx cannot rise, which is what it has to do for high pitches. Some people have so much tongue root tension that you can actually see the tongue vibrating, and the voice develops a wobble or uncontrollable tremolo. This kind of severe tongue root tension cannot be fixed overnight. However, with a bit of time and perseverance, it can be done.

The signs of tongue root tension are that it hurts when you stick it out hard for any length of time, that you have a "furry" tone (although lack of support can also cause this), that you have uncontrollable and excessive rather than natural vibrato, and that high notes are either difficult or impossible, both in head voice and in belt. A tight jaw inevitably means a tight tongue, as they are attached. If you have difficulties with your jaw and your bite, or if your jaw pops in and out, do go and see a good dentist. Jaws are made to go forward and down. Try not to walk around all day with a locked jaw and clenched teeth. This definitely will not help you. It also stops you from raising your soft palate efficiently, which can cause a nasal, metallic tone with "lack of space."

The solution? Stick your tongue out hard, ten times in a row, at least three times a day, if the tongue is overinvolved. When you practice, massage your jaw (the muscles that pop out when you clench your teeth), and at the same time put your two thumbs under your chin in order to feel what your tongue root is doing. Try to keep this area soft. Many singers grip on the tongue root to achieve a high note, rather than using their abdominals and back to support. Make sure the work is happening in the right place. Effort travels, so learn to isolate and avoid excess tension in the neck, tongue root, or jaw.

The Neck: You Are a Human, Not a Turtle

One quick way to spot lack of experience in a singer is when you see her sticking her neck out. This has various negative side effects. When a singer pushes her neck out, it puts excessive strain on the sternocleidomastoid (SCM). The SCM is the big ropey muscle that runs from the mastoid process (the rounded bump be-hind your ear), to the joint between collarbones and sternum at the base of your throat. When the SCM is strained or shortened, the muscle itself rarely hurts, but the problems are referred else-where. A tight SCM inhibits the good function of the laryngeal depressors, the muscles that pull the larynx down. People who stick their necks out tend to have a very high larynx, which can feel as if it just about sits in their chin. This shortens the "tube" and literally turns the voice into an instrument that sounds more like a piccolo than a flute. The larynx should be flexible, rather than permanently held in a fixed place. It should be anchored down with your support, but be free to lift and lower as is re-quired for various pitches and singing styles. You have a much greater chance of achieving this if you lengthen your neck through to the crown of the head. Even when you sing in belt, where a lifted chin can be very useful, the neck should stay long at all times.

There are a few physiotherapists and osteopaths who special-ize in stretching the tongue root and the larynx down for singers who exhibit neck tension and a permanently high larynx. I have learned the technique myself and have found it an invaluable tool over the years. Singers who have a very elevated larynx expe-rience a loss of range (as the larynx literally has nowhere to go and cannot lift any higher), as well as a loss of depth and richness of tone. I have found that a few sessions of gently stretching the larynx and tongue root downward can have an immediate and dramatic effect. Singers sing with greater ease and a fuller tone. I have witnessed singers who were able to add up to five notes to their top range with ease after a little laryngeal manipulation and neck massage. The effects of such a session can be short-lived, however, if postural problems that caused this in the first place are not corrected and permanently addressed by the singer with the correct professional help. Furthermore, the treatment, which is really a little manual encouragement, needs to be repeated a few times.

There are many vocal coaches who advocate a lower larynx. I have found that this is not to be confused with what one does with one's larynx while singing. A singer who has a highly held larynx and then tries to push it down while singing will inevitably exhibit an unstable tone. So "low larynx" refers more to an acquired but relaxed lower resting position. However, a singer with a flexible, relaxed larynx that sits relatively low naturally can lift the larynx when singing and the tone will be beautiful, free, and full of "top." It must also be said that people naturally have different positions. Some have a short neck and therefore a naturally higher larynx, and vice versa.

A note on neck position during performance: take a look at some of the great stars. There is a sense of their "drawing the audience into them." They do not go out to the audience. A performer who sticks his neck out is trying too hard, almost begging for attention from the audience. A confident performer will be poised and almost draw the listener into his energy field. Maintaining a relaxed but long neck and good posture goes a long way toward achieving this. Practice it yourself, in your daily life. Notice the times when you unconsciously start sticking your neck out. It tends to be when you want something from someone else, and when your status is perceived as lower than that of the other person. If you start to observe your habits in this respect, it will go a long way toward fixing the problem. Performing, like it or not, also has to do with charisma. It is impossible to be powerful and charismatic while sticking your neck out.

If you suspect that you have a tendency to stick out your neck, try to locate your SCMs on both sides of the neck and massage them by digging your fingers in fairly firmly. Just be careful not to push on the carotid arteries, which can be felt as a pulsation just anterior to the midpoint of the SCM. If you do have posture problems and suffer from excessive muscular tension in the neck and back, it is extremely important to address this. No amount of vocalizing can make up for some regular massage by an experienced masseur. When I teach my students and notice that the voice is not sounding quite right, I always take a look at the tension in their neck and back and give them a little massage and some strategic painful prodding. The results are often dramatic, as the voice is freed up and flexible again. Singers should exercise, keep their neck long and their back open, and find regular activities such as yoga and Pilates to maintain this physical flexibility on an ongoing basis.

High Larynx vs. Low Larynx: Contemporary vs. Classical Singing

One of the main differences between contemporary singing (musical theatre, pop/rock, jazz) and classical singing is that the former requires a slightly higher laryngeal position than the latter. If you have never experimented with lifting and lowering your larynx I suggest you do so immediately, as it will be a valuable lesson. Try singing an A above middle C in your head voice. First, do it in "mock opera" style. As you imitate an opera singer's voice (if you are an opera singer, then just imitate an older singer's sound), you will find that your larynx will assume a low position in your throat. The more you exaggerate, the more you will be pushing the larynx down, or "digging," as I like to call it. You may find yourself using your tongue root to push it down artificially. Observe that the more you push the larynx down, the more unstable the tone becomes. Now do the opposite. On exactly the same pitch, sing as if you are a small child. Now take this to an even greater extreme and sing the tone as if you are a Disney character. It is quite fun to switch between an extremely high larynx and an extremely low larynx on the same note; it will sound as if you are singing different pitches, even though you are not.

As the larynx's function is to rise when we swallow, we have many more muscles that pull the larynx up than pull it down. This means that if we were to contract all of the elevators and depressors of the larynx with equal force (isotonic contraction), the elevators would win; the depressors are fewer and weaker. Therefore when a singer pushes the larynx down artificially, the voice tends to become unstable and exhibit excess vibrato. Ideally, the larynx should be fairly neutral and flexible. I have come across many young opera singers who push down on the larynx when they sing. This makes them sound as if they are twenty years older and gives the tone a wide and unnatural vibrato. Furthermore, a classically trained singer wishing to shift to singing more contemporary material needs to learn to lift the larynx and sing with a much higher laryngeal position. If you imagine that you are five years old, that is a good start. This alone can fix many a problem, no matter what style you are singing in. You will also find that high notes are suddenly much easier to sing.

It is important to realize that the larynx needs to move up and down freely for different pitches. If you are singing low notes with a very high larynx, then it will probably sound excessively childlike. Especially if you are singing soul or a passionate musical theatre ballad or pop song, it is a nice effect to leave your larynx in a slightly lower position for the lower notes. However, when you approach high notes, you need to start to lift it again. If you leave your larynx in an artificially low position, it will make high notes strained and difficult. The same principle applies to classical singers, although the overall position will always be a little lower, which also gives the voice extra space and more resonance.

Singers who push down on their larynx habitually will hear the sound they are making with a slightly higher larynx from their "inner ear," and feel as if they are singing like Mickey Mouse.

We can hear only 60 percent of our own voice, and the sound is heard very differently from inside the head. I therefore recommend that singers experimenting with this for the first time record themselves. Recording yourself, you will find that your voice sounds better than you imagined, and the tone can become easier, with good high overtones and a lovely ring.

The Soft Palate: Don't Sing Through Your Nose

If you slide the tip of your tongue along the roof of your mouth to the back, you will first feel your hard palate and then the soft palate. This is the soft tissue constituting the back of the roof of the mouth and is responsible for closing off the nasal passages during the act of swallowing. The soft palate acts like a sounding board for your voice. It has two major muscles in it, the tensor palatini (which tenses the soft palate), and the levator palatini (which lifts the soft palate). If your soft palate is lazy and flat, there will be an open cavity at the back of your pharynx that leads to your nasal passages. Your voice will necessarily travel through it, and sound nasal. If your soft palate is lifted and firm however, there will be no nasality, and the sound waves have a nice, hard surface to bounce off, producing a much stronger and more vibrant tone. Good opera singers particularly tend to have a palate that lifts like a dome, giving the voice extra resonance and lovely high overtones. A lifted soft palate lends the voice a sense of "spinning" and vibrancy.

To determine whether you are singing through your nose, sing a song while pinching your nose closed. Although nasal consonants will always be nasal, the vowel sounds should remain the same whether you are holding your nose or not. This is because if the nasopharynx is closed by a lifted palate, pinching the nose makes no difference to the tone. If you find that you are indeed sounding very nasal and feeling the vibrations in your nose, then it is high time to start with some soft palate exercises. You can also hold a small metal mirror in front of your nostrils, to see if it fogs up with nasally exhaled air while you're singing; this is used by speech pathologists to assess hypernasality due to velopharyngeal insufficiency.

Singing scales on a crisp and well-pronounced "Ging," up and down the range, will work the muscles in your palate. You will find it harder on higher pitches, as the palate has to work much harder to lift up there. Jaw and tongue tension make it very difficult for a singer to lift the soft palate efficiently, so endeavor to sort out any such problems. A "sneer" or a smile helps lift the palate (you can see opera singers do it frequently), as does visualizing singing into your ears. Watch out for the tendency to lower the larynx when lifting the palate. Do take note of this and try to isolate. If you place your thumb under your front teeth and push down with your teeth, while lifting up with your thumb, you will feel the palate lift and harden. You can vocalize on vowel sounds while doing this to help find the position. Remove your thumb, but try to keep the "tension and lift" in your palate without tensing anything else. For better or worse, muscular effort travels. Be aware of this and maintain effort in the right places, and not in the wrong ones. As there are very few sensory nerve endings in the soft palate, it is difficult to learn how to control it. Once again, finding a good vocal coach is essential.

Some of the Voice Qualities Used in Contemporary Musical Theatre and Pop/Rock/ Jazz/Soul

Classical singing mostly relies on the head voice. Other genres of singing, however, require the use of different voice qualities. I believe that a healthy, flexible head voice with good range is absolutely essential for any singer, whether he or she is mostly belting in public performance or not.

One of the main challenges affecting pop and musical theatre singers in particular is that they need to learn how to switch voice qualities rapidly, often within the same song. It is important that they master three essential qualities: head voice, speech quality, and belt.

Head voice involves tilting the thyroid cartilage as you do when you cry. This stretches out the vocal folds so that they are vibrating on a thinner edge. Young singers often find it quite difficult to access the head voice, as they speak in a thick-fold style. I have come across many young singers who attend stage schools and have an entirely undeveloped head voice. For girls, this means they sing in speech quality (sometimes referred to as chest voice) and push it up as high as it will go, until they flip into a breathy falsetto. Falsetto is a quality where the vocal folds are "stiff," with lots of air passing through them. The folds are not adducting or meeting, there is no real muscular effort, and the voice sounds breathy and weak. It is a bit like sitting under the folds with a hairdryer. For boys, this means that they sing in their speech quality until they hit their passaggio and then flip into belt. This can be recognized if quiet singing is impossible for the boys up high. Belt is always loud, and boys must be encouraged to find and develop their head voice rather than simply belt in the higher register. High belt tends to be easier for young male singers than true head voice. Girls by contrast have a lower passaggio because their larynx is smaller. Girls cannot take their speech quality as high as boys and must be encouraged to sing in their head voice throughout the range, as well as to learn to belt.

The passaggio, or sense of changing gears at certain points in the range, is an absolutely normal phenomenon. It is the point at which the larynx has to alter position in order to produce a higher pitch. The little click you may hear as you move through the passaggio is no more than a change in the plane of the vibrating vocal fold mass. This is not a "fault." It is a natural point of shift in every voice, and a trained singer is simply better at negotiating it and therefore blending the registers.

If you are a classical singer and singing in your head voice quite low down, there are no real challenges in negotiating voice qualities. However, for a musical theatre or pop singer, negotiating the various voice qualities is an integral part of their challenge.

In my own experience, the best way to negotiate the various voice qualities is to celebrate the difference. Understand your voice well enough to know when you need to "change." As a professional singer, you should know at which point your speech quality sounds pushed, or your head voice sounds too weak. Mezzos can sing much lower down in their head voice in a pop song or ballad, as they have enough strength down there to produce a good-quality tone with a bit of extra twang. Sopranos, however, tend to have to change from speech to belt (in up-tempo contemporary belt numbers and the like) much lower down than the lucky mezzos. The important thing is to know what works for you. There is not one correct way of singing a song. What works for one voice does not work for another. Choose repertoire that shows off the strengths of *your* voice. Isolate the difficult passages where shifts are required, and work them out, practice them, and repeat them.

How long do you need to learn a song? I believe that one week is the absolute minimum amount of time necessary to try to get a song correctly into your muscle memory. Three weeks is ideal. Work out how you should sing a song technically and then stick to it, so that your muscles know what they are doing. Just as a runner specializes in sprint, middle distance, or long distance, so singers are most suited to different material. Get to know what that is, and always lengthen your long rope rather than trying too hard with your short one. Otherwise, like it or not, there will be someone out there who can just sing it better than you can.

Belt

Belt is the quality used in soul or power ballads and lots of pop/musical theatre repertoire. Belt is always loud and requires a very high larynx, and therefore a high tongue position. There is lots of twang. Since the vocal folds are closed for around 60–70 percent of the cycle, very little air is required. Too much air will blow the vocal folds apart. It is very important to go to an experienced vocal coach who works with contemporary singers if you want to learn how to belt. Supporting belt is very different from supporting the head voice, as you are almost coming off your airflow altogether. Support for belt is very high: the muscles in your back and under your armpits widen and there is maximum engagement of the muscles in the torso. It is very useful to slightly lift the chin while maintaining a long neck. This helps prevent the vocal folds from tilting and lengthening, thus maintaining a thicker vocal fold mass, essential for belt.

I have taught many singers how to belt in a healthy way and have never found it damaging. However, there are some important points to consider. When you first learn how to belt, it is advisable to practice it for only five to ten minutes daily. You are simply not strong enough yet, and if you have a longer practice you will ache afterward and hurt yourself. Belt practice at the beginning is a slog. The sound is not attractive and sounds and feels pushed. Singers have to get used to the sensation of lifting their voices into a high twangy place, and to the feeling of "singing through the back of the head." The higher the belt is, the smaller the inner space becomes. Belt should never be pushed. When belt is correctly placed, it feels as if you are lifting the voice, retracting the false folds (a feeling like silent laughter, or a happy surprise) and then throwing the sound behind you. I always teach my singers how to belt on a "Yey!" as it keeps the tongue forward. Back vowels are very hard to belt, and it is important to keep the tongue and the jaw forward. Changing pitches in belt is like rowing in mud as opposed to water; it is much harder work. With short practices over a few weeks, you will find that belt starts "slotting in." It becomes progressively easier and sounds better the more you do it. Through measured, correct practice over time, belt organically changes from an unpleasant, harsh sound to an exciting quality that seems to sit in a place where you get a lot of sound for little effort at the vocal fold level, yet maximum athletic effort in the body. Belt is exciting rather than beautiful. It should be used with discretion.

If you are spending most of your time belting in a show or a pop/rock concert, you must balance the muscular activity of your voice and vocalize using your "thin" folds or head voice every day for at least ten to twenty minutes. I always advise my West End belters and "belty" pop divas to be very disciplined about this. Using your head voice will stretch your folds out again, which is vital, given that you have been belting constantly (which means your vocal folds have been vibrating on a very thick edge). Imagine heavy weight lifting without stretching. The muscles involved become painful if they are not stretched out again after a demanding performance.

Warm up your voice by doing lots of sirens and lip trills before you start belting. Gliding exercises are very good for the voice (make sure there is no tongue and jaw tension). Belting takes at least five minutes to warm up properly. Do not expect the first few notes to be positioned perfectly unless you are a natural belter or speak in a speech quality that closely resembles belt, like some Italians and Americans.

How Your Everyday Speech Affects Your Singing Voice

I am constantly amazed how many professional singers pay no attention to their speaking voice. The way you speak is after all what you do with your vocal folds for most of the day. A badly produced speaking voice contributes to all manner of technical problems in a singer. Your speaking voice should not be husky or raspy or breathy and unsupported. It should have a muscular, round, and clear quality. Sitting in on voice clinics, I have often experienced people who come in and speak in a breathy, weak falsetto and wonder why their voice is wearing out! Such a speech quality is exhausting for the vocal folds. Use the voice properly, with support and energy and a melodious tone, and singing will be so much easier.

Some Practical Tips for Singers

What follows is a list of practical suggestions for vocal performers, pearls that I have gleaned from years of personal experience as a performer and teacher.

- Practice, practice. practice! Practice from the bottom of your range to the top every day. Keep the voice flexible. Practice difficult passages, work them out, and repeat them. Allow yourself to sound bad in order to improve. Practice what you are bad at. Avoid mindless repetition. Practicing is mostly about centrally rewiring your brain; mindless repetition may be technically taxing but does not reach your goal of internalizing and resolving the problems presented by the music.
- Find an excellent vocal coach.

- Learn one song a week.
- Be musical, learn how to read music, and find repertoire you are absolutely passionate about.
- Engage with the text. Read it through without singing it but by speaking it, and understand and absorb it.
- Sing text the way you would speak it. Don't emphasize unimportant words, even if they are on the highest pitch. Such words should be floated and the stress put on the meaningful words. Speak the text through, underline words that you would emphasize in speech, and lean on them when you sing them.
- Allow yourself to fail. Allow at least ten failures for every success. The more you fail, the more you will succeed. When you do have a failure—which you will—have a sense of humor, erase, and continue!
- Practice performing. All great performers have done an awful lot of it.
- Organize concerts and cabarets for yourself at every opportunity.
- Phrase beautifully and always think forward. Music has a forward flow.
- Try to be down-to-earth and practical.
- Treat your singing like an athlete doing his or her training. There will be days when you have to treat your voice gently to encourage it to get back in the right place. Your voice is connected to you. If you are stressed, your voice will be affected.
- Do find a good psychotherapist if you have issues you need to work through. Unresolved problems, burdens, and traumas always slow down a singer's career or make the journey less enjoyable.
- Do listen to a great variety of music. Know what you like and what you don't like. Listen to the greats, and learn from them.
- Use the Internet. Log on to YouTube and Spotify to watch and listen to great performances.

- Organize your music. Have it taped, in a folder with cuts marked correctly and in the right key.
- Have an audition folder with at least eight songs in different styles, which you love and sing well. Have another folder for music that is a work in progress.
- Have an idea what your casting is, and sing songs that suit you. Sing pop songs, rock songs, or arias you can relate to through your own experience.
- Have a regular session with an accompanist or repetiteur, work on your repertoire, and understand it musically.
- Find the emotional truth in a song. Avoid playing the character or playing the cliché. It is not real, and it is not connected to you. You as a person will always be more interesting than any trick or performance. Avoid displaying acting. Be the character. Find connections between the character and your own experience. There is nothing that distances an audience more quickly than seeing a lot of "hard acting" going on.
- "Hear" where you want to go with a song, and then follow with your voice. If a racing car driver focuses on the wall as he drives, he will surely crash into it. Racing car drivers are taught to move the head in the direction they need to go, because the rest will follow. You need to do this with your mind and your "inner ear." If you are on a bicycle and have a narrow entrance to get through at high speed, you need to focus on the gap, on the bit where you want to go. The same applies to singing. Focus on where you want to go, rather than on any anticipated technical difficulties.
- No emotional repetition in songs. It is boring. Find the journey. Go for the positive. Audiences are not interested in victims. They are interested in survivors and heroes and people who find a way to transcend their problems and challenges. An audition panel wants to see your courage.
- Set up the atmosphere before you sing. Don't look into generalized space. Be available as a performer and as a person. Be

specific about your ideas and your choices. Spontaneity takes great preparation!

• Don't fix on your voice. If you listen to yourself with your inner critic, you will not sound as good, and you will ruin the flow and the performance.

• Don't be late, unprofessional, unprepared, narcissistic, neurotic, or precious. If you find you are, laugh about it and snap out of it.

• Don't sing songs publicly or in an audition that you find overly challenging. I have sat on countless audition panels where the singer finishes a poor performance and says, "I sang it because I wanted to challenge myself." Bad idea! Challenges are for practice at home and in singing lessons only. Sing songs you know inside out. A song is never really ready until you have performed it once. Bear that in mind in auditions.

One of the greatest barriers to success is the fear of being judged. Learn to rely on your inner wisdom, and surround yourself privately with people who are true friends and supporters. Get used to the fact that publicly not everyone will be on your side all of the time. It is a normal, unavoidable part of life.

I hope that all of this will help you a little in your journey, or at least help you see the signs of what to look out for. The life of a performer requires commitment and courage. Onward and upward!

33

Musical Theater II:
The View from New York

Surviving Eight Shows a Week on Broadway

JOAN LADER, MA

When Dr. Jahn asked me to write a chapter on "Surviving Broadway," I immediately said yes without thinking about how difficult a topic it really was. The physical and emotional demands of performing eight live shows a week on Broadway are the equal of any athletic event one can think of. For more than thirty years, I have had the privilege of treating and training this extraordinarily complex population of performers. I continue to learn from them every day as I try to provide them with the necessary skills with which to build their craft. It's as true now as it was more than a half-century ago, when Oscar Hammerstein wrote, "It's a very ancient saying, but a true and honest thought, that if you become a teacher, by your pupils you'll be taught."

"Musical theater," as a field, has gone through enormous changes during this time. Performers now have to be able to sing in a wider range of styles than ever before, requiring them to be able to access various vocal qualities. Just look at a recent typical (2008) Broadway season and you'll see how eclectic the field has become: *Rent, Gypsy, In the Heights, South Pacific, Xanadu, Chicago, Wicked, Billy Elliot, Title of Show, Spamalot, Spring Awakening, A Chorus Line, The Lion King,* and *Mary Poppins*—all different, all in their own way difficult. Years ago, voices were defined either as "legit" or "belt." Today, as a result of many more musical genres being included under the umbrella of musical theater, we expect our singers to be able to move easily from one style to another depending on the show's requirements. Belting can no longer be defined as just "brassy, loud, and chesty," à la Ethel Merman. What is considered a "pop" belt sound is decidedly different from a true "Broadway" belt.

With our new generation of composers—Jason Robert Brown, Adam Guettel, Jeanine Tesori, Andrew Lippa, Michael John La-Chiusa, to name a few—styles have become more complex as well as more variable. All are vocally demanding. It is not uncommon to be asked to produce a pop belt sound and to then sustain a high C over heavy orchestration. As a result I think it is essential that the training of a truly healthy singer should include many styles of music, regardless of the singer's "zone of comfort" or the vocal requirements of a particular show. All of my pop singers dabble in art songs, and all of my opera singers can belt. And musical theater performers must do it all. By stretching the highs and lows and mixing styles while training, singers have a chance to perfect their craft, and at the same time to build confidence, flexibility, and endurance.

I recently had a conversation with the noted conductor and musicologist Rob Fisher, who emphasized microphones as the catalyst for the many changes in this field. Orchestras can now be louder, and conversely softer, than they ever were before. Before the 1960s, it was common for the brass and saxophones to "sit it out" or take a rest during soft ballads. With the development and universal usage of the wireless microphone, many new sounds are incorporated into Broadway orchestrations, particularly those of recording studios. Falsetto as well as hard rock became acceptable vocal qualities.

When I began my career as a performer, there were fewer opportunities than there are today. There were no readings or workshops, no City Center Encore Series (our equivalent was a few small-scale productions under the auspices of the Equity Library Theater and some small showcases that were not tiered under Actors' Equity), or opportunities to do television (e.g., "Law and Order") while waiting for a theater job. However, the number of people entering the field today seems to have grown disproportionately to the available jobs. When I applied to college, there were a handful of BFA programs in musical theater. Today, programs are cropping up all over the United States, and the most sought-after are conservatory programs, eliminating much of the liberal arts college experience. When I was starting out, the only summer programs in the United States were Stagedoor Manor and French Woods. Now there are professional three-week intensive programs as well, some of an extremely high caliber, notably the Broadway Theater Project in Tampa, Florida, for students seventeen years of age and up. As a result of the rising costs to run these programs, it is necessary (and the norm) to admit greater numbers of students, all with dreams of a Broadway career.

When I visit these programs and universities, I find it extremely rewarding and nourishing to work with young students who are so full of hope and excitement. I am always amazed at their passion, their talent, and their enthusiasm, but realistically I can't help thinking, How many will actually have careers? It's important to be encouraging, but equally important to prepare them for the tough road ahead . . . in "surviving Broadway"! I usually begin sessions with information regarding vocal hygiene, or in practical terms, "dos and don'ts." I then move on to "How do you know if you've found the right teacher?" I am asked this question over and over again. It is essential that teachers be knowledgeable of anatomy and physiology. However, what is even more important is that they have the tools and the talent to make you a better singer rather than simply conveying to you how smart they are. If the differences and adjustments that are necessary to produce a particular vocal quality are not addressed, that person may not be the right teacher. If you are told that like any other muscle in the body the "vocal muscle" will often fatigue before it gets stronger, once again, move on. Most important, if you have to belt and your teacher thinks it is about dragging up the chest voice or a continuation of your speaking voice, it's time to leave! The bottom line is, of course, vocal health. Are you able to sing consistently over time, without injury?

I often tell young students to prepare two books. The actual audition book should not contain any music they are not prepared to sing. There is nothing worse at this early stage than to have a director go through your book and select a piece of music that is not memorized or fully explored. The audition book should contain material that is age- and type-appropriate as well as vocally appropriate. The second book is more like a workbook. It may contain works in progress as well as material that will stretch you in various ways, including material that will force you to cross over. Students should be aware of red flags that signal vocal distress, they should know where to get help, and most important they should understand and be committed to the idea that prevention is better than treatment.

As a vocal coach, working with musical supervisors on several Broadway shows, I've had to address many of the problems that are encountered during the rehearsal process, or with performers running into trouble during a long run. The troubleshooting includes topics such as:

- Vibrato vs. straight tone (very fast vibrato, tremolo; nonexistent vibrato, straight tone; wobble). Shows such as *Spring Awakening* are adamant with regard to no vibrato.
- Tense breathing patterns
- Breathing for belting versus legit singing

- Intonation (sharp or flat)
- Nasal versus de-nasal
- Intensity (loud versus soft)
- Muscle tension issues
- Possible psychological and emotional issues affecting the voice
- Pressed or constricted versus hypo-functional production
- General roadblocks to breath support, i.e., raked stages, heels, cumbersome costumes (bulky costumes, high collars, tight corsets, shoulder pads), hats and wigs, old habits and ideas, mike packs, etc.

Just recently a student reported that a physical therapist was hired by the producers of the Broadway play *Boeing-Boeing* to instruct actors on core support in order to deal with a very raked stage. More and more, producers are recognizing the relationship between injury and repetitive stressful movements and are hiring physical therapists as well as massage therapists as consultants. Singers, however, are expected to perform day after day and remain in top condition regardless of extraordinary demands, sometimes complicated by an unhealthy performance space (stage smoke, fog, dust, etc.). Singers are not robots, and no matter how healthy their technique they can easily be derailed by situations such as these.

The most important issue is endurance. I am often put in the uncomfortable position of evaluating singers before they are actually given a role. The flip side, and not an uncommon scenario, is the panicked phone call from a singer who has just opened in a Broadway show and recently been diagnosed with some form of "vocal fold swelling." The rehearsal period on Broadway is intense, and the concept of "marking" is often misunderstood or not allowed at all. The singer's only hope is to have a doctor intercede, thereby leaving the door open for possible dismissal. As is often the case, the cast album is scheduled during previews on the "supposed" day off, when even the "healthy" singer is totally exhausted. I am clearly the actor's advocate, but there is always a bit of a dance when dealing with management. As coaches and therapists, we are often asked to make judgments that have more to do with bargaining than protecting the vocal health of our clients.

It's never easy. The actor's job is always to be "getting a job," and once they've got a job, it's creating the proper balance between the stress of performing a live show "eight times a week" while enduring the ups and downs of daily living, whether psychologically induced or the result of the inevitable illnesses and medical problems. So the circle of events becomes, "Oh God, I need this job; Oh God, I got this job; Oh God, I need this job!" Is it any wonder that the voice has often been referred to as the barometer of human emotion? Dr. Gwen Korovin, a noted otolaryngologist, and I, in conjunction with psychologist Dr. Julio Rosario, have been investigating this phenomenon. We hypothesize that emotional states can cause a malfunction in the vocal instrument, thereby limiting vocal range and flexibility; the voice is out of control. At times the emotional state of an individual may actually contribute to a vocal pathology. Medical conditions limiting vocal production may in turn exacerbate and heighten emotional states, thereby affecting the voice. The bottom line is that the actors or singers are left in a state where they are unable to access the full range of their instrument. None of these points exist in isolation. They form a loop; one thing feeds into another, somewhat akin to a dog chasing its tail. It is therefore important for all performers to have a team that they can rely on. It is not the job of the voice therapist, teacher, or coach to diagnose, but it is essential to have some understanding of the order of events and be able to make proper referrals, whether to a psychologist, otolaryngologist, osteopath, acupuncturist, massage therapist,

Pilates or yoga instructor, or Alexander, Feldenkrais, or Gyrotonics practitioner.

We all pray for a "hit" and a long run of a show, but the glamour and notoriety wane after a few short months. The actor is forced to come to the realization that it's his job to make sure that he's always at the "top of his game" no matter how he's feeling. There must be constant vigilance in terms of physical stamina and vocal health. Routines vary from performer to performer, but it is this individual discipline that enables the actor to get through a long run. A good routine will include some type of daily physical exercise, as well as hands-on work with a qualified body worker, vocal warm-ups before a show, and cool-downs following heavy vocal use. When working full-time, performers often become aware of their dietary habits and simply what and when they can eat or drink. This is a time of increased sensitivity. I have seen many performers, unaware of their limitations, agree to an added load of benefit performances, interviews, and workshops, which ultimately result in unnecessary wear and tear of their instrument while they're doing eight shows a week. The long run is especially exhausting for performers not trained specifically for Broadway. Television and film, although extremely demanding, are rarely are as depleting as sustaining eight live shows a week. I seldom have enough time with these actors before they begin a run, and the work is much more intense once they are in performance.

If I had to pick one word as the key to prolonged vocal health and success, it would be "balance": in preparation, in routine, and in one's personal life. Life for the Broadway performer is like a big pie. How it is sliced may vary, but all of the pieces are important. For some, the task is too difficult, no matter how great the talent. For others, it is a way of life, and there is nothing else they would want to do.

34

Perils of the Stage (and Backstage)

An Insider's View

ANTHONY LACIURA

Opera singers are notoriously cautious about their health. They will make the extra effort to avoid every germ that comes their way. Along with scores and sheet music, the singer's bag probably contains vitamins and supplements, teabags, herbal remedies, and whatever else is purported to prevent or lessen congestion, scratching, hoarseness, or any other threat to the sung vocal line. A sneezing or coughing fellow traveler on a plane, train, subway, or bus will send the singer scurrying to the most distant seat. If a singer has a rehearsal period or performance imminent, just try to persuade him or her to attend a crowded movie or a family dinner where young children may be harboring the latest playground virus! A singer will take extreme measures to avoid any threat to the vocal apparatus and to their overall general health.

Besides these precautions, there is the "twenty-four, seven" process of preparation. Wake up—is the voice there? A little test, one or two notes. Sinuses too dry—try the saline solution or the humidifier. Not too much coffee or juice—too much acid could cause reflux; better have herbal tea. Go to the piano, vocalize, study the music, have a voice lesson, or a coaching session. Get sufficient sleep, make lighter schedules on performance days, have just the right types of meals at just the right time before curtain, take a nap, don't talk too much, stay out of drafts, exercise. It seems endless. Singers do know how to prepare; each will develop a pre-performance ritual that is as important as the performance itself.

Then it's time for the performance, and the singer has to walk onto the stage to do the job. There awaits a virtual minefield: dangers and risks totally distinct from those the singer has so carefully avoided to be in top condition for this performance. Some of the dangers lie totally beyond the singer's control, but others can be anticipated and avoided.

Rehearsals are, importantly, a time to familiarize oneself with the stage; its layout, sets, and props; all the potential hazards that the singer must navigate around. During the rehearsal period, the singer must be aware of anything that can go wrong; if and when it does go wrong, the singer will be ready. It goes almost without saying that the singer must absolutely know his job, having internalized not only his own part but also the parts of others. A singer who is vocally and dramatically secure can deliver a performance in spite of falling props, nonsecured flats, doors that won't open, darkened stairways or any other unexpected event that can otherwise send a performance into a disturbing downward spiral.

During the rehearsal period, the singer needs to be aware of the stage environment, even if the rehearsals aren't onstage yet. Walk on stage, check to see that the environment is safe for what you will be expected to do. This is the time to get to know your colleagues and your crew. Although only the director can correct a performer's position on stage, each performer can get a sense of other performers' movements or "meanderings" and thus avoid unexpected collisions with chorus members, dancers, or set pieces. Nothing disturbs a dramatic moment more effectively than the domino effect of performers nudging one another out of the way or awkward grasps at falling items once a set piece has been jostled.

The regular regimen of performance preparation—voice lessons, vocal coaching, physical exercise, and rest—should give the singer a solid foundation of vocal health to rely on for the run of a production. But everyday stress can offer challenges to vocal health, and the start of a production period presents the singer with numerous opportunities for additional stress. At the very beginning of the rehearsal period, the singer will meet fellow cast members and the production staff. Getting to know all the members of the ensemble is generally a wonderful experience through which lasting collegial relationships are forged. But the singer must now begin to adapt to the demands and the eccentricities of this new microcosm. Generally, a collaborative team effort diffuses any stressful situations and everyone involved will participate in a successful run.

Directors, conductors, choreographers, and costumers come with their own demands, to offer the singer a few more opportunities for stress. The singer naturally works to accommodate the director's staging and the conductor's musical subtleties, but there are other details to be concerned with. These details need to be tended to early on; otherwise, the singer's vocal performance will suffer. This is the time for the singer to make the effort to work patiently and collaboratively with all members of the production staff. Be prompt for coachings and costume or wig fittings. Work with the person whose job it is to make the singer look and sound best. Anticipate what might happen if a wig is not secured properly or if a hem is a bit too long. Ask the costumer to insert an easily accessible pocket for a mini-flashlight. This is a backup if a crewmember cannot be there at that moment. Practice walking in platform thongs over that raked stage surface of bamboo poles. If, after you have practiced and tried to iron out any problems, there are still difficulties maneuvering through the stage business or attending to the conductor's cues, consult with the appropriate member of the staff to ensure a comfortable performance. In my experience, letting the staff know early on what the anticipated difficulties might be allows the rehearsal period to proceed smoothly and the performances to come off without a hitch. Of course, it goes without saying (which is why I am repeating it) that optimal vocal health and solid preparation will serve the singers well, and they can continue to sing well in spite of whatever comes their way.

Equally as important as the singer's business onstage is the singer's business backstage. The rehearsal period is also the time to get to know the stage crew. Be assured that the stagehands do know their business backstage, and they can be very helpful in keeping the performers safe. The unions representing the stage crew are very safety-conscious and will have emphasized compliance with all safety regulations and policies. They are accustomed to working in small areas in the dark, usually surrounded by a clutter of set pieces, cables, and other equipment. The stage crew knows what is in their way, but until the rehearsals begin on stage the performers do not. A professional stage crew is generally very willing to work with the singers to make them aware of the hazards lurking. Here are some points to discuss with the crew: where to walk and to wait for entrances; what path to follow after exits; where cables are laid; where light poles will be placed; where sharp objects or jutting set pieces will be stored during acts or intermissions; the existence of escape steps from stage platforms or elevated pieces; the use of backstage lighting or railings when necessary; an assistant to lead the performer safely on or off the stage for tricky entrances or exits; a lit crossover area, etc.

Being aware of what can trip up a singer backstage can keep the singer from being tripped up vocally during the course of the performance. Also, since wing space has the potential for danger, never invite friends or family to watch the performance from the wings. Most theaters strictly prohibit this practice, but there is always the temptation to let someone sneak in "just for a minute." An unauthorized person's presence really impedes the stage crew's work, and it is simply too dangerous.

With the end of the rehearsal period, the singer should feel comfortable and familiar with every aspect of the stage and backstage experience. The performance itself brings more challenges. The adrenaline rush that usually accompanies a performance cannot overpower the singer's concentration and control. The singer must be particularly cautious since elevated physical energy can easily disrupt a smooth vocal line. When the staging calls for the singer to run or climb, or carry, reposition, or throw hand props on stage, an additional layer of concentration is required. The singer must therefore know every inch of the set well, what and where every other movable prop is positioned, where the other performers, including chorus, dancers, and supers, are moving throughout the scene. It might be necessary to adjust to unexpected movements or performers' memory lapses on staging.

For scenes involving stage combat, it is important to insist on special rehearsal time and follow the choreography and the musical cues assiduously. Even such simple moves as a "thrust-parry" in a swordfight need multiple repetitions and rehearsal sessions, so that the singer will memorize and internalize the movements and not be tempted to ad lib à la Errol Flynn.

Vocal and dramatic control should prevail so that the audience sees only a seamless performance. Energy levels can escalate, and the singers have to remember that they are not actually chasing someone or hurling objects at another performer, only acting as if they are. Once an audience realizes that something has gone awry on stage, the production value plummets.

Some personal experiences and incidents related from fellow singers might help to illustrate the importance of stage safety or lack thereof. I was privileged to work with the wonderful character artist Andrea Velis for many years at the Metropolitan Opera. One of his many memorable roles was as the Witch in *Hansel and Gretel*. As I was preparing to perform the Witch for the first time, Andy asked me if I were going to fly. He then related this story. For the performances at the Met, he agreed to fly; and for every rehearsal and performance, the same technician was there to connect the wires to the harness in preparation for the Witch's flight. But for one performance, a different technician appeared and asked him, "What do I do?" Andy replied, "Absolutely nothing!" That night the Witch did not fly; Andy entered from stage right, running, not flying, but holding the Witch's broom, menacingly as ever. His message was clear.

On another occasion, I was in Mexico for the Cervantino Festival, performing the role of Jaquino in *Fidelio*. In Act II, the upstage set is the wall of the prison, constructed of very heavy oak and iron materials. As I entered through the double oaken doors with Marcelline, speaking the lines of dialogue, I heard a sound similar to applause. Applause made no sense at that moment. I then noticed colleagues in the wings gesturing frantically to continue to move forward. That also made no sense until I noticed the conductor staring upward, his face as pale as his white tie, his baton frozen, his expression, one of shock. Glancing over my shoulder, I realized the cause of their alarm. The entire set was falling forward. I led Marcelline downstage with me as the set crashed to the floor a few inches from our heels. There was total silence in the theater until everyone realized no one was hurt. Rocco entered, spoke his lines, the maestro resumed, and the band played on. Oddly enough, the well-rehearsed prisoners, as shocked as everyone else, refrained from making an early escape until their musical cue. This is clearly one of those occasions where

singers could not have prevented the mishap, but the vocally prepared cast managed to keep the performance afloat.

Singing well is always the singer's primary concern, and singing well in a performance requires the singer's concentrated effort
and attention to the stage environment. Thoroughly preparing a
role, vocally and dramatically, staying healthy, and collaborating
with colleagues will enable a singer to have a successful and a safe
performing experience. The key is to expect the unexpected and
to carry on!

35

Secrets of a Long Career

MARNI NIXON

As I sit down and write this, I look back on a lifetime of music, one that really began in my early childhood and continues to this day. I have been fortunate in my career choice, and in retrospect would not change too many things.

What are the secrets of a long career? Well, it is a combination of many factors: talent and aptitude, opportunities, and hard work. During childhood, parental guidance to help make the right choices is essential. Throughout a professional lifetime, it is important to prioritize the right things and step around potential pitfalls.

I began my musical training as a violinist in 1934, when I was four years old, in Los Angeles. This meant a life of discipline at an early age, reading music before kindergarten. Later, when I was in grammar school, I had to practice at least one hour before I left the house in the morning. We *all* played instruments and practiced, and we had a family orchestra. Practicing and playing wasn't a conscious decision; I just didn't realize we had any choice other than to do what the family did! My teacher-mother was of German descent, after all, and my Scottish dad got a kick out of it all; he was a good musician and singer, and besides it was fun and we got my parents' attention!

I first started to sing, in addition to playing the violin, because my sisters and I had to earn money for our music lessons. We learned to sing and harmonize, and I in particular began to sing solos at PTA meetings and Kiwanis clubs and churches. My mother always insisted that we get paid when we performed, even for a charitable organization, even if just a little. Before I was a teenager, I started acting lessons and was coached by my mother in monologues she'd written, which somehow always included my violin playing. When later in life I began teaching, I would reflect on the fact that I had begun to pay for my own training very early in my life. Most children don't have this arrangement, and I wonder whether paying for one's own lessons is in itself a lesson!

In addition to singing, I also did straight plays at various theaters, including the famed Pasadena Playhouse—with many now-famous actors and directors. Since I was trustworthy, my mom would put me on a bus from school (I dutifully spent the time learning my lines) and a fellow actor would bring me home at night; I would do my homework at breaks during the rehearsals in the day and performances in the evening. I had to be responsible or else! *Doing* was the teacher. Performing imparted experiential wisdom. I learned to trust and obey my instincts.

We also played in Meremblum's training orchestra. This youth orchestra was founded in 1936 by the Russian-born conductor Peter Meremblum.[1] I was asked to sing arias I'd learned, using standard arrangements and accompanied by my own orchestra! One of my first coaches in foreign languages and operatic music was Charlie Previn (the uncle of the then-young recent émigré André Previn, who was almost just my own age). So besides being "in music," we were also "in Hollywood."

Visitors to our Saturday morning orchestra rehearsals included guests who were department heads at the various film studios. While I was still in high school, I became a messenger girl at MGM. I was given voice lessons by the voice teacher at the studio then (as was Jane Powell too). I was supposed to be groomed to become a young starlet . . . or at least that was ostensibly the informal plan concocted by the secretary of Louis B. Mayer, Ida Koverman, who had visited this little training orchestra.

I was inventive and curious and a good musician, and I had acquired experience in performing and acting since I was about eight years old. I had fun doing this job as a messenger and discovered that I was not only good at delivering mail but also had the chutzpah to give visitors back-lot tours, where the sets and streets of the films were built. I made tip money and it was fun, but after a while I began to lose interest in the studio, even though I sneaked into many stages and watched the shooting of films.

At age fourteen, I became one of the original members of the now-well-known Roger Wagner Chorale. I loved choral music. Many evenings we'd sit around the kitchen table, read madrigals and vocal music of many countries, and make glorious music, enjoying the literature of past and present, secular and religious cantatas and motets, requiems and chants, as well as contemporary music. These were the war years, and many European musicians had settled in California. Igor Stravinsky, Ernst Krenek, and Arnold Schoenberg were all residents of Los Angeles. Stravinsky would often give us first crack at new compositions. In Los Angeles at that time, there were the famed Monday Evening Concerts, where we'd perform and premiere classical contemporary music along with all types of ancient as well as romantic music, from all over the world, in various combinations with first-rate musicians. There were often visiting intendants and directors on the faculties of the music and opera departments of USC, UCLA, and Los Angeles City College.

I am relating all this early training only to let you know how necessary and valuable those early years are in setting priorities and awareness, and in developing focus. We had our goals and we had our physical strength, our emotional joy of discovery, and our respect for music and art and its continuance through participation in that cultural world. We were a *part* of it. Why aren't we aware of the great value of that aspect of child rearing today?

So this exposure to all kinds of art forms, and especially classical music, was a necessary and vital part of our growth as kids. It was a history lesson and a perspective that opened up our own creativity, too. To be immersed in the world of *all* kinds of music, especially classical and ancient, gave us our foundation, and that led to personalization and to contemporary classical music, as well as modern contemporary, popular, and folk music. I also believe that having started out as an instrumentalist was valuable, since a singer is, first and foremost, a musician who needs to have exposure to and understanding of many forms of music.

At a certain point (when we could sneak a listen or peek), I became interested in popular music. (This was a no-no, in our pre-teen years.) I soon discovered that popular music was harder to perform than classical music. I had to be more *personal* about it. This is why it fascinated me. This was the time when I discovered that theater per se was a part of the musical world also. Or, let's say that musicals, though more "vernacular," were also a part of the *cultural* scene and not separated from the world of music, but could be considered another form of the combinations of theater and music. I began to realize that music of the popular kind was not just something we were *not* supposed to listen to because it was beneath us and vulgar or commonplace.

I soon discovered that there was a cultural bias against popular music. It was generally known, in my vocal schooling at the time in California, and indeed in academic circles, that popular music was "not good for the voice." And indeed, we know now that certain kinds of vocal pressures are not healthy if misdirected and misused.

But now I wanted to take the time to do things *my* way. I had always been getting top grades and followed directions, but that personal side was not as developed as it could have been. I think I also was into a little teenage rebellion against all the rules I'd had. I was disciplined and had learned how to practice my violin and learn the music, but nobody taught "popular" music in my surroundings. I had to just listen privately and let it sink in. It was an individual, personal experience. Since then, I have of course realized that this is true for all music. I think eventually one has to let any kind of music, on whatever level, sink into one's self, if one is to perform it. But back then, I hadn't experienced that, nor matured into this realization in those days when I'd performed classical music. I realized later that I was in fact doing it all along, the personalization, but I'd not known it at the time. This was the issue: I had to do it myself, in my own way, *and* I had to not ruin one discipline while discovering the other.

The "school" for popular music, then, was to imitate. There were many great singers to listen to. The phrasing of Bing Crosby, Anita O'Day Ella Fitzgerald, and Frank Sinatra was impeccable. At the same time, I was beginning to trust my instincts and to keep my classical chops too.

This was a time of liberation for me. In my new emergence of independent thinking at this time, I wanted to try things out; use my intuition, my musicality, my acting skills; have the nerve to throw away rules; *and* not ruin one type of singing for the other. But in order to do this, I had to become aware of *each* "discipline." The differences became apparent after a while.

Nowadays I can clarify the *technical* differences for me between the approach to pop singing and the approach to classical singing.

Although many technical issues are common to all good singing, some are especially important for popular music. The mindset, the openness to making different sounds and the development of certain muscles, in the throat and the tongue, has to be present. The flows, the aligned body, the Alexander approach, the yoga fluidity, the centeredness and flexible grounding, the athletic strength, the ease of delivery, and the awareness of shapes and spaces within the vocal mechanism have to be experienced. The freedom one can finally experience and the simplicity when all is working together, from the activating brain to the responsive muscles, is an incomparable experience.

There is a saying: "The art is to hide art." Although the artistry and interpretation has to be studied, the apparent spontaneity and joy in the process must be there to make it all seem natural and intuitive, free of extraneous and distracting things like twitches, postures, and distortions. The coloring and flavors and accents can all be incorporated, but the main thing is that the performance completes its particular mission: to reach the heart and soul and perception, and bring enjoyment of the listener . . . to elicit a response from the listener, internally or externally. This is the goal. Various depths and levels can be present in the response.

What am I saying here? I think I'm saying that in a good performance everything simply *is*. I did not initially know this was the essence of Zen. I just read it in Isaac Bashevis Singer, and I didn't think of him as being "Zen." I guess it's a significant insight, that this can come out of the mouths of both Eastern philosophers and Jewish writers!

We must include, and try to not exclude. In the developmental aspect of using the voice, the comprehensive process is active on many levels: physical, mental, spiritual, experiential, practical. We have to be aware of the learning curve, the maturity of the person's body and mind. Then we can, and indeed must, make our *choices* as to which part of what particular discipline to use for whatever aesthetic reason. Some people just seem to *do* it, this "singing," and others have to be spoon-fed at first, but at some point the inevitable happens: "I want to become a singer/performer/actor, and so I will proceed."

I am a firm believer in widening our perceptions and then focusing our efforts to match our particular talents. This means working hard to obtain all the skills and abilities of a performer, but also knowing what our particular choices are and then going for it. The dilemma is whether to go early where your natural aptitudes lead you, at the risk of neglecting other aspects, or in a disciplined way to push in every direction until, over time, your own personality emerges. Whatever itinerary your career takes, to be a *part* of that process, no matter what, is the main thing. The chips will fall, but we must single-mindedly keep at it, pursue, gather our forces and resources, and charge ahead. This is not in blind pigheadedness, but being aware of the things that we need individually to succeed. With continuous self-awareness, we are able over time to regroup realistically, if necessary. Investigating as we proceed with ever-growing knowledge and realistic aims, we will arrive at every goal with renewed vigor and success.

Over a long career, many opportunities have come my way. How to choose? First of all, I think I tried to do everything that I possibly could fit in, if I felt it was practical to be able to complete it. I said yes to as much as I could, and I felt that if they asked me to do it, or if I got the audition, then *they* knew I could do it, and I just sort of tried to do it! Foolhardy, maybe, and in retrospect my eyes were sometimes bigger than my stomach, as they say. But the scrambling out of a mistake made me invent, and prevent a future mistake, even if it was not really a mistake, but just knowing that I could do better next time. This testing of the limits is in some ways just as important as doing what you do well, since it clarifies and defines the parameters in your career.

My choices, my path, reflect advice I have received over the years, but more importantly what the craft itself has taught me, about music, about performing, about people. My teachers probably had good influence on me and kept me from doing anything totally stupid. But it was a combination of things. Mostly it was doing anything and everything in the hope that I would acquire some knowledge of what to accept, or even go out for. If I wanted to do something, I cajoled my way into doing it and made it all come out right, if possible. My mother's old adage—that I could probably do anything if I put my mind to it—gave me a completely innocent but unshakeable sense of self-trust. Later, of course, I had a manager and agents who "saw" me and thought I would be right for a particular part.

Auditioning is an important process, on many levels. Remember that one does not just accept things at first; one "goes out for them," that is, auditions. If I didn't get the audition, in self-preservation I had to learn that it was not a *personal* rejection, but in their mind, I simply wasn't right for it—no matter what I really thought!

When considering a role, my first thought always was, Do I *want* to do it? If the answer was yes, then no matter how it turned out I would have learned something. It's worth it. We are talking about choices in the early days of development, which meant not being exposed to the whole world on every decision, for heaven's sake!

Did I make any mistakes? It is inevitable that you *have* to make mistakes, and hopefully early on. If you are too careful, you do nothing. And you have to *do*. You find out about yourself by *doing* mistakes, and then, as you learn your strengths and limitations, you can start to ferret out the right roles and opportunities.

The second consideration was, Could I *afford* to do it? I mean, later on I had three kids and I couldn't afford to do things that were not paid, or that didn't develop me in some way, or didn't lead to a step up the ladder. And finally, could I miss the opportunity of working with some of the greatest people I knew? Would you have turned down Bernstein, or Previn, or Stokowski, or Stravinsky if they offered something to you? No, if they offered it to you, of course you could do it—and I did!

A career is about making some choices and turning down others. Choices are not necessarily good or bad, since so much depends on mitigating circumstances and issues that are not clear at the moment. Things are always clearer in retrospect, not only because you see how they turned out but also because (you hope) you have greater wisdom. If I'd known that the San Francisco Opera was going to offer me opening night as Nanetta in Verdi's *Falstaff* (with Elisabeth Schwartzkopf) just after I had signed a year's contract to do the *Tennessee Ernie Ford Show* at NBC as a performer (solos once in a while) and with the Voices of Walter Shuman as his backup group every show . . . would I have turned down the whole year of work when I had young kids and the need to make a living? When I was offered the role, I would have had to leave the TV show for maybe two weeks only. NBC said if I took that offer, I would not have my job when I returned. I had to make our living then; my husband had no composing jobs at that point. We had a house and three kids. What do you say? Was it a mistake? Who knows? I might have been not very good, and not had the career that I've had, because I might have gotten "bad" reviews. Who thinks of that, though, at such a time, and who knows? I think I would have been terrific, and it would have led to more focus in another direction. As it turned out, I did subsequently sing with the San Francisco Opera anyway. . . . But who knows?

Touring is a big part of a career in musical theater, and books could be written about maintaining your health and sanity while on tour. I will list just a few points, based on personal experience.

First, you have to have a very good contract and an experienced agent. Try to have a good manager (!) who knows the answers to questions ahead of time, such as travel arrangements, days off, rooms, drivers and transportation, meal arrangements, and interviews. On a recent tour I did with Cameron MacIntosh for *My Fair Lady*, I had first-class transportation all the way, which saved my life. First-class hotels (there were choices one could make), and transportation to and from the theater, really reduce the general stress level. Seemingly minor things become important: private dressing rooms, easy access to the theater and steps, etc. How many interviews and after-show discussions am I *required* to attend? On tour, these small items have a cumulative effect and need to be considered.

Over the years, as one matures and becomes successful, the career changes. I gradually began to get offered more and more assignments, and not have to try to *get* auditions. I could cull from these offers and make some choices on the basis of various matters (as stated above). I no longer need to audition, but this aspect doesn't change things much, actually. Now they say: "Come in for a meeting with the producer and director, and incidentally have a bit of music with you to sing." Not an audition in name, but they want to hear what you *still* can do, related to their job.

The whole field of musical theater has also changed over the years. Much is different, as you know, in style of singing and hiring practices. It's gone from Gilbert and Sullivan and *Oklahoma!* to *Spamalot*. You are required to dance, sing, and do anything else, unless they think they know you and can tailor a role to suit your particular talent, which may not always be possible.

I am sometimes asked how I would practically advise a young singer who is hoping for a long career in musical theater. The audition is usually the focus of the first big question. These points I would consider important:

• You need to have a good, varied audition book with numbers that you can sing with authority and in their own style. By varied, I mean varied in era, style, range, etc.
• Be in good dancing and athletic shape.
• Be able to have an attitude of willingness and "yes-ness," and curiosity to try to find out what they think they are looking

for. This may not be easy, as they sometimes don't really know! At the same time, you must know what *your* best points are, and have the varied material in a condensed version to show them—on the spot. This means preparing many things well. It means even having monologues and some dance routines available.

• Look your moderately informal best, with an open and cheerful attitude about the investigation, as it is fun for you to share with them what you can give them and show them! Give them choices up front, if need be: "I have this and this from this and this show—which material do you think best suits for me to sing for you, according to what you are looking for?" If they say "It's up to you. Anything" then choose what you feel the most comfortable and easiest and happiest with, and they can guide you from there. Answer their questions, look them in the eye, be happy to share what you can (but not too close physically, so they can gaze at the whole you), but be simple and have a sense of humor. And always be in the moment, of course! If they say "Thank you very much" and don't seem much interested, be gracious and leave without questioning that. Their lack of interest may have nothing to do with what you've done per se, but something like height, coloring, the range of your particular voice, or just personal prejudice . . . you can't outthink them, and it is pointless to self-flagellate over an unsuccessful audition.

As an example of this last point, I once was eager to accept an invitation to a very important audition, but then I had to wait about an hour before singing. I got into the audition, but they were hardly listening, and they cut me off after a few measures. Afterward, in the hallway outside, the monitor came running out and apologized because they'd found out, just during that hour while I was waiting, that the *need* to replace the original girl was no longer relevant. They were embarrassed and the audition panel hadn't quite all gotten the right message, until and during my first few bars. Which was embarrassing to them and to me. My attitude and professional acceptance of their confusion was helpful to me, and to them in subsequent negotiations later on other projects.

By contrast, I've had occasion to be cut off at the beginning, and thanked (thinking I was dismissed) them and then found I'd gotten the job by the time I returned home! Go figure! I guess if you are right for it, in their mind, no need to gild the lily, as they say.

So there are things you can prepare for, and other things are out of your hands. It is good to know the difference.

Overall, regarding the audition process, just know that in it-self it is forever confusing for both sides, and the more you real-ize this—the more you know and allow yourself to *be* yourself—the more you can be helpful to yourself and the listener. They want to find what they need, even if they don't quite know what they need ahead of time! They have to be free to observe what's there in front of them. Centering and happiness and the discov-ery of the moment at hand leads to confidence and is a powerful magnet.

Other than that, the main thing in musical theater is that you have to know yourself and what types you are able to project. Be prepared to show that, in as many ways as possible. Be profes-sional and dependable. Learn your lines, and practice your craft always. Draw the character to you and through you. Be sturdy and observant as to how you can help any situation, be consistent and open to direction, and respond as yourself.

And finally, on the job, always be a good colleague.

Notes

1. For film aficionados: this children's orchestra was featured in the 1939 movie *They Shall Have Music*, with Jascha Heifetz and Walter Brennan.

36

Coda

Personal Reflections on the Treatment of Singers

ANTHONY F. JAHN, MD

The elderly woman sat in front of me, anxious and quiet, listening to my analysis of her illness. As I went through a measured discussion of her problem and her treatment options, she suddenly looked up and, almost inadvertently, blurted out: "I don't want medications and I don't want surgery. I just want to get better!"

Well, yes. Any normal person just wants to feel well, function fully, live a healthy life, and treatments be damned! And yet, as physicians, nurses, and therapists of all descriptions, treatment is what we have to offer, to guide patients back to good health, ideally with the focus not on a specific pill, exercise, or operation but squarely on the individual seeking our help.

The Three Aspects of Treatment

In order to be maximally effective as we care for vocal professionals, we need, in every clinical situation, to consider not one but three factors: the *disease*, the *patient*, and the patient's *environment*.

Much of modern medicine has focused on the first of these. Certainly, as we continue to investigate the cause and the pathophysiology of an illness, we get a better idea of what has gone wrong, and a clearer idea of how to defuse or abort the abnormal sequence of events that has made our patient ill. Modern medical science, driven by research and technology, addresses the disease directly, and the spectacular advances in this area account for the success of modern medicine in dealing with life-threatening illnesses. It is due to our understanding of disease processes that we have come to this juncture: never in the history of humankind have so many lived so well, and for so long.

However, understanding the disease process is only one part of the picture. Diseases don't develop in a vacuum. A strep infection can be asymptomatic, mildly unpleasant, or a major illness—and the bacterium responsible may be identical in all these cases. The difference often lies not in the pathogen but in the patient. How diseases manifest, their clinical course, and the ultimate outcome often vary greatly from one patient to another. And that variation is a reflection of the patient, his general health, his immune system, his psychologic makeup.

Clinically we get to know a disease through its manifestations, its signs and symptoms. But these signs and symptoms can convey only an idea of the "essence" of that disease, as reflected through the many facets of the one individual patient. When we ask "How do you feel?" we get a sense of the problem not in isolation, but as it affects this particular individual, an organism made up of bones, muscles, sensory organs, thoughts, and emotions. An appreciation for her as an individual is the second aspect of effective therapy.

It is here, of course, that preventive care comes in, specifically the need to maintain the individual's general good health in order to minimize the impact of any illness. Healthy habits, diet, adequate sleep, and exercise, as well as dealing with stress, whether by yoga, meditation, or counseling, focus squarely on the second aspect of our therapeutic approach. Although this is true for all patients, it has particular relevance for singers: most of the problems we encounter in the singing community are not life-threatening and do not require drastic medical measures, but rather a rebalancing of the patient's underlying healthy constitution to help in overcoming medical problems.

The third aspect of effective treatment is to understand the world in which the patient must function. This is again especially important in the case of a singer: we need to know how she lives and what she does (vocally and otherwise), what the physical and emotional demands of her profession entail.

Thirty-five years ago, as young resident I attended a presentation on treatment of opera singers, given by the eminent New York phoniatrist Dr. Friedrich Brodnitz. After the lecture, I was convinced that this is what I wanted to do as well! I cornered the lecturer in the hallway and blurted out: "Dr. Brodnitz, I'm just starting my studies in otolaryngology and want to work with singers. What advice would you have for me?" He looked up and said, simply, "Know the roles!"

Knowing the roles, as well as understanding other aspects of a performer's life, including the physical aspects of the theaters and the productions, rehearsal schedules, travel, and of course the stress, personal, professional, financial—this is the third important part of our therapeutic approach. What does a singer with lower back pain feel when standing for three hours on a steeply raked opera stage? How about singing while hanging upside down in a Cirque de Soleil production? Or running around with a heavy and elaborate load on your shoulders as the hyena in *Lion King*? And what about the actual vocal task? Several years ago I was treating the cast of *Miss Saigon* and was told, by some exhausted singers, that the vocal part was purposely written to be difficult to sing, in order to convey the pain the girls were feeling.

A cold can be a trivial inconvenience or a major disaster, depending on whether you can rest, or can afford to cancel, or must record. Treatment of even such minor illnesses should be informed by not only understanding the condition but also knowing the patient, and appreciating the demands of his or her personal and professional life.

Which Treatment Is Best?

Actuality trumps theory. I recall, as a young medical student in the 1960s, finding something during cadaver dissection that was not in the anatomy manual. Confused, I sought out the demonstrator, an old English doctor with years of experience. "Sir," I said anxiously, pointing to the structure in question, and then to the book, "This is not supposed to be here!" He looked at me calmly and uttered words that have continued to resonate ever since: "My boy, never argue with the specimen!"

What is, is. So the challenge for both diagnosis and therapy is to remain open to what is new, what is unique, and what *is*, even while guided by books and the accumulated experience of others. Medical models, whether Western, Eastern, or otherwise, have no intrinsic value. Theories gain their value from how they reflect reality. So long as they guide us, they are beneficial. If they fall short, they need to be examined and reformulated, not unquestioningly enshrined.

For the person administering treatment, this may at times be an uncomfortable position. We feel more secure when guided by books and dogma. But although it would be foolish to disregard the accumulated wisdom of the past, the reality is that no single treatment is best. The surgeon whose answer to every problem seems to be a procedure needs to remain open and inquisitive just as much as the herbalist who has been taught that all problems can be solved with the right combination of grasses and decoctions. And a traditional medicine practitioner who disparages

Western medicine to his patient projects a narrow and defensive attitude just as a Western doctor who refuses to consider alternative medical models does. Such self-serving behavior ultimately diminishes the effectiveness of treatment, and it is the patient who loses.

The truth is, every school of treatment has shortcomings. There are multiple realities, and no one has all the answers. We need to openly consider all that is beneficial and therapeutic, regardless of the therapeutic model it is based on.

Treatment on Multiple Levels

A common but false assumption is that every disease consists of a specific pathogenic process that produces a unique fingerprint of signs and symptoms. Though comforting to the scientist, this paradigm does not hold in every clinical situation. Nature is profligate and messy: a single disorder can manifest in many seemingly unrelated ways. Conversely, a single sign or symptom can result from many causes, and often from the combination of several simultaneous diseases. Furthermore, as an illness progresses the signs and symptoms will change, depending on the body's response. What we see in the office is in fact not just the disease but the individual's reaction to that process, and at that particular instant in time.

Good treatment needs to address the entire condition, both cause and effect—or, as Chinese medicine would have it, root and branch. Consider a singer with vocal fold nodules. She is hoarse, and has neck strain after singing. Treating the nodules with cortisone or treating the discomfort with analgesics or muscle relaxants is the lowest level of intervention; it addresses the branch. But what has caused the nodules? Treating the cause, be it excessive singing, inadequate vocal training, emotional issues, interpersonal conflicts, or a stressful environment, enhances the effectiveness of therapy. And to simultaneously treat both the cause and the effects (in this example, medication, voice rest, vocal retraining, acupuncture, meditation or relaxation techniques, environmental modification, and psychologic support), makes therapy most effective.

Our books guide us, but our patients teach us. There is no cookbook recipe for the single best therapy, and life does not follow the textbook.[1] Each clinical situation is a unique combination of pathogen, individual, and environment. It is only by looking, listening, and appreciating the patient in the context of his or her daily life, and open mindedly considering all available treatments, that we will be most effective in caring for our patients.

And finally, we need always to leaven our treatment with love and respect, humor and humanity. As one of my mentors, Dr. Eugen Grabscheid, a well-known laryngologist who practiced for many years in New York, once told me (in his thick Viennese accent): "Keep in mind three things when treating singers: (1) treat everyone, (2) do not try to get rich on any patient, and, *perhaps most important of all*, (3) remember: not every singer is crazy."

Well put, Dr. G!

Notes

1. Although, hopefully, a good textbook will more or less follow life!

About the Contributors

Jean Abitbol, MD, a French otorhinolaryngologist, specializes in phoniatrics and voice surgery. He has published extensively on voice medicine and is recognized internationally for his contributions to voice surgery and care of the professional voice. A lifelong student of the intricacies of the human voice, Dr. Abitbol practices otolaryngology, phoniatry, and laser voice surgery in Paris, where he is Ancien Chef de Clinique at the University of Paris. His interest in the human voice led him to develop innovative diagnostic and therapeutic techniques, including vocal dynamic exploration, a method that allows physicians to look at the vocal folds of a patient speaking or singing and, more recently, the use of three-dimensional imaging of the larynx. His research has centered on the effects of hormones on the human voice. Among many other honors, Dr. Abitbol is a recipient of the coveted Legion d'Honneur.

Pedro de Alcantara (www.pedrodealcantara.com) is a prolific and multifaceted teacher and performer. After growing up in São Paulo, Brazil, he studied cello at the State University of New York's Purchase College (BFA in music, 1981) and the Yale School of Music (MM in music performance, 1983). De Alcantara trained as an Alexander teacher in London, with Patrick Macdonald (who was himself trained by Alexander in the 1930s) and Shoshana Kaminitz. After obtaining his certification in 1986, he taught for three years at the Alexander Institute (directed by Dr. Wilfred Barlow, who was also trained by Alexander) before moving to Paris in 1990, where he currently resides. De Alcantara is the author of numerous books dealing with performance, practice, and the Alexander technique.

Maris Appelbaum, AuD, is a clinical and academic audiologist with a special interest in noise-induced hearing loss and its rehabilitation. She is on the graduate faculty of Montclair State University (New Jersey), where she is clinical preceptor and director of the Hearing Aid Center.

Steven K. H. Aung, MD, OMD, PhD, FAAFP, CM (www.aung.com), is a master teacher and practitioner of traditional Chinese medicine. A former Buddhist monk in Myanmar, Dr. Aung is a pioneer in the integration of TCM into Western medical practice. He has written extensively and lectures around the world on integrated medicine. Dr. Aung is clinical associate professor, Faculty of Medicine and Dentistry, University of Alberta, Canada; adjunct professor of extension, rehabilitation medicine, public health, and pharmacy and pharmaceutical sciences at the University of Alberta, Edmonton, Alberta; and associate clinical professor, College of Dentistry, New York University.

Andrew Blitzer, MD, DDS, an internationally renowned otolaryngologist, is professor of otolaryngology at Columbia University. Widely recognized as a founder of Botulinum toxin (Botox) therapy for functional and cosmetic problems in the head and neck area, Dr. Blitzer has written numerous books and more than three hundred articles in his specialty. He holds numerous national and international honors and is former president of the American Laryngological Association.

Ory Brown, a New York–based mezzo soprano, is a versatile performer with an active career as an operatic and concert soloist.

Judith E. Carman, DMA, RYT, has taught singing for forty years, practiced yoga for almost twenty years, and taught yoga classes especially designed for singers for a decade. Dr. Carman has conducted Yoga for Singers workshops in university settings, for choral groups, in yoga studios, and for the National Association of Teachers of Singing and National Opera Association national conferences and at national workshops. She is on the editorial board of the *Journal of Singing* and has written widely on the subject of yoga for singers, and she is the author of *Yoga for Singing: A Developmental Tool for Technique and Performance*, recently published by Oxford University Press.

Marshall Chasin, AuD (www.musiciansclinics.com), is a Toronto-based audiologist who specializes in the diagnosis and remediation of hearing problems in musical performers. He is director of auditory research at the Musicians' Clinics of Canada in Toronto, the coordinator of research at the Canadian Hearing Society, and the director of research at ListenUp Canada. He is the author of numerous articles and textbooks, including *Musicians and the Prevention of Hearing Loss*.

Youngnan Jenny Cho, MD, is a board-certified otolaryngologist and head and neck surgeon in New York, with a special interest in the professional voice. Dr. Cho is assistant clinical professor of otolaryngology at Columbia University, as well as medical director at Lincoln Center's New York State Theater and New York City Opera. She is also on the medical staff of the Metropolitan

Opera, and of Jazz at Lincoln Center. Her busy practice includes vocal performers from both the classical and popular musical fields.

Tom Cleveland, MA, PhD, is director of vocology at the Vanderbilt Voice Center and associate professor of otolaryngology in the School of Medicine, Vanderbilt University, Nashville, Tennessee, where he conducts research and is involved in team management and care of the singing voice. Dr. Cleveland holds a Ph.D. from the University of Southern California and conducted graduate and postgraduate research with Dr. Johan Sundberg at the Royal Institute of Technology, Stockholm, Sweden, as a Fulbright scholar, and as the recipient of a grant from the Voice Foundation of America. Dr. Cleveland has lectured in Australia, Brazil, England, France, Italy, the Netherlands, Portugal, Sweden, Turkey, and the United States. He is the author of more than seventy articles and research papers.

David Goldfarb, MD, is a board-certified otolaryngologist and head and neck surgeon practicing in Toronto, Canada. His interests include general otolaryngology and hearing disorders, as well as the management of sleep disorders. He is lecturer at the University of Toronto Department of Otolaryngology, and chief at North York General Hospital in Toronto.

Boyan Hadjiev, MD, is a New York–based physician who is double-board-certified in internal medicine (ABIM) and allergy and immunology (ABAI). He specializes in allergy immunology, asthma, sinusitis, and allergic skin diseases.

Leontine Hass, BA, Dip RAM (www.leontinehass.co.uk), is a singer, actor, and master vocal coach who completed her undergraduate training in her native Australia, and her graduate studies in London, where she now works and resides. She is the artistic director and founder of the Associated Studios Group. Hass facilitates and devises the development of new writing in plays, musical theatre, and opera. She was producing two shows in 2011: *Londonstani* (book by Gautam Malkani, music by Rishi Rich) and *I'm a Rainbow Too* (book by Benjamin Zephanaia and Clint Dyer). She also played the lead role in a Channel 4 sitcom called *Extra*, comprising thirteen episodes, which won a BAFTA and an RTS award. As a vocal coach, she teaches workshops and lectures internationally. She has given numerous lectures and workshops on voice and performance, including at the Old Bailey, to an audience of High Court judges and QCs, at La Salle in Singapore, and at the VCA, Melbourne. Hass is a vocal consultant to various music management companies. She is the regular Voice Clinic columnist at www.voicecouncil.com.

Len Horovitz, MD, known to his patients as "Dr. H.," is one of the premier internists and pulmonary specialists in the country. His client list reads like a "Who's Who" of Broadway and film. He is in private practice in New York City, where he is the director of Carnegie Medical P.C., focusing on care of the professional performer. In addition to his medical practice, Dr. Horovitz is a an accomplished concert pianist.

Anthony F. Jahn, MD (www.operadoctor.com), is a New York–based otolaryngologist with a special interest in vocal performers. In addition to otolaryngology, Dr. Jahn also practices medical acupuncture as applied to ear, nose, and throat disorders. He is professor of clinical otolaryngology at Columbia University (New York) and adjunct professor of vocal pedagogy at Westminster Choir College (Princeton). Dr. Jahn is also director of medical services at the Metropolitan Opera and consultant otolaryngologist to the Juilliard School and St. Thomas Choir School, all in New York. He is a frequent medical contributor to *Classical*

Singer Magazine and writes a medical blog for nonclassical singers at www.voicecouncil.com.

Anat Keidar, MA, PhD, is a speech and language therapist and voice expert. She obtained her undergraduate training as a singer in her native Israel and then completed her graduate training in psychology and speech sciences at the University of Iowa, under the direction of the renowned voice scientist Dr. Ingo Titze. Dr. Keidar has worked in a variety of academic and clinical settings and is currently in private practice in Manhattan. In addition to voice therapy, she is a master teacher. She mentors vocology students and is an active lecturer at Westminster Choir College in Princeton, New Jersey, as well as the New York Singing Teachers' Association.

Maurice M. Khosh, MD, FACS (www.facedoctornyc.com), is a fellowship-trained facial cosmetic and reconstructive surgeon. He is also a board-certified otolaryngologist and head and neck surgeon, and he holds academic and clinical appointments at Columbia University and at St. Luke's/Roosevelt Hospital Center in New York.

Karen H. Kim, MD, is a board-certified dermatologist practicing in Boston. She has a special interest in cosmetic dermatology and laser skin surgery. Dr. Kim has published widely in the field of dermatology. She is a member of several prestigious associations, including the American Society for Laser Medicine and Surgery, the American Society for Dermatologic Surgery, and the Women's Dermatologic Society.

Gertrude Kubiena, MD, is an Austrian physician and an internationally renowned teacher, practitioner, and author on the subject of traditional Chinese medicine. Dr. Kubiena began her career as an otolaryngologist but then developed expertise in TCM, with a special concentration on acupuncture and Chinese herbal medicine. One of the leading teachers of TCM in Europe, Dr. Kubiena is a founder of the Austrian Society for Controlled Medical Acupuncture and has trained hundreds of physicians in acupuncture and Chinese herbal medicine. She lectures widely in Europe, the United States, and Asia, and she is the author of numerous textbooks on acupuncture, acupressure, and Chinese herbal therapy.

Anthony Laciura has an international reputation as an operatic comprimario. Born in New Orleans, he studied voice there with Charles Paddock. He made his operatic debut as a boy soprano in New Orleans in 1965. In 1982 he joined the Metropolitan Opera in New York. After his first performance, as the Majordomo in *Der Rosenkavalier*, with Dame Kiri Te Kanawa he continued a distinguished career that spans than three decades, giving more than eight hundred performances. In addition to his many performances at the Metropolitan Opera, Laciura has appeared with companies in Geneva, Amsterdam, Montreal, Mexico City, Tokyo, San Francisco, Los Angeles, Chicago, and especially Santa Fe. He teaches and gives workshops throughout the United States. In recent seasons, Mr. Laciura has turned to stage direction as well. As of 2010, he is seen in the Emmy-nominated HBO television series *Boardwalk Empire*, which is produced by Martin Scorsese.

Joan Lader, **MA**, has been, for the past thirty years the go-to resource for Broadway performers. As a New York voice coach, she has worked with the top performers in musical theater in New York. Her client list includes a number of international musical theater stars. Trained as a master's-level speech and language pathologist, Ms. Lader specializes in working with professional singers and, in collaboration with New York's top otolaryngologists, rehabilitation of injured voices.

Nancy Kleemann Menges, MA, is a twenty-year veteran of the middle and high school choral classroom. She is currently the director of vocal music at Garden City (New York) Middle School, where she conducts three choruses, provides vocal direction for the Spring Musical, and directs the Guitar Ensemble. Menges graduated summa cum laude from Adelphi University with a BS in music education and received her master's degree in music history from the Aaron Copland School of Music, Queens College, New York. She is listed in "Who's Who in American High School Teachers" (1998, 1999). She is a member of both NMEA and NYSSMA. In addition, Menges serves as a mentor and cooperating teacher to undergraduate music education majors.

Marni Nixon, singer and actor (www.marninixon.com), is an American soprano and playback singer for featured actresses in movie musicals. Among her many other credits, Marni will always be known as the voice of Audrey Hepburn in the film version of My Fair Lady. She has also spent much of her career performing in concerts with major symphony orchestras around the world and in operas and musicals throughout the United States. After playing the violin as a child, Nixon began singing at an early age in choruses. At fourteen, she became part of the newly formed Los Angeles Concert Youth Chorus under conductor Roger Wagner; this choir evolved into the Roger Wagner Chorale in 1948, and later into the Los Angeles Master Chorale in 1964. She went on to study singing and opera with Carl Ebert, Jan Popper, Boris Goldovsky, and Sarah Caldwell. She embarked on a varied career, involving film and musical comedy as well as opera and concerts.

She appeared on American television; dubbed the singing voices of film actresses in *The King and I*, *West Side Story* and *My Fair Lady*; and acted in several commercial stage ventures. She has performed works by Anton Webern, Igor Stravinsky, Charles Ives, Paul Hindemith, and Alexander Goehr, many of which she has also recorded. Her opera credits include performances at Los Angeles Opera, Seattle Opera, San Francisco Opera, and the Tanglewood Festival, among others. In addition to giving recitals, she appeared with the New York Philharmonic under Leonard Bernstein, the Los Angeles Philharmonic, the Cleveland Orchestra, Toronto Symphony Orchestra, the London Symphony Orchestra, and the Israel Philharmonic Orchestra, among others. She taught at the California Institute of Arts from 1969 to 1971 and joined the faculty of the Music Academy of the West, Santa Barbara, in 1980, where she taught for many years.

Annette Osher, MD (www.oshermd.com), a New York cardiologist, is a diplomate of the American Board of Internal Medicine and an associate fellow of the American College of Cardiology. She is a voluntary attending physician at Mount Sinai Medical College Center and holds a teaching appointment with the Mount Sinai Medical School of the City University of New York. Dr. Osher is on the medical advisory board of various sports training centers and lectures in the New York area on cardiovascular response to exercise. She was also the founder of Women's Medical Practice, P.C., a medical practice specializing in the health care of professional women.

Fred Plotkin (www.fredplotkin.com) is a noted author, lecturer, and expert in the field of music and opera. The author of nine books, including *Opera 101* and *Music 101*, he writes a popular blog on opera for WQXR in New York. He has traveled and lectured extensively, and has worked in association with numerous theaters, including the Metropolitan Opera House in New York and La Scala in Milan.

Jackie Presti, MA, CCC-SLP (www.jackiepresti.com), is a voice teacher and speech pathologist practicing in New York. Presti completed her undergraduate training in music at the University of Miami and obtained her M.A. in speech and language pathology at Columbia University. In addition to her work as a speech and voice pathologist, Presti is a professional singer who has worked on Broadway and in films. She is also in demand as a conductor and contractor. As a voice teacher and therapist, Presti specializes in combining the science of the voice with her practical, professional singing experience. Her studio is filled with working singers from all backgrounds, including theatre, jazz, recording artists, actors and on-camera personalities. She has taught on the faculties of New School of Social Research (1983–1989) and Manhattan School of Music (1994–2000).

Mitchell S. Roslin, MD (www.nycbariatrics.com), has dedicated his professional career to the treatment of morbid obesity. Dr. Roslin has been performing obesity surgery in New York City since 1994; in 1996 he became director of bariatric surgery at the Maimonides Medical Center. In 2000 he was appointed the chief of obesity surgery at Manhattan's Lenox Hill Hospital and has supervised its growth into one of the most prestigious programs in the United States. Considered one of the best bariatric surgeons in New York, Dr. Roslin is also the president of Manhattan Minimally Invasive and Bariatric Surgery, P.C.

Rebecca J. Scott, PhD (www.nysleepinstitute.com), is a clinical psychologist and sleep specialist at the New York Sleep Institute of New York, and assistant research professor in the NYU School of Medicine. She is associate director of the Sleep Disorders Center at Columbia University. Additionally, she holds a medical staff appointment at Rockefeller University Hospital, where she is part of a team investigating the relationship between sleep and cancer. She has presented research on insomnia, sleepwalking, and other areas of sleep at national conferences. Her primary areas of interest include the psychophysiological, behavioral, physiological, and neurochemical underpinnings of various sleep disorders, cognitive behavioral therapy as a treatment modality for sleep problems, and help in reduction or elimination of sleeping aids in those who feel they have dependency issues.

David M. Sherman, MD, is a board-certified psychiatrist with a humanistic and eclectic orientation. He is on the faculty of New York Presbyterian Hospital, and in private practice in Manhattan. He trained at the University of Illinois and Columbia University. Dr. Sherman is consultant in psychiatry to the Juilliard School in New York.

Phillip C. Song, MD, is an otolaryngologist with subspecialty training in laryngology and neurolaryngology. He holds an academic appointment at Harvard University and treats disorders of the voice as well as swallowing and TMJ dysfunction at the Massachusetts Eye and Ear Infirmary in Boston.

Richard A. Stein, MD, a cardiologist, is professor of medicine at New York University, and co-director of the Cardiology Consult Service at NYU-Langone Medical Center, NYU Cardiology Associates, and NYU Cardiac Rehabilitation Associates.

Sharon Zarabi, RD, CDN, CPT (www.sharonzarabi.com), is a registered nutritionist and dietitian, as well as a fitness specialist and personal trainer. Ms. Zarabi directs the Bariatric Nutrition program at Lenox Hill Hospital in New York, where she works with both internists and surgeons who care for overweight patients.

Steven M. Zeitels, MD, FACS, is a board-certified otolaryngologist who subspecializes in laryngeal laser and microsurgery. Dr. Zeitels is Eugene B. Casey Professor of Laryngeal Surgery at Harvard University, and director of the Center for Laryngeal Surgery and Voice Rehabilitation at Massachusetts General Hospital in Boston. He has successfully treated thousands of vocal performers from both the United States and abroad. A pioneer in the surgical treatment of laryngeal disorders, Dr. Zeitels's innovative research continues to advance our understanding of benign and malignant laryngeal disease.

Index

CPSIA information can be obtained
at www.ICGtesting.com
Printed in the USA
BVHW041551050122
624979BV00001B/3